To our parents
Evelyn and Raymond Franks
Ellen and the late Patrick Howley

Fitness Leader's Handbook
Second Edition

B. Don Franks, PhD
Louisiana State University
at Baton Rouge

Edward T. Howley, PhD
University of Tennessee
at Knoxville

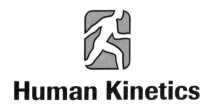

Human Kinetics

Library of Congress Cataloging-in-Publication Data

Franks, B. Don
    Fitness leader's handbook / B. Don Franks, Edward T. Howley. -- 2nd ed.
        p. cm.
    Includes bibliogtaphical references (p.) and index.
    ISBN 0-88011-654-4
    1. Physical fitness. 2. Exercise. 3. Physical fitness--Physiological aspects.   I. Howley, Edward T.,
    1943-   . II. Title
    GV481.F727 1998
    613.7'1--dc21   97-38458
                                                                                                           CIP

ISBN-10: 0-88011-654-4
ISBN-13: 978-0-88011-654-1

Acquisitions Editor: Scott Wikgren; **Managing Editor:** Coree Schutter; **Assistant Editors:** Erin Sprague and Jennifer Jackson; **Copyeditor:** Bonnie Pettifor; **Indexer:** Mary G. Neumann; **Graphic Designer:** Nancy Rasmus; **Graphic Artist:** Doug Burnett; **Cover Designer:** Nancy Rasmus; **Photographer (cover):** International Stock/ © Mark Bolster; **Illustrators:** Joe Bellis (Mac art); Kristin Mount (medical art); Tim Stiles (line drawings); **Printer:** United Graphics

Printed in the United States of America   10   9   8   7   6   5

Human Kinetics
Web site: www.HumanKinetics.com

United States: Human Kinetics, P.O. Box 5076, Champaign, IL 61825-5076
800-747-4457
e-mail: humank@hkusa.com

Canada: Human Kinetics, 475 Devonshire Road, Unit 100, Windsor, ON N8Y 2L5
800-465-7301 (in Canada only)
e-mail: info@hkcanada.com

Europe: Human Kinetics, 107 Bradford Road, Stanningley
Leeds LS28 6AT, United Kingdom
+44 (0) 113 255 5665
e-mail: hk@hkeurope.com

Australia: Human Kinetics, 57A Price Avenue, Lower Mitcham, South Australia 5062
08 8372 0999
e-mail: info@hkaustralia.com

New Zealand: Human Kinetics, Division of Sports Distributors NZ Ltd.
P.O. Box 300 226 Albany, North Shore City, Auckland
0064 9 448 1207
e-mail: info@humankinetics.co.nz

Contents

Part II Who Should Be in a Fitness Program?

Part III Fitness Components

Chapter 7 Desired Aerobic Fitness

Chapter 8 Muscular Strength and Endurance

Chapter 9 Flexibility

Chapter 10 Preventing Low-Back Problems

Chapter 11 Coping With Stress

Part IV The Fitness Program

Part V Scientific Foundations

Chapter 16 Basic Exercise Science

Chapter 17 Measurement and Evaluation

Part VI Safe and Effective Programs

Chapter 18 Preventing and Treating Injuries

Chapter 19 Special Personal Conditions

Chapter 20 Environmental Problems

Chapter 21 Program Organization

Chapter 22 Human Relations

Preface

We have written this book, *Fitness Leader's Handbook, 2nd edition (FLH-2)*, to help the exercise leader who provides appropriate and safe fitness activities day after day. It deals with practical aspects of health-related fitness components, evaluation, and ways to improve health and fitness. *FLH-2* also suggests ways to change other heath-related behaviors and prevent injuries. It includes practical competencies for the fitness leader as identified by ACSM and other fitness organizations. A companion book, *Fitness Facts: The Healthy Living Handbook,* is for fitness participants. Participants in your fitness program or those you work with individually might benefit from reading *Fitness Facts.*

We are pleased with the very positive response to our first edition of *FLH.* This second edition continues to provide practical information written in a straightforward manner. The major changes in our recommendations for fitness testing and prescriptions are based on the latest research and major position statements, such as the *Surgeon General's Report: Physical Activity and Health.* The third edition of *Health Fitness Instructor's Handbook (HFIH-3),* published in August, 1997, offers information to assist fitness professionals in understanding the bases for fitness programs. *HFIH-3* includes all of the competencies for the American College of Sports Medicine (ACSM) Health Fitness Instructor certification. However, much of the material in *HFIH-3* assumes formal education in kinesiology and related fields.

Here's to improved health and fitness for you and your clients.

Acknowledgments

Thanks to David Bassett, Jr., Vernon Bond, Jr., Janet Buckworth, Sue Carver, Jean Lewis, Wendell Liemohn, Daniel Martin, and Dixie Thompson. Their contributions to the 3rd edition of the *Health Fitness Instructor's Handbook* were invaluable to us as we developed this book.

We would also like to thank the many fitness professionals who have provided helpful suggestions for the revised edition. We appreciate authors and publishers who were kind enough to allow us to use materials from their articles and books. We are indebted to our former professors, our students, and professional colleagues in AAHPERD, ACSM, and AAKPE, too numerous to list, who have educated us over the past 3 decades.

Finally, thanks to the folks at Human Kinetics: Rainer Martens, Julie Martens, Scott Wikgren, and Coree Schutter, who have provided encouragement and assistance in many ways.

PART I
Bases For Fitness Programs

Fitness Defined
Fitness Program Described

The first part of the *Fitness Leader's Handbook* deals with the fundamentals. What is physical fitness? How does it differ from performance? What are the components of a physical fitness program?

Much of the material in this text is also covered in our fitness participant's handbook, *Fitness Facts*, though in a less technical fashion. You may suggest that your fitness participants read particular sections or complete certain forms as they progress through the program. Remember that the two books do not cover the topics in the same order since the needs of the instructor preparing a program and those of the participant starting one are quite different.

Chapter 1 defines physical fitness. The fitness leader must clearly understand the distinction between fitness and performance, because many fitness participants associate any type of exercise with the performance goals they may have experienced in athletics or the military. Chapter 2 outlines what the fitness program is designed to do (and, by inference, not do). It also includes the new recommendations for moderate-intensity physical activity found in the *Surgeon General's Report on Physical Activity and Health*. The exercise leader can help participants understand the reasons for the tests and activities based on this understanding of fitness programs.

Chapter 1
Fitness

Fitness Goals
Disease, Movement, and Performance
Characteristics of Fitness
Control of Health Status

The people entering your fitness class, or asking you to be their personal fitness trainer, have taken an important first step toward improving their fitness levels. It is your responsibility to help them in several ways:

1. To understand the components of fitness
2. To analyze their current fitness status
3. To begin or continue appropriate physical activity habits
4. To determine other health behaviors that they need to change
5. To take appropriate steps to change behavior

In this text, we occasionally refer to forms and charts that are in *Fitness Facts*. Encourage your fitness participants to complete these forms and give a copy to you so you can assist them in their programs. Many of the same tables and figures are included in this book for your information. You have permission to copy and use the forms in this book for educational purposes.

Setting Goals

Participants should indicate their satisfaction with their current fitness level (table 1.1) as well as things that bother them (table 1.2) as a start in deciding what areas of life they should consider changing. You can have participants use the forms from *Fitness Facts*, or you can copy the forms from this book for them to use.

Although you can help people make healthy changes in their lives, the individual has to decide what changes to make. Honest answers concerning the participant's plans for changing behavior (table 1.3) will assist you and the participant in establishing the goals of a fitness program.

Table 1.1	Degree of Satisfaction With Different Aspects of Fitness			
Circle the best number for each aspect of your fitness level, using this scale: 4 = Very satisfied 3 = Satisfied 2 = Dissatisfied 1 = Very dissatisfied				
Amount of energy	4	3	2	1
Cardiovascular endurance	4	3	2	1
Blood pressure	4	3	2	1
Amount of body fat	4	3	2	1
Strength	4	3	2	1
Ability to cope with tension and stress	4	3	2	1
Ability to relax	4	3	2	1
Ability to sleep	4	3	2	1
Posture	4	3	2	1
Low-back function	4	3	2	1
Physical appearance	4	3	2	1
Overall physical fitness	4	3	2	1
Level of regular medication	4	3	2	1

Note. From *Fitness Leader's Handbook* (2nd ed.) by B.D. Franks and E.T. Howley, 1998, Champaign, IL: Human Kinetics. This form may be copied by the fitness leader for distribution to participants.

Table 1.2	Things That Bother Me

List the things that bother you about yourself:

Specific physical problem:

Appearance of particular part of body:

Ability to play a specific sport:

Risk of a health problem:

Other:

Note. From *Fitness Leader's Handbook* (2nd ed.) by B.D. Franks and E.T. Howley, 1998, Champaign, IL: Human Kinetics. This form may be copied by the fitness leader for distribution to participants.

Table 1.3	Plans to Change Behavior

Circle your plans to change each area:

Behavior		Plan to change	
Exercise	Now	Soon	No plans
Weight	Now	Soon	No plans
Use of drugs and medications	Now	Soon	No plans
Pattern of sleeping	Now	Soon	No plans
Use of tobacco	Now	Soon	No plans
Handling of tension and stress	Now	Soon	No plans
Diet	Now	Soon	No plans
Use of seat belts	Now	Soon	No plans
Other (list) _____	Now	Soon	No plans
_____	Now	Soon	No plans

Note. From *Fitness Leader's Handbook* (2nd ed.) by B.D. Franks and E.T. Howley, 1998, Champaign, IL: Human Kinetics. This form may be copied by the fitness leader for distribution to participants.

Fitness Defined

Total fitness is striving for the capacity to achieve the optimal *quality of life*. This dynamic, multidimensional state has a positive health base and includes individual performance goals. Total fitness includes healthy mental, social, spiritual, and physical behaviors resulting in positive health that exceeds the state of simply being free from disease. The fit person has high levels of cardiorespiratory function and mental alertness; meaningful social relationships; desirable levels of fat, strength, and flexibility; and a healthy low back.

Total fitness is realized by exercising regularly, eating a healthy diet, and developing the ability to cope with stress without substance abuse. Being fit means being able to enjoy a full life and having a low risk of developing major health problems. Figure 1.1 illustrates the quality of life continuum, showing various stages from *known illness* to *absence from disease* to *life* in the fullest sense of the word. The first criterion for a fitness component is evidence that it is related to positive health. Change in any fitness characteristic causes movement along the quality of life scale.

Total fitness is *dynamic*—the optimal quality of life involves striving, growing, developing, and becoming. It can never be "achieved" in the fullest sense; the fit person is continually approaching the highest quality of life possible.

Total fitness is *multidimensional*. It is difficult to imagine the highest quality of life without including intellectual, social, spiritual, and physical components. Mental alertness and curiosity, emotional feelings, meaningful relations with other humans, awareness and involvement in societal strivings and problems, and the physical capacity to accomplish personal goals with vigor and without undue fatigue appear to be essential elements of life. These aspects of fitness are interrelated in that a high level of fitness in one area enhances all other areas, and, conversely, a low fitness level in any area restricts the accomplishments possible in other areas.

Fitness also includes *unique aspects* for each individual dependent on particular interests and aims in life. Maintaining certain body positions and postures for extended periods of time or different levels and types of physical activity may be a part of a person's vocation. The things a person enjoys doing during leisure time may also have different physical characteristics and

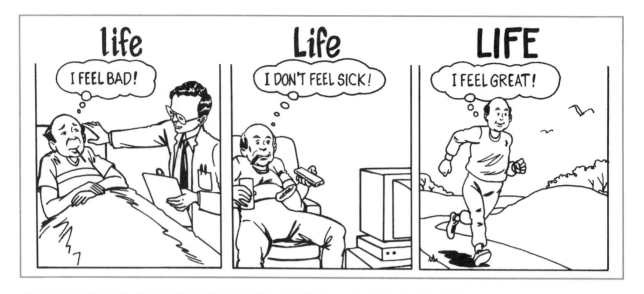

Figure 1.1 Quality of life continuum.

requirements. A careful analysis of regular activities at work, at home, and during leisure, along with potential problems that need to be changed, can chart the course toward a healthier life.

People can achieve fitness goals up to their *genetic potential*—an individual's inherited capacity for both health and performance. It is impossible, however, to determine exactly how much of your health or performance is due to heredity and how much to development. You should help the fitness participant understand that some aspects of fitness are inherited, but a particular genetic background neither dooms a person to low, nor guarantees high, fitness levels.

Certain aspects of our *environment* can be controlled—many of the mental and physical exercises we do are a matter of choice. But we are all limited in various ways by our past and current environments. For example, some children have inadequate diets as a result of their environments; obviously, they can't think about other aspects of fitness until their basic food needs are fulfilled.

Interrelationships of Health, Physical Fitness, and Performance

Regular exercise, a healthy diet, living without substance abuse, and coping with stress effectively can influence many of the primary and secondary risks to health. In addition to helping pre-

vent health problems, these behaviors provide the basis for a higher level of fitness. One of the confusing aspects of "fitness" is that the term has been used for many different goals of life; for example, the avoidance of disease, the ability to do a day's work without fatigue, the ability to perform in different activities at desired levels, and the achievement of mental and social goals. This section of the chapter presents the layers of health, physical fitness, and performance (see figure 1.2).

Lack of Disease

The first layer of health, fitness, and performance is the medical diagnosis that we are free from disease (unfortunately referred to as "apparently healthy"). This is the minimum goal for all of us. We try to prevent sickness, illness, and known diseases. You have probably assisted in health fairs to help people identify signs, symptoms, and test scores that may indicate a possible medical problem. Freedom from disease is an important first step, but as terms such as "positive health" and "wellness" attempt to communicate, there is much more to health than simply being without disease.

Everyday Efficiency

The second layer deals with a person's ability to carry out typical activities at work, at home, and in leisure pursuits without undue fatigue. The characteristics necessary for this level differ

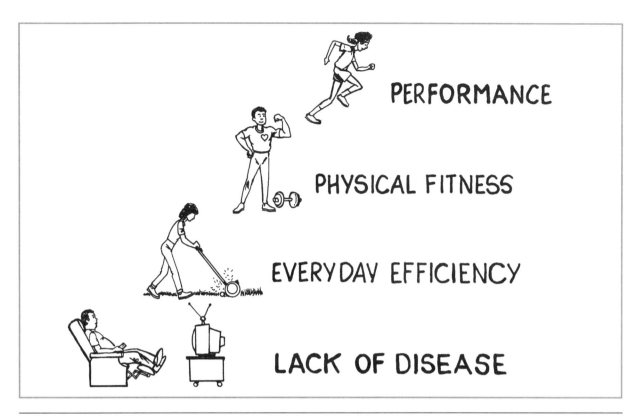

Figure 1.2 Health, fitness, and performance: the layered look.

depending on vocation and lifestyle and vary among individuals. The emphasis here is not on how well the physical tasks are done, but that they *can* be done.

Physical Fitness

This book will focus on the *physical fitness* aspects of positive health. Physical fitness is the physical well-being that is related to optimal health. It includes having appropriate levels of the components of fitness that provide dynamic health and a low risk of developing major health problems.

Performance

The last layer recognizes that many individuals choose to participate in certain sport activities. The performance element involves developing those skills and underlying abilities needed to do the activity well enough to compete with others (or self) at the individual's desired level. The activities and desired level will, of course, vary among different persons. Some will be happy to break 100 in golf while others may want to play in the "A" division of the adult soccer league. The underlying performance abilities (e.g., agility, balance, coordination, power, speed) and skills will, of course, vary, depending on the desired activity.

Control of Health Status

This chapter has presented the broader picture so that you can help fitness participants put physical fitness into perspective with other aspects of health, fitness, and performance.

The knowledge that health status and risk of major health problems can be modified is an exciting yet frustrating aspect of fitness programs. It is exciting because individuals can actually gain control of their health. It is frustrating in that it may be difficult for some people to change unhealthy lifestyles. Participating in a fitness program puts a person at the cutting edge of health. You can help fitness participants gain control of their lives, beginning with an evaluation of risk factors and behaviors related to health.

Summary

Physical fitness is defined as those aspects of an ultimate quality of life that are related to positive physical health. Physical fitness is a necessary ingredient of fitness, but fitness includes much more than simply the physical aspects. On the one hand, people cannot achieve total fitness without a good physical health base. On the other hand, having a high level of physical fitness without the other aspects of fitness would be a sterile existence. The relationship between physical fitness, health, and performance is depicted by describing the different goals of being free from disease, having sufficient energy to achieve one's goals, and competing in specific activities at desired skill levels.

Chapter 2
Fitness Program

Principles
Workout Format

As we said in chapter 1, you, as the fitness leader, are in an important position to assist participants to define their goals and set up the kind of program that meets these goals (figure 2.1).

Principles of Fitness Improvement

Some general principles can guide you in helping participants improve their cardiorespiratory function, relative leanness, flexibility, muscular strength and endurance, and low-back health.

Overload

For any tissue to increase in function, it must be exposed to a "load" greater than that to which it is accustomed. The tissue then gradually adapts to this load by increasing its size or function. The process of *overload followed by adaptation* is the basis of fitness and performance programs. A good example of this principle is seen in figure 2.2, which shows how a muscle is made stronger. The subject lifts a light weight and over a period of time the muscle adapts to that weight. He or she then lifts a heavier weight and, once again, the muscle adapts. The process continues as he or she proceeds through the training program. In order to maintain the tissue at any size or function, the person must continue to work against the load appropriate to that level. In fact, if he or she stops working against that load, the system returns to its former "untrained" state. This is sometimes referred to as the Principle of Reversibility. In short, use increases function; disuse decreases function.

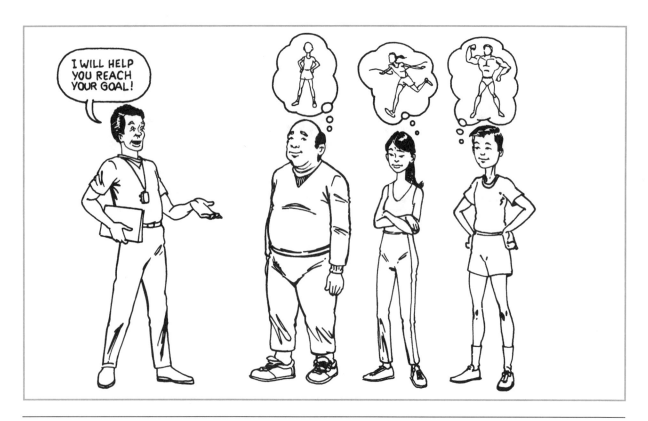

Figure 2.1 Different fitness goals.

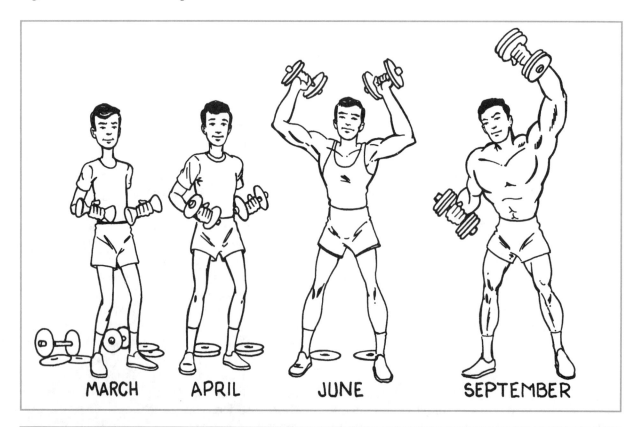

Figure 2.2 Strength and endurance progression.

Specificity

The second major principle of training is *specificity*, which means that the type of adaptation that occurs is related to the type of exercise used in the fitness program. Figure 2.3 shows what happens when one identical twin participates in cardiovascular endurance exercises while his brother participates in a weight-training program. The first twin shows signs of a leaner body (less fat) and increased heart function, with the muscles having an increased capacity to work without fatigue. The other twin shows an increase in muscle mass and strength, with little change in heart function. In each case the muscles were "overloaded," but the type of load was different: endurance activity for one and resistive work for the other. The muscles respond to these unique overloads by adapting in specific ways. The emphasis for persons in your health and fitness programs is on cardiovascular function, but the program also includes specific strength-building and flexibility exercises to allow people to participate in everyday activities without undue strain.

New Recommendations for Physical Activity

The 1978 American College of Sports Medicine (ACSM) guidelines for improvement of cardiorespiratory function have been widely used. At least 20 min of continuous vigorous (60% to 90% of maximal capacity) aerobic activity, 3 to 5 days per week, with a warm-up and cool-down, has been the standard exercise prescription for the past 2 decades.

In the early 1990s, the ACSM, Centers for Disease Control and Prevention, and the President's Council on Physical Fitness and Sports recommended that sedentary individuals engage in at least 30 min of moderate-intensity physical activity daily, based on evidence that moderate aerobic activity can reduce the risk of heart disease.

These two recommendations have caused some confusion. However, as the 1996 *Surgeon General's Report on Physical Activity and Health* indicates, there is a way to harmonize them. Generally, sedentary individuals should be encouraged to engage in at least 30 min of some sort of physical activity every day. Persons who

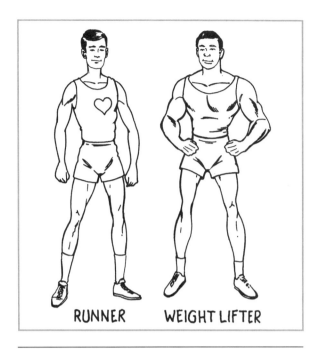

RUNNER   WEIGHT LIFTER

Figure 2.3 Training is specific.

are already doing this can achieve additional health and fitness improvements by doing more, or more intense, activity. Part IV of this book will provide more specific recommendations.

Components of Physical Fitness

Part III of this book includes a separate chapter on each of the fitness components (figure 2.4) discussed below, as well as a chapter on coping with stress. Chapters in part IV provide more detail concerning the fitness activities. This section provides an overview of the important aspects involved in improving each of these components.

Cardiorespiratory Function

Encourage the participant to improve cardiorespiratory function by engaging in activities that use large muscle groups. Examples include walking, jogging, swimming, dancing, and cycling. These activities require the heart and the muscles involved in breathing to work harder to deliver the oxygen that the muscles need. In this way the heart and the respiratory muscles increase their ability to do work and to do that work more efficiently.

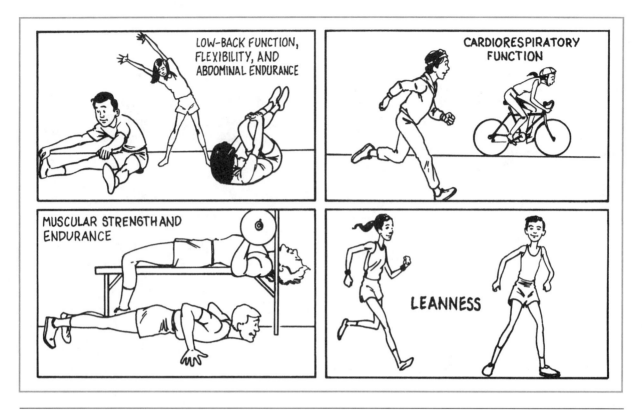

Figure 2.4 Fitness components.

Relative Leanness

Body fatness is usually expressed as a percent—for example, 30%. If a person weighs 200 lb and is 30% fat, it means that there are 60 lb of fat tissue and 140 lb of fat-free, or lean, tissue present. Participants can decrease their body fat percentage by decreasing the number of pounds of fat tissue, increasing the number of pounds of lean tissue, or both. Lean tissue can be increased by strength training, in which case the individual may become heavier but leaner (having a lower body fat percentage). In order to lose 1 lb of fat, the participant has to use about 3500 kilocalories (kcal) of energy. You can help the individual accomplish this by increasing the amount of exercise, decreasing the number of calories eaten per day, or both. The best way to lose body fat is to use a combination of diet and exercise. A small percentage of participants have less than the essential level of fat. You should encourage them to increase caloric intake (especially carbohydrates).

Muscular Strength and Endurance

People need a certain amount of strength and endurance to perform many tasks in daily life. Doing regular strengthening exercises that appropriately overload all the muscle groups can maintain muscular strength and endurance. Most participants can achieve this with calisthenics that use their bodies as the resistance. For those who want more strength and endurance, increase the overload. Strengthening activities also help individuals maintain bone density, thus preventing osteoporosis.

Flexibility

Being able to move one's joints through a full range of motion is helpful as one does daily tasks. Flexibility can be maintained by including static stretching exercises as part of the warm-up and the cool-down, and by doing activities that move joints through a full range of motion during workouts.

Low-Back Function

Low-back pain is responsible for a great deal of human suffering, but it can often be avoided. The incidence of low-back pain in this country has increased over the past several decades in relation to the increasingly sedentary lifestyles adopted by many Americans. To deal with this problem, attention has been focused on ways to prevent or relieve the problem. Most people know that pregnant women experience an increase in low-back pain in the months before the baby is due. The growth of the fetus (along with the associated support tissue) enlarges the abdomen, stretching the abdominal muscles and pulling the spine forward. A similar situation can occur in someone who is not pregnant. *One of the major contributors to low-back problems is weak abdominal muscles* that allow the abdominal contents to "stick out." One way to deal with this problem is to help the participant strengthen abdominal muscles through special "curl-up" exercises that focus the overload on the abdominal muscles.

Another factor related to low-back pain is *lack of flexibility* in the low back due to tight muscles in the hip area. One way to alleviate this problem is to help participants stretch the muscle groups involved (see chapter 10). When a person is not coping well with stress, various muscle groups tighten and can contribute to low-back pain. A physician may prescribe a muscle relaxant to treat this problem; however, there are a variety of ways to relieve tension without medication (see chapter 11).

Format for the Fitness Beginner

Individuals without major health problems or symptoms can begin moderate-intensity activities (e.g., walking a few minutes at their own pace) with very low risk. If moderately active individuals want to increase their vigorous-intensity physical activity, then you as the fitness leader can help the person set up a fitness program. You need to consider some important points related to the overall fitness program as you help establish the individual's program to improve flexibility, cardiorespiratory function, strength, and leanness.

Screening and Testing

Chapter 3 helps you determine a person's health status, and chapter 4 shows you how the fitness director uses this information to judge whether a potential fitness participant should begin a vigorous-intensity exercise program. A fitness program should allow for periodic testing of the various fitness components. This enables you to provide feedback about how the participant is progressing toward individual goals. A general rule of thumb is to have participants aim at making about a 10% change over a 3-month period in the areas that need improvement. Once the participant achieves his or her goal, periodic testing demonstrates maintenance of fitness status.

Encouraging a Routine of Exercise

If an individual is judged able to participate in a fitness program, you need to help her recognize the importance of staying active as part of a lifelong habit. Fitness changes are both gained and lost quickly. The only way your participants can hold onto the fitness they develop is by maintaining a regular program of physical activity. In addition, if exercise is to be useful in a weight control program, it must be done on a regular basis.

Starting Slowly

For many people it has been several years since they were active and fit. If it took years to get out of shape, it is reasonable to suggest that the participant allow some months to get back into shape. You will find it does not take a great deal of activity for a sedentary individual to overload the body and experience a training effect. Knowing that and the desire to minimize the likelihood of muscle soreness or an injury, you should encourage each participant to begin an exercise program slowly. *It is better to do too little than too much.* Figure 2.5 indicates that though the idea of "no pain, no gain" may be appropriate for athletes training for championship competition, it is irresponsible nonsense when applied to fitness programs.

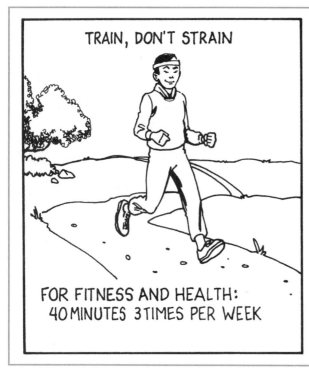
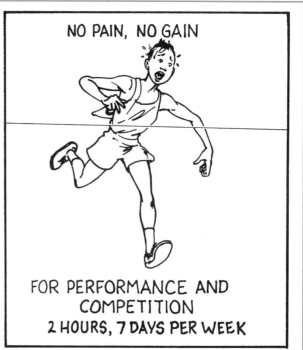

TRAIN, DON'T STRAIN

FOR FITNESS AND HEALTH:
40 MINUTES 3 TIMES PER WEEK

NO PAIN, NO GAIN

FOR PERFORMANCE AND
COMPETITION
2 HOURS, 7 DAYS PER WEEK

Figure 2.5 Fitness programs versus performance training.

Teaching Fitness Guidelines

The fitness leader can help participants learn the basic guidelines for developing and maintaining fitness. The recommendations are different for the sedentary individual doing daily moderate-intensity activity, the moderately active individual engaging in vigorous-intensity activity for health and fitness goals, and the athlete performing in competition.

Warm-Up and Cool-Down.   Begin each exercise session with some low-intensity activities, including some appropriate stretching exercises to develop a healthy low back. The warm-up provides a smooth transition from the resting state to the higher level of energy expenditure and effort experienced in the main part of the workout. At the end of the exercise session, gradually diminish the intensity to allow the body to make the transition back to rest. This reduces the chance that participants will experience the light-headedness that can occur when suddenly stopping an activity and standing idle. The cool-down can also include some of the same stretches used in the warm-up. If an exercise session must be shortened due to lack of time, keep the warm-up and cool-down periods and reduce the time spent in the main part of the workout. Increasing amounts of warm-up and cool-down are needed as one moves from moderate-intensity activity (very little), to fitness-related vigorous-intensity activity (5 to 10 min), to athletic performance (20 to 40 min or more).

Frequency.   Moderate-intensity activity should be done every day. The recommended frequency of vigorous-intensity exercise sessions to achieve cardiovascular fitness, as well as weight loss goals, is 3 or 4 times per week—about every other day. Exercising fewer than 3 times a week requires very high-intensity activity to achieve a cardiovascular training effect; this higher intensity is associated with more injuries. In addition, it is difficult to achieve a weight loss goal when exercising fewer than 3 times per week. If a previously sedentary person begins to exercise strenuously more than 4 times per week, his or her risk of injury increases. The day-on, day-off routine seems to be optimal and makes an exercise program easy to schedule. Athletes training to a high performance level will often train 6 to 10 times per week.

Total Work and Duration.   Moderate-intensity physical activity emphasizes getting the person up and moving, engaging in at least 30 min of activity each day. For fitness-related vigorous activity, one should aim at setting up a program that allows the participant to expend 200 to 300 kcal per exercise session in order to achieve a cardiovascular training effect and meet body composition goals. The total caloric cost of a workout is determined by the *duration* and the *intensity* of the workout.

Generally, a person needs about 30 to 40 min of activity (including warm-up and cool-down) to achieve a 200 to 300 kcal expenditure when working at the appropriate intensity. The duration of lighter activities has to be extended to achieve the 200 to 300 kcal goal. Athletes will expend a larger amount of energy as they prepare for specific performances.

Progression.   As we mentioned previously, it is important to progress from light to more intense exercise sessions. We feel that you should encourage the participant to be able to walk about 3 mi briskly before he or she undertakes more strenuous activity. By achieving this goal the individual will have established a regular pattern of activity and made some body composition changes that will ease the transition to more strenuous exercise. Figure 2.6 shows that the progression from walking to jogging to running occurs over a period of months.

Intensity.   There is little emphasis on intensity for the daily 30 min of activity recommended for sedentary individuals. The individual does activity well within the comfort zone (e.g., slight increase in breathing, little or no sweating). For fitness-related vigorous activity, the intensity of exercise is best described by the overload it places on the cardiorespiratory system during a workout. The threshold needed to achieve the training effect is lower for the very sedentary (60% of maximal heart rate) compared to the very fit (90% of maximal heart rate). The primary way to judge exercise intensity is to see how high the heart rate goes during the activity, since heart rate increases in a regular manner with exercise intensity. (If you are interested in learning more about intensity, read chapter 14 in the *Health Fitness Instructor's Handbook*, 3rd edition.) You can determine the appropriate exercise intensity by calculating a *target heart rate* (THR) *zone.* The THR zone represents the range

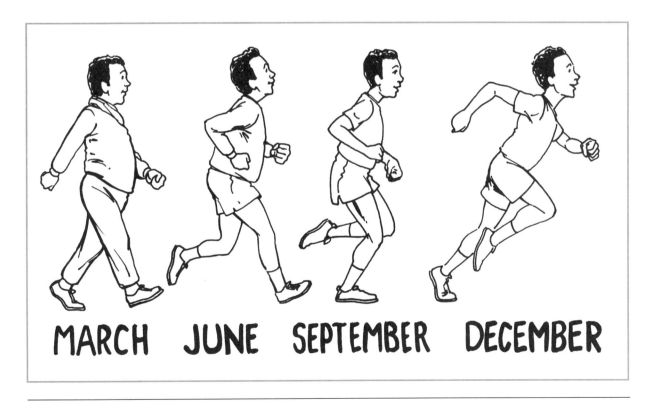

MARCH   JUNE   SEPTEMBER   DECEMBER

Figure 2.6 Cardiorespiratory progression.

of heart rate values that are *high enough to cause a training effect yet low enough to allow the participant to exercise long enough* to achieve the total work (200 to 300 kcal) needed for a training effect. For the average participant, the THR zone is 70% to 85% of maximal heart rate. Athletes will exercise at much higher intensities in preparation for high-level performance.

The first step in calculating THR is to estimate maximal heart rate (HR). Complete the following:

---

220 – age (years) = age-adjusted maximal HR

Example: For a 50-year-old person,
$220 - 50 = 170$ beats·min^{-1}

Now use the participant's age:

$220 - $ _____ (years) = _____ beats·min^{-1}

The second step is to calculate the THR zone:

70% maximal HR = low end of THR zone

Example: 70% of 170 beats·min^{-1} = 119 beats·min^{-1}

Participant: .70 x _____ beats·min^{-1} = _____ beats·min^{-1}

85% maximal HR = high end of THR zone

Example: 85% of 170 beats·min^{-1} = 145 beats·min^{-1}

Participant: .85 x _____ beats·min^{-1} = _____ beats·min^{-1}

As you can see from our example, the 50-year-old person does not have to exercise at a very high heart rate to have a training effect. This is a very important point. You need to educate the participant to begin a fitness program at the low end of the THR zone and concentrate on doing activity for a longer duration at a lower intensity. Furthermore, we strongly recommend that sedentary persons be able to walk 3 mi at a brisk pace before they become concerned about the intensity of their workout. Walking may be all the exercise some individuals need to reach the THR.

This leads to an important question: How can one measure heart rate during exercise? Electronic devices can be used to measure heart rate

"on the go," but they are not really necessary. If HR is monitored immediately after an individual stops exercising, that value is a good estimate of what the heart rate was during the exercise. Monitor heart rates (or teach participants to monitor their own) within 5 s after exercise ends by counting the pulse rate on the wrist or neck for 10 s. Heart rate decreases so fast after exercise is stopped that it must be monitored quickly if one is to make a good estimate of the exercise heart rate. Multiply the 10-s heart rate value by 6 to calculate the heart rate in beats·min^{-1}. Table 2.1 lists THR values for people of different ages, based on present activity status. The THRs are listed as 10-s values because that is the way people commonly refer to THR. Check participants' heart rates at various times during the workout, frequently enough so they learn what it feels like to work in their target heart rate zone.

Types of Activities.   At the beginning of a fitness program, we recommend activities that are easily controlled in terms of intensity, provide an adequate means of expending calories, and have a low probability of causing injury. Walking, cycling, and swimming are examples of such activities. Emphasize lower intensity and longer duration at the start of the program, progressing to more and varied activities as the participant becomes more fit. We recommend a progression in movement from walking to jogging to running to games (see figure 2.6). The direction is from low- to high-intensity, from more to less controlled activity, and from activities with a low risk of injury to those representing a slightly greater risk.

Individualizing the Workout

We have presented these guidelines for improving fitness based on what each individual needs. In some programs, however, you will be working with fitness participants in a group setting. It is important to plan group activities so that each person maintains an appropriate intensity while exercising with others. Continually encourage all participants to exercise in their target heart rate zones. Remember, it is the combination of intensity and duration that caus-

Table 2.1   Estimated 10-Second Target Heart Rate

Population	Intensity % CRF[a]	Age (years)						
		20	**30**	**40**	**50**	**60**	**70**	**80**
Inactive with several risk factors	50	22	21	20	18	17	16	15
	55	23	22	21	19	18	17	16
	60	24	23	22	20	19	18	17
Normal activity with few risk factors	65	25	24	23	21	20	19	18
	70	26	25	24	22	21	20	18
	75	28	26	25	24	22	21	19
	80	29	28	26	25	23	22	20
Very active with low risk	85	30	29	27	26	24	23	21
	90	31	30	28	27	25	24	22

Note. To be used only for people whose max HR is unknown.

[a]CRF = cardiorespiratory fitness (aerobic fitness).

Adapted from Howley and Franks 1997.

es the training effect and the expenditure of calories. During the early phases of the fitness program, people who reach the low end of their THR zone at similar speeds should walk and jog together. In the later phases of the program, participants can work in the middle of the THR zone. It may be necessary for you to modify rules of games and provide encouragement to keep the participants in the THR zone. After a THR check, encourage those who are too low to work harder and those who are too high to slow down.

Maintenance

For some people, long walks may be the first and last step of an exercise program that satisfies their needs and accomplishes their goals. Others may desire a higher level of fitness to enjoy recreational interests that might include racquetball, basketball, soccer, tennis, or 10K runs. When participants have achieved the level they desire, they can maintain that status by daily moderate-intensity physical activity and by including vigorous-intensity physical activity three or four times per week, 30 to 40 min per session at their THR.

You need to help fitness participants assign a high priority to the routine of regular exercise. By doing so they will find it very easy to maintain their fitness over the years and minimize the "aging effect" experienced by a sedentary population.

Summary

Everyone's health is enhanced by finding ways to engage in at least 30 min of moderate-intensity physical activity daily. Fitness changes are made by placing an overload on a tissue (muscle) or system (cardiovascular) and allowing an adaptation to occur over time. Fitness improvements are specific to the type of training used. Body fatness can be changed by both diet and exercise. To lose 1 lb of fat requires a caloric deficit of 3500 kcal. A fitness program should also try to improve low-back function by providing exercises to strengthen abdominal muscles and stretch muscles in the hip area. A fitness program begins with an evaluation of health status and emphasizes the need to exercise on a regular basis and start slowly. After achieving 30 min of moderate-intensity activity daily, then plan three or four workouts per week at about 70% to 85% of maximal heart rate for 30 to 40 min per session to result in the expenditure of about 200 to 300 kcal per session. Each session begins with a warm-up, concludes with a cool-down, and includes exercises to improve low-back function and muscular endurance. We recommend that you set up a progression from walking to jogging to running to games.

PART II

Who Should Be in a Fitness Program?

Health Status
Screening

Part II of the *Fitness Leader's Handbook* deals with one of the primary responsibilities of any fitness leader: helping potential participants determine their current health status and decide on the first steps toward fitness.

Chapter 3 describes the bases for evaluating health status. Chapter 4 outlines the bases for screening persons for medical referral or entry into a supervised or unsupervised fitness program. Although fitness program policies determine exactly how persons will be evaluated and screened, the exercise leader needs to know why these decisions are made.

Chapter 3
Health Status

Risks of Health Problems
Known Problems
Characteristics
Behaviors
Signs and Symptoms

The primary responsibility of the fitness leader is to supervise physical activity. Participants may have a variety of potential health problems, and a knowledgeable fitness leader must be alert to signs and symptoms that may indicate such problems. This chapter provides information to help you understand the factors related to the risks of health problems.

Risks of Health Problems

Many characteristics and behaviors are related to positive and negative health. Most studies of risk factors for health problems have dealt with some aspect of cardiovascular disease. That is the focus of this chapter, although we also include factors related to low-back problems.

Health risks are normally divided into primary and secondary risk factors. (Participants may refer to *Fitness Facts* for a discussion of this material.) Primary risk factors are those characteristics that are strongly associated with a particular health problem independent of all other variables. For example, a fitness participant who smokes (a primary risk factor for heart disease) has a high risk of heart disease even if no other risk factors are present. Secondary risk factors, however, have a high relationship with the health problem only when other risk factors are present. For example, if someone is in a stressful situation (a secondary risk factor), that individual is not at high risk if no other risk factors are present. Inability to cope with stress, however, does increase the risk of heart disease when other risk factors are present. Another way to classify risk factors is to distinguish inherited risk factors that cannot be altered from lifestyle behaviors that can be modified.

Unavoidable Risks

Some risk factors are easily identified but unfortunately can't be altered. The following segments of the population have a greater risk of heart disease, especially if they adopt unhealthy behaviors:

- Those with a family history of the disease
- Older people
- Men
- African-Americans

It is important to point out that these are secondary risk factors for heart disease. They cause a person to be at high risk only when added to one or more other risk factors. In addition, part of the risk associated with family history and age results from behaviors that can be changed. Family history risks include unhealthy dietary, activity, smoking, and stress behaviors that tend to be transmitted from parents to children. These types of behaviors can be corrected with proper attention throughout life, especially in early childhood. In terms of aging, explain to participants that though many fitness characteristics get worse as people grow older, a portion of the deterioration seen in aging curves results from many individuals becoming less active as they get older—not from aging itself. If participants maintain active lifestyles, they can minimize the fitness decline seen in typical aging curves.

Alterable Risks

Many of the risks for heart disease (as well as for back problems) can be modified.

Primary Risk Factors. Some characteristics and behaviors create a higher risk for coronary heart disease (CHD), even in the absence of other risk factors. The independent, primary risk factors are as follows:

- Smoking
- Physical inactivity
- High concentrations of serum low-density lipoprotein cholesterol (LDL-C)
- Low concentrations of serum high-density lipoprotein cholesterol (HDL-C)
- High blood pressure

Secondary Risk Factors. Some characteristics and behaviors cause increased risk of CHD only when other risk factors are present. In addition to the factors that cannot be altered (age, family history, gender, and race), there are other secondary risk factors:

- Obesity
- High-fat diet
- Inability to cope with stress
- Coronary-prone personality
- High triglyceride levels

Physical Activity and CHD Risk Factors

Regular physical activity can decrease many of these risk factors for heart disease. Table 3.1 describes the effects that regular physical activity has on the risk factors for heart disease.

Low-Back Factors

Various orthopedic problems can develop with exercise (see chapters 18 and 19). A major health problem that affects many people is low-back pain. Clinical evidence indicates that there are several risk factors associated with low-back problems:

- Lack of abdominal muscle endurance
- Lack of flexibility in the midtrunk area and back of upper legs (hamstrings)
- Poor posture—lying, sitting, standing, moving
- Poor lifting habits
- Inability to cope with stress

Evaluation of Health Status

The first step for a potential fitness participant is to determine current health status. Health status includes five major categories (see figure 3.1):

- Diagnosed medical problems
- Characteristics that increase the risk of health problems
- Signs or symptoms that indicate health problems
- Lifestyle behaviors related to positive or negative health
- Test scores

Table 3.1   Effect of Physical Activity on Risk Factors

Risk factor	Effect of regular physical activity		
	Improve	May improve	No effect
Older age			X
Smoking		X	
High total cholesterol	X		
High low-density cholesterol	X		
African-American			X
Low high-density cholesterol	X		
Fibrinogen	X		
Male			X
High very low-density cholesterol	X		
Family history			X
High blood pressure	X		
Physical inactivity	X		
Low cardiorespiratory fitness	X		
High-fat diet		X	
Obesity	X		
Diabetes		X	
Inability to cope with stress		X	

Reprinted from Howley and Franks 1997.

Have the fitness participant complete the Health Status Questionnaire (use a copy of table 3.2 on pages 24-26) to provide information about health status. Use questions 12 to 14 to review known health problems that may affect an exercise program.

Characteristics Related to Health

As we mentioned earlier in this chapter, a person has a higher risk of cardiovascular disease if his or her relatives (especially parents and grandparents) died before age 50 from cardiovascular disease. Male and African-American participants are also at higher risk. Everyone has increased risk of major health problems as they grow older. Any of these characteristics can motivate persons to adopt healthy behaviors and change unhealthy practices.

Signs and Symptoms Related to Health

Question 15 on the Health Status Questionnaire includes some of the major signs and symptoms that could indicate a major health problem. Participants with any of these signs or symptoms should check with their physicians to determine if they reflect some problem that needs medical attention. They should not begin a fitness program until these signs or symptoms have been checked.

Table 3.2 Health Status Questionnaire

Instructions

Complete each question accurately. All information provided is confidential if you choose to submit this form to your fitness instructor.

Part 1. Information about the individual

1. _____   _____
   Social security number   Date

2. _____   _____
   Legal name   Nickname

3. _____   _____
   Mailing address   Home phone

   _____   _____
                                                                             Business phone

4. *EI* _____   _____
   Personal physician   Phone

   _____
   Address

5. *EI* _____   _____
   Person to contact in emergency   Phone

6. Gender (circle one):   Female   Male (RF)

7. *RF* Date of birth: _____
                       Month   Day   Year

8. Number of hours worked per week: Less than 20   20-40   41-60   Over 60

9. *SLA* More than 25% of time spent on job (circle all that apply)

   Sitting at desk   Lifting or carrying loads   Standing   Walking   Driving

Part 2.   Medical history

10. RF Circle any who died of heart attack before age 50:

    Father   Mother   Brother   Sister   Grandparent

11. Date of

    Last medical physical exam: _____
                                Year

    Last physical fitness test: _____
                                Year

12. Circle operations you have had:

    Back *SLA*   Heart *MC*   Kidney *SLA*   Eyes *SLA*   Joint *SLA*   Neck *SLA*

    Ears *SLA*   Hernia *SLA*   Lung *SLA*   Other _____

13. Please circle any of the following for which you have been diagnosed or treated by a physician or health professional:

Alcoholism *SEP*	Diabetes *SEP*	Kidney problem *MC*
Anemia, sickle cell *SEP*	Emphysema *SEP*	Mental illness *SEP*
Anemia, other *SEP*	Epilepsy *SEP*	Neck strain *SLA*
Asthma *SEP*	Eye problems *SLA*	Obesity *RF*
Back strain *SLA*	Gout *SLA*	Phlebitis *MC*
Bleeding trait *SEP*	Hearing loss *SLA*	Rheumatoid arthritis *SLA*
Bronchitis, chronic *SEP*	Heart problem *MC*	Stroke *MC*
Cancer *SEP*	High blood pressure *RF*	Thyroid problem *SEP*
Cirrhosis, liver *MC*	Hypoglycemia *SEP*	Ulcer *SEP*
Concussion *MC*	Hyperlipidemia *RF*	Other _____
Congenital defect *SEP*	Infectious mononucleosis *MC*	

14. Circle all medicine taken in last 6 months:

Blood thinner *MC*	Epilepsy medication *SEP*	Nitroglycerin *MC*
Diabetic *SEP*	Heart rhythm medication *MC*	Other _____
Digitalis *MC*	High blood pressure medication *MC*	
Diuretic *MC*	Insulin *MC*	

15. Any of these health symptoms that occurs frequently is the basis for medical attention. Circle the number indicating how often you have each of the following:

5 = Very often
4 = Fairly often
3 = Sometimes
2 = Infrequently
1 = Practically never

a. Coughing up blood *MC*
   1   2   3   4   5

g. Swollen joints *MC*
   1   2   3   4   5

b. Abdominal pain *MC*
   1   2   3   4   5

h. Feeling faint *MC*
   1   2   3   4   5

c. Low-back pain *MC*
   1   2   3   4   5

i. Dizziness *MC*
   1   2   3   4   5

d. Leg pain *MC*
   1   2   3   4   5

j. Breathless with slight exertion *MC*
   1   2   3   4   5

e. Arm or shoulder pain *MC*
   1   2   3   4   5

k. Palpitation or fast heartbeat *MC*
   1   2   3   4   5

f. Chest pain *RF MC*
   1   2   3   4   5

l. Unusual fatigue with normal activity *MC*
   1   2   3   4   5

(continued)

Table 3.2 *(cont'd)*

Part 3.　　**Health-related behavior**

16. *RF* Do you now smoke?　　Yes　　No

17. *RF* If you are a smoker, indicate number smoked per day:

    Cigarettes:　　　40 or more　　20-39　　10-19　　1-9
    Cigars or pipes only:　　5 or more or any inhaled　　Less than 5, none inhaled

18. *RF* Do you exercise regularly?　　Yes　　No

19. How many days per week do you accumulate 30 minutes of moderate activity?

    　　0　　1　　2　　3　　4　　5　　6　　7　　days per week

20. How many days per week do you normally spend at least 20 minutes in vigorous exercise?

    　　0　　1　　2　　3　　4　　5　　6　　7　　days per week

21. Can you walk 4 miles briskly without fatigue?　　Yes　　No

22. Can you jog 3 miles continuously at a moderate pace without discomfort?　　Yes　　No

23. Weight now: _____lb.　One year ago: _____lb.　Age 21: _____lb.

Part 4.　　**Health-related attitudes**

24. RF These are traits that have been associated with coronary-prone behavior. Circle the number that corresponds to how you feel:

    6 = Strongly agree　　　　　I am an impatient, time-conscious, hard-driving individual.
    5 = Moderately agree
    4 = Slightly agree　　　　　　1　　2　　3　　4　　5　　6
    3 = Slightly disagree
    2 = Moderately disagree
    1 = Strongly disagree

25. List everything not already included on this questionnaire that might cause you problems in a fitness test or fitness program:

Code for Health Status Questionnaire

The following code will help you evaluate the information in the Health Status Questionnaire.

EI = Emergency Information—must be readily available.

MC = Medical Clearance needed—do not allow exercise without physician's permission.

SEP = Special Emergency Procedures needed—do not let participant exercise alone; make sure the person's exercise partner knows what to do in case of an emergency.

RF = Risk Factor for CHD—educational materials and workshops needed.

SLA = Special or Limited Activities may be needed—you may need to include or exclude specific exercises.

OTHER (not marked) = Personal information that may be helpful for files or research.

Reprinted from Howley and Franks 1997.

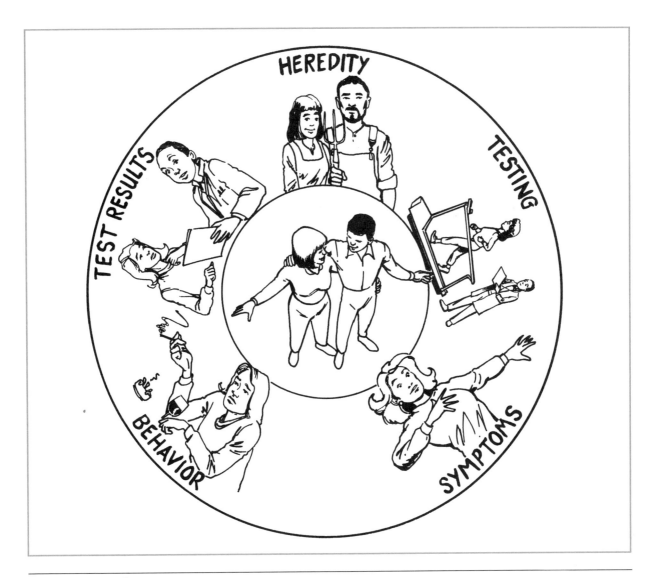

Figure 3.1 Health status.

Behaviors Related to Health

Questions 16 to 24 are related to healthy (and unhealthy) behaviors, such as smoking, physical activity, body weight, and personality type.

Test Scores Related to Health

Finally, as an initial part of the fitness assessment, you will administer a number of physical fitness tests. It is not important for an individual to perform better than everyone else on these tests, but it is important for the participant to be in the healthy range for body fatness, have adequate levels of cardiorespiratory

fitness, and develop sufficient abdominal strength and endurance and midtrunk flexibility to minimize the risks of low-back problems. These tests and health standards will be covered in part III.

Summary

Unavoidable risks of heart disease include family history, aging, and being male or African-American. Primary risks of heart disease include smoking, physical inactivity, high concentrations of serum low-density lipoprotein cholesterol (LDL-C), low concentrations of serum high-density lipoprotein cholesterol (HDL-C), and high blood pressure. Secondary risk factors include obesity, inability to cope with stress, a coronary-prone personality, high-fat diet, and high triglyceride levels. Regular physical activity can decrease many of these risk factors for heart disease.

Causes of low-back problems include lack of abdominal muscle endurance; poor flexibility in the low back and hamstrings; poor posture in lying, sitting, standing, and moving; poor lifting habits; and inability to cope with stress.

One of the responsibilities of a fitness program is to evaluate participants' current health status. This information includes known medical problems; characteristics that put the fitness participant at risk; and signs, symptoms, and behaviors that are related to a healthy lifestyle.

Chapter 4
Screening

Information
Decisions

If the potential fitness participant is under treatment for a major health problem, you must rely on guidance from the fitness program director and medical professionals to determine appropriate fitness programs. A fitness participant whose health status has been carefully analyzed by a physician and who has no health problems or unhealthy behaviors can continue a fitness program, modifying it based on his or her particular interests. Most people, however, fall between these two extremes. They do not have a major health problem, but they have not carefully checked their health status.

The Health Status Questionnaire (HSQ) in chapter 3 provided information concerning illness, characteristics, symptoms, and behaviors that are related to health problems. Part 1 provides *personal and emergency* information about the individual. Keep the emergency information readily available in case you need to call the participant's physician or family. Part 2 includes a *medical history* of the participant and the participant's family. This information will aid the director of the fitness program in deciding appropriate activity and educational programs. Part 3 deals with *behaviors* known to be related to safety and health. You may be able to help the participant modify these behaviors for a healthier lifestyle. Part 4 includes some of the *psychological aspects* of fitness and attitudes that are associated with the healthy life. This section will help you better understand how to deal with the individuals in your program.

Testing is the other source of information about an individual's health status. Table 4.1 outlines the items included in fitness testing. Part III of this book includes detailed recommendations for fitness testing.

Table 4.1	Physical Fitness Test Items	
Minimum battery		**Additional variables**
Rest		
Heart rate (beats · min^{-1})		12-lead ECG[a]
Blood pressure (mmHg)		Blood profile[b]
Percent fat (%)		Overall flexibility
Sit-and-reach (cm)		Pulmonary function
Submaximal		
Heart rate		ECG
Blood pressure		Blood profile
Rating of perceived exertion (RPE, 0-10)		
Maximal		
BP		$\dot{V}O_2$
RPE		Blood profile
Time to max (min)		ECG
Functional capacity (METs)		Modified pull-ups or push-ups
Curl-ups (number/min)		

Adapted from Howley and Franks (1986).

[a]ECG abnormalities are medically evaluated to determine appropriate referral or placement of person.

[b]Includes total cholesterol, HDL, triglycerides, and glucose.

Adapted from Howley and Franks 1997.

Decisions

You must decide whether each potential fitness participant should have medical clearance prior to beginning a fitness program. The standards in this area are changing. Several years ago, it was recommended that everyone undergo a complete medical examination before beginning a fitness program. Three factors have caused that standard to change.

1. Health and fitness professionals increasingly recognize that being active is healthier than being inactive (some have suggested it is the folks who plan to remain inactive who need a complete physical examination!).

2. There is mounting evidence that beginning a good fitness program involves a very low risk of health problems for the vast majority of people.

3. We cannot justify spending the time and money for every individual to have a medical examination.

Apparently healthy individuals (those with no known major health problem) can begin moderate-intensity activities with minimal risks based on self-screening (use table 4.3). The current standard for those interested in vigorous-intensity physical activity is to require medical clearance for people who either have known health problems or signs or symptoms that indicate potential health problems or who intend to engage in very strenuous activities (athletic performances where the intensity is much higher than that needed for fitness gains).

The health status form and fitness testing allow the fitness program director to recommend one of the following actions regarding an individual's desire to enter a fitness program:

1. Deny the request to enter the fitness program, or make immediate referral for medical attention.

2. Begin daily moderate-intensity activities.

3. Admit to a fitness program that is
   - medically supervised,
   - carefully prescribed and supervised by an exercise leader, or
   - unsupervised.

This chapter outlines procedures to help you decide on appropriate placement or referral based on an individual's health status (see figure 4.1).

Medical Referral

All persons indicating illness, characteristics, or symptoms coded MC (medical clearance) in the HSQ (table 3.2) must be referred to an appropriate medical professional. With the permission of the appropriate physician, the individual can begin a medically supervised (MS) or Health Fitness Instructor (HFI)–supervised fitness program. Table 4.2 lists the conditions that require medical clearance, as well as the test scores from

the fitness tests that serve as the basis for medical referral. The characteristics and test scores for supervised programs and special attention are also included in table 4.2.

Supervised Program

Table 4.2 lists conditions that may require medical referral if they are severe; however, an individual who experiences mild or moderate levels of difficulty can participate in a carefully supervised fitness program. It is important that the program director check to determine if any of the participants have these or other conditions that might affect their ability to exercise.

Several problems (listed in table 4.2) call for special attention. Your adaptation of activities will be based on common sense regarding the particular condition. You can talk with the participant about how to deal with the situation or consult with the fitness director and physician concerning the limitations that should apply to specific problems.

Although we recommend screening of all fitness participants prior to their participation in an exercise program, we know that you may be in a position to lead exercise for persons who have not been screened. Table 4.3 provides a simple checklist that can be completed either by each individual before exercise, or by your asking for answers from the group as the first part of the exercise session. We suggest that you refer all those who answer "yes" to any of these questions to the director of the fitness program prior to exercise.

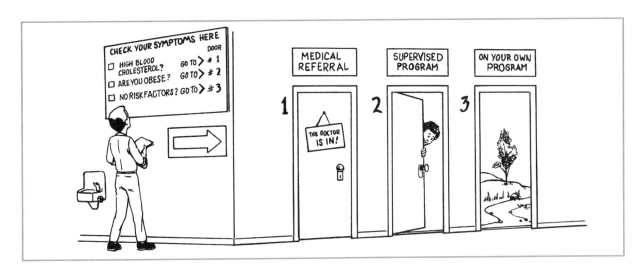

Figure 4.1 Decision based on health status.

Unsupervised Program

People with none of the problems that are coded MC, SEP, or RF (risk factors for CHD) in the HSQ can be admitted to any of the fitness activities. Table 4.2 lists results from the fitness tests that are cause for concern. Encourage individuals with these scores to include in their fitness programs special activities aimed at improving the component or components of fitness reflected by the low score or scores.

Additional Guidelines for Decision Making

Note that the values listed for medical referral and for supervised programs are guidelines for the individual and the fitness program director to use along with other information. Because some of the variables may be influenced by pretest activities and reaction to the testing situation itself (especially in people unaccustomed to being tested), borderline scores, especially at rest and during light work, should be replicated before medical referral. For example, if a high resting heart rate or blood pressure is measured, it may have been because the participant ate,

smoked, took medicine, or participated in physical exercise immediately before the test. Was the person anxious about taking the test? Were there unusual conditions during the test (lots of people, noise, and so on)? The individual should relax for a few minutes, be reassured about the purpose and safety of the test, and then be measured again. If the person is still anxious, you might schedule the test session for another day. If the questionable test result is repeated, the program director may refer that individual to a physician.

Other factors may indicate that a person with the characteristics we have listed as warranting a supervised program should actually be medically referred; for example, multiple risk factors, each close to the referral value. Or the medical consultant may recommend that someone in our "refer" category enter a supervised program, based on a recent medical examination or conversation with the personal physician. Programs with excellent and accessible medical and emergency facilities may use higher values for referral than do programs isolated from medical and emergency facilities. We recommend that each program, in consultation with its medical advisors, establish its own standards.

Table 4.2	Conditions and Test Score Criteria for Physical Activity Decisions

Basis for medical referral

Conditions	Test scores[a]
Breathlessness with slight exertion	Resting HR > 100 bpm
Cirrhosis	Resting SBP > 160 mmHg
Concussion	Resting DBP > 100 mmHg
Cough up blood	% fat > 40 female; > 30 male
Current medication for heart, blood pressure, or diabetes	Cholesterol > 240 mg/dl
Faintness or dizziness	Cholesterol/HDL > 5
Heart operation, disease, or problem	Triglycerides > 200 mg/dl
Pain in the abdomen, leg, arm, shoulder, or chest	Fasting glucose > 120 mg/dl
Phlebitis	Vital cap < 75% predicted
Stroke	FEV_1 < 75%
Swollen joints	

Basis for a supervised program

Conditions (currently under control)[b]

Alcoholism	Diabetes
Allergy	Emphysema
Anemia	Epilepsy
Asthma	Hypoglycemia
Bleeding trait	Mental illness
Bronchitis	Peptic ulcer
Cancer	Pregnancy
Colitis	Thyroid problem

Test scores[c]

Hypertension 140-155/90-95 mmHg

Hyperlipidemia (cholesterol) 240-255 mg/dl

Cholesterol/HDL 4.5-4.8

Obesity 32%-38% female; 25%-28% male

Waist-to-hip ratio > 0.8 female; > 0.9 male

Smoking > 20 cigarettes/day

Exercise < 1.5 hr/week at or above moderate intensity

Basis for special attention

Conditions

Arthritis

Back, eye, joint, lung, or neck operations

Eye problems

Gout

Hearing loss

Hernia

Lengthy time spent driving, lifting, sitting, or standing

Low-back pain

Test scores

Values of risk factors approaching those in supervised programs

Any of the reasons for stopping a maximal test that occur at light to moderate work

Max RPE < 5 (15 on 6-20 scale)

Max METs < 8

Max $\dot{V}O_2$ < 30

% fat < 15% or > 30% females; < 6% or > 25% males[d]

Curl-ups < 10

Sit-and-reach < 15 cm

Modified pull-ups < 5

Push-ups < 10

Note. Any condition or test value that causes the person or the HFI to be concerned for the person's health or safety is the basis for medical referral. FEV_1 = forced expiratory volume in 1 s; RPE = rating of perceived exertion.

[a]Any of these individual scores would be the basis for referral. A person might also be referred if more than one test score approached these values.

[b]Severe or uncontrolled levels should be referred for medical attention.

[c]Persons with higher scores should be referred for medical attention.

[d]Participants who have either too little fat or too much fat may have health problems that need special attention. If there is any question, refer them to the program director.

Reprinted from Howley and Franks 1997.

Education

The HSQ and fitness test results also give the fitness leader information about appropriate education and workshops for the participants. You should give all persons with risk factors for CHD information about their increased risk. We have not provided any quantification of risk—there is only limited basis for assigning a specific risk number. However, there is sufficient evidence to warrant indicating areas of potential health problems, assisting individuals in becoming aware of risk characteristics that cannot be changed, and helping persons with health-related behaviors

Table 4.3		**Checklist for Self-Screening and Walk-In Exercisers**

_____ Yes _____ No — Have, or have had, cardiovascular disease (i.e., heart problems)

_____ Yes _____ No — Have pains or pressure in the left or midchest area, neck, or left shoulder or arm at rest or in response to exertion

_____ Yes _____ No — Often feel faint or have spells of dizziness

_____ Yes _____ No — Experience extreme breathlessness after mild exercise

_____ Yes _____ No — Have high blood pressure

_____ Yes _____ No — Have high cholesterol

_____ Yes _____ No — Smoke more than a pack of cigarettes a day

_____ Yes _____ No — Am over 60 years of age and not accustomed to vigorous exercise

_____ Yes _____ No — Have bone or joint problems that would interfere with or be aggravated by exercise

_____ Yes _____ No — Have two or more of the following (check which ones):
   a. Family history of premature coronary heart disease
   b. Obesity
   c. Type A behavior with stressful occupation and (or) lifestyle
   d. Diabetes

_____ Yes _____ No — Have a medical condition not mentioned here that might need special attention in an exercise program

_____ Yes _____ No — Taking medication for a cardiorespiratory problem

Reprinted from Howley and Franks 1997.

that can be modified. Chapter 15 assists the fitness leader in using behavior modification to help participants achieve desired behavior changes indicated in the HSQ, part 3. In addition, a number of questions indicate a need for education in terms of exercise, nutrition, alcohol, smoking, and stress management. This information will be useful for the program director in deciding what workshops and educational materials to offer to the participants.

Summary

One of the first responsibilities of a fitness program is to help people evaluate their current health status. This information can be used to refer potential participants to appropriate professionals, to an exercise program, or for additional tests. The health status form in chapter 3 (table 3.2) and suggested fitness test items presented in this chapter help you identify characteristics that indicate medical referral. Use of this information helps distinguish among those conditions and risk factors that suggest a supervised versus an unsupervised exercise program. Special conditions needing attention, extra caution, and special or limited activities are described. Finally, fitness participants who are at higher risk of developing serious health problems need additional education.

PART III
Fitness Components

Desired Weight
Desired Aerobic Power
Prevention of Low-Back Problems
Desired Flexibility, Strength, and Endurance
Coping With Stress

Part III of the *Fitness Leader's Handbook* provides a more complete analysis of each of the components of fitness.

Chapter 5 deals with body composition and exercise related to body weight. Chapter 6 provides information on healthy nutrition. Chapter 7 analyzes cardiorespiratory fitness. Chapters 8 and 9 deal with muscular strength and endurance and flexibility. Chapter 10 summarizes the causes of low-back problems and recommends activities to help prevent this problem. Chapter 11 suggests ways to cope with stress.

Chapter 5
Desired Weight

Weight Analysis
Test for Body Fat Percentage
Weight Loss

You will find that many potential fitness participants have a full-time preoccupation with losing weight. Part of the reason for this is social pressure to have a certain "look," but part is related to the health consequences of carrying too much fat. People who are too fat are more likely to have high blood pressure, heart disease, and diabetes. In contrast, some may get carried away with the need to be thin, with serious and potentially deadly consequences. The purpose of this chapter is to help you separate fact from fiction regarding body composition and weight control.

Weight-to-Height Ratio

A variety of weight-to-height tables have been used over the years to classify a person as being "overweight" or "underweight" by comparing the person's body weight to values obtained from people who are the same gender and height. One central problem with these tables is

that they do not distinguish between a person who is heavily muscled from weight lifting and someone who is fat due, in part, to a sedentary lifestyle. In spite of these limitations these indexes can be useful because so many individuals fall into the category of being sedentary.

One of the most common of these weight-to-height ratios is the body mass index (BMI). The BMI is the ratio of the person's weight (in kilograms) to height (in meters) squared ($kg \cdot m^{-2}$).

For example, for a 70-in tall person weighing 154 lb, you would calculate BMI as follows:

154 lb / 2.2 $lb \cdot kg^{-1}$ = 70 kg

70 in x 2.54 $cm \cdot in.^{-1}$ = 177.8 cm, or 1.778 m

$$\frac{70 \text{ kg}}{[1.778\text{m}]^2} = \frac{70 \text{ kg}}{3.161\text{m}^2} = 22.14 \text{ kg} \cdot \text{m}^{-2}$$

The BMI value is interpreted as follows:

- 20 to 24.9 kg·m⁻²—Desirable for adult men and women
- 25 to 29.9 kg·m⁻²—Grade 1 obesity
- 30 to 40 kg·m⁻²—Grade 2 obesity
- >40 kg·m⁻²—Grade 3 obesity

This method is easy to use. However, because it does not provide information about body composition, other techniques are needed.

Components of Body Composition

The human body is composed of a wide variety of tissues and organs, such as muscle, bone, heart, liver, brain, and fat. To simplify our discussion of body composition, we will divide the body into fat-free mass and fat mass and express each as a percent of total body weight. For example, a woman who is 30% fat and weighs 150 lb is carrying 45 lb of fat (30% of 150 lb). Fat-free mass includes all tissues and organs other than fat. Fat mass includes *essential fat,* the fat that is necessary for survival, and the "extra" that we carry along. Fat is found in all cells, surrounds most nerves, and is associated with specific tissues. Essential fat totals about 3% to 5% of body weight for men and 11% to 14% of body weight for women. The higher value for women allows for the fat that is deposited in the breasts and hips at puberty and is related to the production of estrogen. You must understand the nature of essential fat, because it sets the lower limit of body fatness for men and women. What, then, is a reasonable amount of fat? Does it matter where it is located (e.g., hips or abdomen)?

Recommended Fatness Values

Body fatness values associated with good health are *neither too low nor too high.* In the past, most fitness books were concerned solely with people at the high end of the scale; that is no longer true. Our country has experienced an increase in the number of eating-disorder problems associated with those (primarily teenage girls and

young women) who strive to be as thin as possible. *Anorexia nervosa* is an eating disorder in which people have a distorted view of their body fatness; they see themselves as fat even if they are emaciated. *Bulimia* is a ritual of overeating followed by vomiting to help keep body weight low. Concern about these eating disorders has led to the identification of both low and high body fatness values that are consistent with good health.

You should recognize that recommended body fatness values will be different for the athlete interested in world-class performance than for the average person participating in a health-related fitness program. Figure 5.1 lists body fatness values that bracket the healthy range. Your goal should be to help participants achieve that healthy range. Keep in mind the fact that body fatness normally fluctuates some amount during the year, as physical activity and food consumption patterns vary with the season and holidays.

Distribution of Body Fat

Individuals who store a large portion of their body fat in the trunk area ("apple-shaped obesity") have a higher risk of heart disease and diabetes than those who carry the fat on the hips and buttocks ("pear-shaped obesity"). A simple measurement to evaluate the degree to which an individual is shaped like an apple or a pear is the waist-to-hip ratio. Women with values above 0.86 and men with values above 0.95 are at a very high risk of these diseases. To measure the waist-to-hip ratio use the following procedure:

1. The subject should wear little clothing, allowing the tape to be placed at the proper location.
2. The subject stands with feet together, arms at the side. The measurer faces the subject.
3. With the subject's abdomen relaxed, place the measuring tape around the narrowest part of the torso, between the umbilicus and the bottom of the sternum. Keep the tape parallel to the ground. Record to nearest 0.1 cm.
4. Measurer squats at subject's side and places tape around the subject's buttocks where it has its greatest size. Keep the tape in the horizontal plane, and measure to the nearest 0.1 cm.

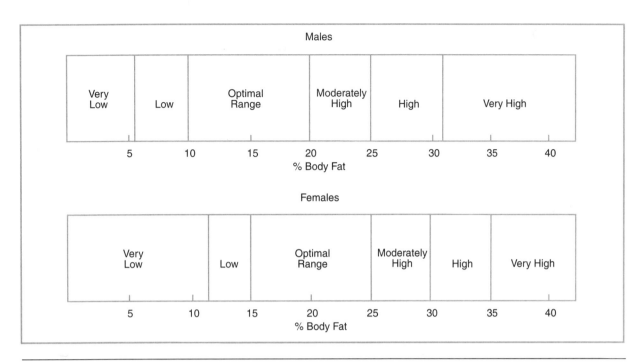

Figure 5.1 Body fatness values.

This article is reprinted with permission from the *Journal of Physical Education, Recreation & Dance* 68 (9), 1987, 98-102. *JOPERD* is a publication of the American Alliance for Health, Physical Education, Recreation and Dance, 1900 Association Drive, Reston, VA 20191.

5. Divide the measurement in step 3 by the measurement in step 4. For example, if a male has a waist circumference of 96.5 cm (38 in.), and a hip circumference of 99.1 cm (39 in.), then his waist-to-hip ratio is 0.97 and he is at a high risk of developing cardiovascular and metabolic disease.

Measurement of Body Fat Percentage

The major aspect of body composition related to fitness and health is the amount of fat a person has in relation to total body weight. Although a person's weight compared to height provides some information, it is better to estimate the amount of fat more directly. Body fat percentage can be estimated in a variety of ways. The best field method is to use skinfold measurements that have been validated against underwater weighing techniques. Table 5.1 describes, and figure 5.2 illustrates, the technique used to obtain and score skinfold measurements. Table 5.2 lists the things you need to measure skinfolds.

Estimation of Fat in Men

A good estimate of body fat for men uses the chest, abdomen, and thigh skinfolds. Figure 5.3 shows these locations. Refer to table 5.3 to determine a man's percent fat using the sum of these three skinfolds. The *chest* skinfold is measured with a diagonal fold halfway between the nipple and the junction of the arm and shoulder (see figure 5.3). The *abdominal* skinfold is taken as a vertical fold about 1 inch to the right of and level with the umbilicus, and the *thigh* skinfold is taken as a vertical fold half way between the top of the knee cap and the hip on the midline of the thigh.

Estimation of Fat in Women

Body fat is estimated for women in the same manner, except that the exercise leader uses skinfolds from the *triceps* (a vertical fold halfway between the shoulder and elbow), *suprailiac* (a slightly diagonal fold lifted to follow the natural contour just above the crest of the hip bone in the midline on the side of the body), and the thigh, as described above (see figure 5.3). Use table 5.4 to estimate body fat percentage in women in the same way you use table 5.3 for men.

Table 5.1   Technique in Taking Skinfold

Steps	Technique
1	Explain the purpose of the test—to determine the amount of fat in relation to total body weight.
2	Take the skinfolds in a private setting where the score will not be shared with others.
3	Always use the right side of the body.
4	Grasp the least amount of skin that will make a fold between the thumb and forefinger.
5	Lift the skinfold firmly and hold (do not let go when measuring with calipers).
6	Place the jaws of the caliper 1/2 inch above or below fingers.
7	Slowly engage the calipers to measure the fold.
8	Read the dial to the nearest 0.5 millimeter (mm) when the needle stops or the calipers have been taken to the designated point.
9	Remove the calipers prior to letting go with the fingers.
10	Repeat measurement 3 times—if within 1 to 2 mm, take middle score. If greater than a 2-mm difference exists, repeat procedure.

Scoring

11	Record number of mm for each site on the score card.
12	Sum the scores from the sites.
13	Go to appropriate chart to determine percent fat.

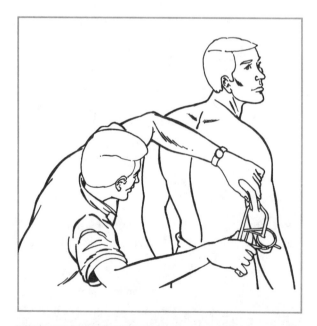

Figure 5.2 Using skinfold measurements to evaluate body fatness.

Reprinted from Howley and Franks 1986.

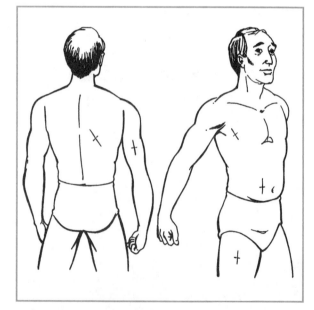

Figure 5.3 Skinfold sites.

Reprinted from Howley and Franks 1986.

Table 5.2	Items Needed for Skinfolds
Skinfold calipers	
Trained administrator	
Score sheet or card	
Area where test can be conducted in private	

Note. The following calipers are recommended:
   Harpenden (Quinton Instrument Co., Seattle, WA)
   Lange (Cambridge Scientific Industries, Cambridge, MD)
Less expensive calipers are available and have been found to be reliable when used by experienced testers.

Calculation of Desired Weight

The steps for determining desired weight are listed in table 5.5.

For example, if you measure the thickness of the triceps, suprailiac, and thigh skinfolds on a 140-lb, 35-year-old woman as 18, 22, and 26 mm respectively, perform the following steps to estimate her percent fat and determine her desired weight:

1. Add the skinfold measurements (18 mm + 22 mm + 26 mm = 66 mm).

2. Read across the top of table 5.4 until you find the appropriate age (in this case, 33-37).

3. Follow down the 33-37 years of age column until you reach the total of the skinfolds (in this case, 65-67 mm).

4. Read the number that represents the estimated percent fat (26.4% in this example).

5. Now go to table 5.5.
   Fat weight = (body wt × % fat) = (140 lb × .264 [26.4%]) = 37 lb.

6. *Fat-free weight (FFW)* = (wt – fat wt) = (140 lb – 37 lb) = 103 lb.

7. Assume that desired percent fat = 23%.

8. *Desired weight* = FFW/(1 – desired % fat) = 103 lb/(1 – .23) = (103 lb/.77) = 133.8 lb.

9. *Desired weight loss* = 140 – 133.8 = 6.2 lb.

Estimation of Fat in Children and Youth

You may be asked to help test or set up a fitness testing program for children and youth. This section outlines how you can use skinfolds to estimate fat in the younger population. Use a vertical fold for both the triceps skinfold and the medial calf skinfold (taken on the *inside* of the calf at the point of the largest muscle mass, with subject's foot on a bench and knee slightly bent; see figure 5.4). Then compare the sum of the skinfolds to the chart for boys (figure 5.5) or girls (figure 5.6) to determine whether they are in the optimal range for body fat percentage.

Changing Fat Levels

The previous sections described the difference between body weight and body fat and showed you how body fatness can be estimated by a very simple procedure. This section deals with issues related to changing body weight and body composition.

Caloric Balance and Weight Control

When we discuss weight control and body composition we are dealing with the issues of *gaining and losing fat and lean tissue.* There is no question that a person can lose body weight through excessive sweating or with the use of diuretic drugs that cause the kidneys to produce lots of urine. However, water weight is easily replaced and does not represent the fat weight that is linked to diabetes and heart disease. Therefore, in our discussion of this topic, we will refer to methods that alter the fat mass and the fat-free mass of the body. This is how to alter body composition to improve health status.

Table 5.3	Percentage Body Fat[a] Estimation for Men From Age and the Sum of Chest, Abdominal, and Thigh Skinfolds

Sum of skinfolds	Age to the last year								
(mm)	Under 22	23-27	28-32	33-37	38-42	43-47	48-52	53-57	Over 57
8-10	1.3	1.8	2.3	2.9	3.4	3.9	4.5	5.0	5.5
11-13	2.2	2.8	3.3	3.9	4.4	4.9	5.5	6.0	6.5
14-16	3.2	3.8	4.3	4.8	5.4	5.9	6.4	7.0	7.5
17-19	4.2	4.7	5.3	5.8	6.3	6.9	7.4	8.0	8.5
20-22	5.1	5.7	6.2	6.8	7.3	7.9	8.4	8.9	9.5
23-25	6.1	6.6	7.2	7.7	8.3	8.8	9.4	9.9	10.5
26-28	7.0	7.6	8.1	8.7	9.2	9.8	10.3	10.9	11.4
29-31	8.0	8.5	9.1	9.6	10.2	10.7	11.3	11.8	12.4
32-34	8.9	9.4	10.0	10.5	11.1	11.6	12.2	12.8	13.3
35-37	9.8	10.4	10.9	11.5	12.0	12.6	13.1	13.7	14.3
38-40	10.7	11.3	11.8	12.4	12.9	13.5	14.1	14.6	15.2
41-43	11.6	12.2	12.7	13.3	13.8	14.4	15.0	15.5	16.1
44-46	12.5	13.1	13.6	14.2	14.7	15.3	15.9	16.4	17.0
47-49	13.4	13.9	14.5	15.1	15.6	16.2	16.8	17.3	17.9
50-52	14.3	14.8	15.4	15.9	16.5	17.1	17.6	18.2	18.8
53-55	15.1	15.7	16.2	16.8	17.4	17.9	18.5	19.1	19.7
56-58	16.0	16.5	17.1	17.7	18.2	18.8	19.4	20.0	20.5
59-61	16.9	17.4	17.9	18.5	19.1	19.7	20.2	20.8	21.4
62-64	17.6	18.2	18.8	19.4	19.9	20.5	21.1	21.7	22.2
65-67	18.5	19.0	19.6	20.2	20.8	21.3	21.9	22.5	23.1
68-70	19.3	19.9	20.4	21.0	21.6	22.2	22.7	23.3	23.9
71-73	20.1	20.7	21.2	21.8	22.4	23.0	23.6	24.1	24.7
74-76	20.9	21.5	22.0	22.6	23.2	23.8	24.4	25.0	25.5
77-79	21.7	22.2	22.8	23.4	24.0	24.6	25.2	25.8	26.3
80-82	22.4	23.0	23.6	24.2	24.8	25.4	25.9	26.5	27.1
83-85	23.2	23.8	24.4	25.0	25.5	26.1	26.7	27.3	27.9
86-88	24.0	24.5	25.1	25.7	26.3	26.9	27.5	28.1	28.7
89-91	24.7	25.3	25.9	26.5	27.1	27.6	28.2	28.8	29.4
92-94	25.4	26.0	26.6	27.2	27.8	28.4	29.0	29.6	30.2
95-97	26.1	26.7	27.3	27.9	28.5	29.1	29.7	30.3	30.9
98-100	26.9	27.4	28.0	28.6	29.2	29.8	30.4	31.0	31.6
101-103	27.5	28.1	28.7	29.3	29.9	30.5	31.1	31.7	32.3
104-106	28.2	28.8	29.4	30.0	30.6	31.2	31.8	32.4	33.0
107-109	28.9	29.5	30.1	30.7	31.3	31.9	32.5	33.1	33.7
110-112	29.6	30.2	30.8	31.4	32.0	32.6	33.2	33.8	34.4
113-115	30.2	30.8	31.4	32.0	32.6	33.2	33.8	34.5	35.1
116-118	30.9	31.5	32.1	32.7	33.3	33.9	34.5	35.1	35.7
119-121	31.5	32.1	32.7	33.3	33.9	34.5	35.1	35.7	36.4
122-124	32.1	32.7	33.3	33.9	34.5	35.1	35.8	36.4	37.0
125-127	32.7	33.3	33.9	34.5	35.1	35.8	36.4	37.0	37.6

[a]Percentage of fat is calculated by the formula of Siri: percent fat = $[(4.95/D_b) - 4.5] \times 100$, where D_b = body density.

Reprinted from Pollack, Schmidt, and Jackson 1980.

	Body Fat[a] Percentage Estimation for Women
Table 5.4	**From Age and Triceps, Suprailium, and Thigh Skinfolds**

Sum of skinfolds	Age to the last year								
(mm)	Under 22	23-27	28-32	33-37	38-42	43-47	48-52	53-57	Over 57
23-25	9.7	9.9	10.2	10.4	10.7	10.9	11.2	11.4	11.7
26-28	11.0	11.2	11.5	11.7	12.0	12.3	12.5	12.7	13.0
29-31	12.3	12.5	12.8	13.0	13.3	13.5	13.8	14.0	14.3
32-34	13.6	13.8	14.0	14.3	14.5	14.8	15.0	15.3	15.5
35-37	14.8	15.0	15.3	15.5	15.8	16.0	16.3	16.5	16.8
38-40	16.0	16.3	16.5	16.7	17.0	17.2	17.5	17.7	18.0
41-43	17.2	17.4	17.7	17.9	18.2	18.4	18.7	18.9	19.2
44-46	18.3	18.6	18.8	19.1	19.3	19.6	19.8	20.1	20.3
47-49	19.5	19.7	20.0	20.2	20.5	20.7	21.0	21.2	21.5
50-52	20.6	20.8	21.1	21.3	21.6	21.8	22.1	22.3	22.6
53-55	21.7	21.9	22.1	22.4	22.6	22.9	23.1	23.4	23.6
56-58	22.7	23.0	23.2	23.4	23.7	23.9	24.2	24.4	24.7
59-61	23.7	24.0	24.2	24.5	24.7	25.0	25.2	25.5	25.7
62-64	24.7	25.0	25.2	25.5	25.7	26.0	26.2	26.4	26.7
65-67	25.7	25.9	26.2	26.4	26.7	26.9	27.2	27.4	27.7
68-70	26.6	26.9	27.1	27.4	27.6	27.9	28.1	28.4	28.6
71-73	27.5	27.8	28.0	28.3	28.5	28.8	29.0	29.3	29.5
74-76	28.4	28.7	28.9	29.2	29.4	29.7	29.9	30.2	30.4
77-79	29.3	29.5	29.8	30.0	30.3	30.5	30.8	31.0	31.3
80-82	30.1	30.4	30.6	30.9	31.1	31.4	31.6	31.9	32.1
83-85	30.9	31.2	31.4	31.7	31.9	32.2	32.4	32.7	32.9
86-88	31.7	32.0	32.2	32.5	32.7	32.9	33.2	33.4	33.7
89-91	32.5	32.7	33.0	33.2	33.5	33.7	33.9	34.2	34.4
92-94	33.2	33.4	33.7	33.9	34.2	34.4	34.7	34.9	35.2
95-97	33.9	34.1	34.4	34.6	34.9	35.1	35.4	35.6	35.9
98-100	34.6	34.8	35.1	35.3	35.5	35.8	36.0	36.3	36.5
101-103	35.3	35.4	35.7	35.9	36.2	36.4	36.7	36.9	37.2
104-106	35.8	36.1	36.3	36.6	36.8	37.1	37.3	37.5	37.8
107-109	36.4	36.7	36.9	37.1	37.4	37.6	37.9	38.1	38.4
110-112	37.0	37.2	37.5	37.7	38.0	38.2	38.5	38.7	38.9
113-115	37.5	37.8	38.0	38.2	38.5	38.7	39.0	39.2	39.5
116-118	38.0	38.3	38.5	38.8	39.0	39.3	39.5	39.7	40.0
119-121	38.5	38.7	39.0	39.2	39.5	39.7	40.0	40.2	40.5
122-124	39.0	39.2	39.4	39.7	39.9	40.2	40.4	40.7	40.9
125-127	39.4	39.6	39.9	40.1	40.4	40.6	40.9	41.1	41.4
128-130	39.8	40.0	40.3	40.5	40.8	41.0	41.3	41.5	41.8

[a]Percentage of fat is calculated by the formula of Siri: percent fat = $[(4.95/D_b) - 4.5] \times 100$, where D_b = body density.

Adapted from Pollock, Schmidt, and Jackson 1980.

Table 5.5	Steps in Estimation of Desired Weight
Step	**Measurement or calculation**
1	Body weight (wt)
2	Estimation of percent fat (% fat, expressed as decimal)
3	Decision concerning appropriate level of percent fat (desired % fat)
4	Fat weight (fat wt) = body wt x % fat
5	Lean body weight (LBW) = body wt – fat wt
6	Desired weight (des wt) = LBW / (1 – desired % fat [expressed as fraction])
7	Desired weight loss = wt – des wt

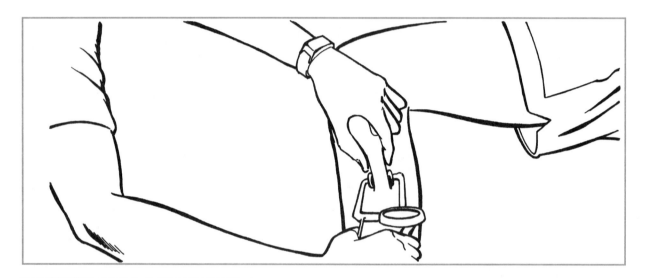

Figure 5.4 Medial calf skinfold.

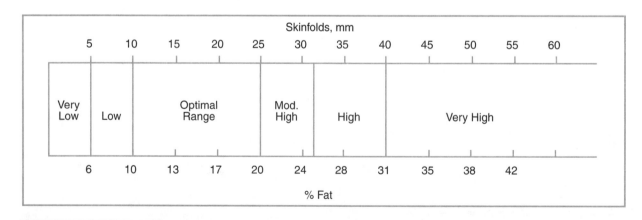

Figure 5.5 Triceps plus calf skinfolds—boys.

This article is reprinted with permission from the *Journal of Physical Education, Recreation & Dance* 68 (9), 1987, 98-102. *JOPERD* is a publication of the American Alliance for Health, Physical Education, Recreation and Dance, 1900 Association Drive, Reston, VA 20191.

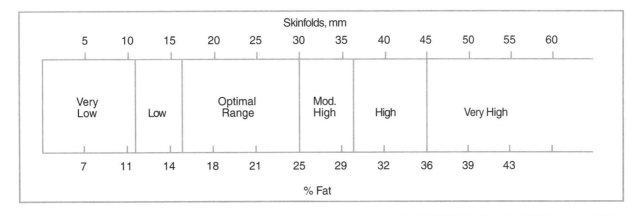

Figure 5.6 Triceps plus calf skinfolds—girls.

This article is reprinted with permission from the *Journal of Physical Education, Recreation & Dance* 68 (9), 1987, 98-102. *JOPERD* is a publication of the American Alliance for Health, Physical Education, Recreation and Dance, 1900 Association Drive, Reston, VA 20191.

The central concept that affects weight control is found in the *energy balance equation:*

If caloric intake *is equal to* caloric expenditure, then energy balance exists → no change in weight

If caloric intake *is greater than* caloric expenditure, then *positive* energy balance exists → weight gain

If caloric intake *is less than* caloric expenditure, then *negative* energy balance exists → weight loss

The total amount of energy expended each day is related to the following:

- Resting metabolic rate—the amount of energy we use while lying or sitting. What is surprising to most people, is that resting metabolic rate represents about 60% to 70% of a person's total daily energy expenditure.

- Thermic effect of food—the amount of energy required to process the food we eat. This equals about 10% of total daily energy expenditure.

- Physical activity associated with work, recreation, and sports represents the balance, and equals about 20% to 30% of total daily energy expenditure.

Since resting metabolic rate makes up such a large portion of each day's energy expenditure, it is important to maintain that value as high as possible to help balance the calories we eat. In addition, the energy expenditure associated with physical activity is quite low in sedentary individuals and must be the focal point of the fitness leader in helping participants achieve energy balance.

Caloric intake refers to the number of kilocalories (kcal) of food that a person consumes. You need to help the participants understand that when you refer to *diet* for calorie and nutrient intake, it does not necessarily mean depriving oneself of food. Diet may also be called a "food plan." If participants wish to maintain body weight then they must balance intake and expenditure, and if you wish to help participants lose weight, you must work with them so they create a negative energy balance by expending more kcal than they consume.

A person can achieve negative energy balance by keeping energy expenditure the same and simply reducing caloric intake. In this case the focus is on trying to eat a nutritionally sound diet while consuming fewer kcal. A person can also lose weight by keeping the diet the same but increasing energy expenditure. In this case, the caloric cost of activity must be taken into account. In either case, 3500 kcal must be expended from the body's energy store to lose one pound of fat. A person who creates a negative energy balance of 500 kcal per day would lose about one pound of fat per week. The recommended rate of weight loss is a maximum of 1 to 2 lb per week, so the total negative energy balance should be no more than about 1000 kcal per day.

Details on evaluating weight loss diets are in the next chapter. Weight loss behaviors should focus on the following:

- Increasing aerobic and resistance physical activity
- Decreasing calorie and fat intake
- Changing eating habits

Interaction of Diet and Exercise for Weight Management

Even though a person can lose weight by reducing the number of calories consumed or by increasing exercise, for reasons illustrated in figure 5.7 and listed next, you should recommend that participants use a combination of the two to achieve their goals.

1. When an individual reduces caloric intake, the body responds as if it is beginning to starve. One of the body's adaptations is to decrease energy production to save its energy stores. This means that a very low-kcal diet can become counterproductive to weight loss; the more you cut back on caloric intake, the more the body responds by decreasing its energy expenditure.

2. When weight is lost by *diet alone* 35% to 45% of the weight lost is lean tissue, not fat tissue. Therefore, one could actually lose weight but not change percent of body fatness (body composition) very much. This loss of lean tissue also contributes to the body's reduction in resting energy expenditure, making it more difficult for a person to lose weight. Resistance training can increase muscle mass and help maintain the resting metabolic rate.

The overall consequence of a weight loss program that uses diet alone is a slower rate of fat loss. It should be no surprise, then, that a combination of diet and exercise is the recommended way to achieve weight loss and body composition goals. Exercise helps to maintain lean tissue (muscle) while more fat is being lost; in this case the body actually makes changes in body fat percentage faster than it can through diet alone. We have seen this in many individuals who begin an exercise program: Body weight may not change for several weeks but clothing sizes do. Why does this happen? The exercise is *increasing* fat-free body mass while fat mass is decreasing slightly. With time, body weight will decrease in proportion to the change in energy balance.

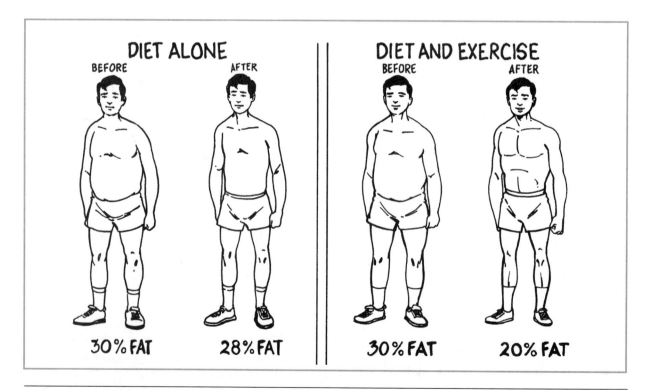

Figure 5.7 Reduction of fat: diet alone versus diet and exercise.

We have already stated our recommendation regarding weight loss: Use a combination of diet and exercise to achieve the goal. We'll now discuss some facts about exercise and weight loss, and also present additional information to show participants that exercise is a very beneficial part of their lifestyle, whether they are losing weight or not.

Caloric Cost of Activity

The body expends energy whether at rest, work, or play. A person must take in and use oxygen (O_2) for this to occur. In fact, if we know how much oxygen is being used we can calculate how many kcals of energy the body expends. Figure 5.8 shows that the body's use of 1 L of oxygen causes the expenditure of 5 kcal of energy. This is a very important point in understanding the role of exercise in weight loss. We have already indicated that a negative caloric balance of 3500 kcal is necessary to lose 1 lb of adipose (fat) tissue. Figure 5.9 shows two people trying to lose weight—one by sitting in a sauna and the other by running around a track. The person sitting in the sauna expends only 72 kcal per hour, because the body uses very little

oxygen while sitting at rest; however, the person running around the track expends 600 kcal per hour, because the body requires a great deal of oxygen to run. It would take 50 hours of sitting in a sauna to expend the caloric equivalent of 1 lb of fat (3500 kcal) but only 6 hr of running. Fortunately, one need not do all that exercise at one time! Remember, a combination of diet and exercise results in a steady reduction in body weight and leaves the participants with diet and activity habits they can incorporate into their lifestyles.

Caloric cost refers to the amount of energy required to perform a particular activity and is usually given in kilocalories (kcal). The kcal value may be given in whole numbers; for example, a person can expend 400 kcal per hour by jogging. It may instead be given as the number of kcal required per kilogram (1 kg = 2.2 lbs) of body weight; for example, a person expends about 0.36 kcal per pound (0.8 kcal per kg) per mile when walking. This information tells you how many calories are going to be used in an activity and is very important for people using physical activity as part of a weight loss program. Because you already

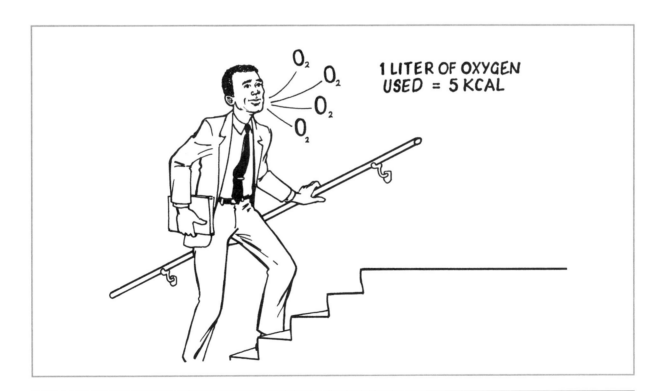

Figure 5.8 Oxygen consumption.

know that the energy values of various foods are also stated in kcal, it is possible to state the energy cost of an activity in terms of food. For example, eating 10 potato chips is equivalent to the energy required to run 1 mi. You will find a more extensive discussion of caloric cost of activities in chapter 14.

Diet, Exercise, and Cholesterol

Exercise and a diet that provides an appropriate number of calories influences more than just weight loss. It has been shown that a low-fat diet like the one recommended in chapter 6 (30% fat, 55% to 60% carbohydrate, and 10% to 15% protein) is associated with low levels of serum cholesterol, one of the major risk factors of heart disease. In addition, exercise appears to have a separate effect of raising levels of "good," high-density lipoprotein (HDL) cholesterol. The result of lowering total cholesterol and raising HDL cholesterol levels is a reduction of the risk of heart disease.

Summary

Help participants strive for a healthy level of body fat, which is between 10% and 20% for men and between 15% and 25% for women. Too little fat may reflect an eating disorder that may call for professional help. Too much fat is a risk factor for several major health problems. An individual's body fatness and healthy weight range can be estimated from skinfold measurements, with different skinfold sites used for children, men, and women. The best way to reduce excess fat is by modest changes in exercise and dietary patterns, resulting in a loss of 1 lb of fat (a negative caloric balance of 3500 kcal) every week.

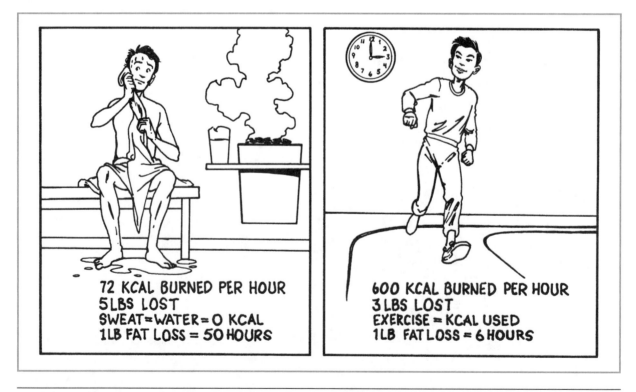

72 KCAL BURNED PER HOUR
5 LBS LOST
SWEAT = WATER = 0 KCAL
1 LB FAT LOSS = 50 HOURS

600 KCAL BURNED PER HOUR
3 LBS LOST
EXERCISE = KCAL USED
1 LB FAT LOSS = 6 HOURS

Figure 5.9 Energy cost of sitting in a sauna versus running.

Chapter 6
Healthy Nutrition Plans

```
Nutritional Goals
Healthy Food Choices
Evaluation of Diet
Diets and Weight Loss
```

Caloric intake is clearly one of the major factors in our weight loss equation. The fitness leader, however, needs to help participants understand that following a healthy diet means more than counting calories. The types of food a person eats have a major bearing on overall health and well-being. This chapter presents some basic information concerning the dietary and nutritional goals that you can help fitness participants achieve.

Dietary Goals

We now have clear evidence that the typical American diet has adversely affected our health. There are clear links between overconsumption of saturated fats and cholesterol and the rate of heart disease in this country. In addition, lack of dietary fiber has been tied to a variety of intestinal health problems. Because of this information, the United States Senate Select Committee on Nutrition and Human Needs held hearings in 1977 to determine dietary goals that would point the way toward improved health status for Americans. The current guidelines, which have changed little over the years, are shown in figure 6.1. In general, the recommendations call for the following:

- Increasing carbohydrate intake (55% to 60% of total calories) while simultaneously decreasing intake of simple sugars to less than 10% of total calories

- Decreasing total and saturated fat intake to ≤ 30% and ≤ 10% of total calories, respectively

- Maintaining a protein intake equal to 10% to 15% of total calories

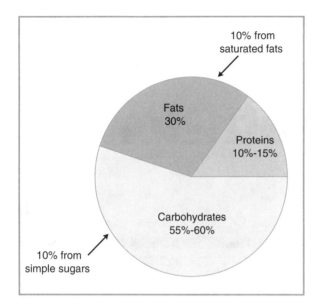

Figure 6.1 Recommended intake of carbohydrates, fats, and proteins.

Reprinted from Howley and Franks 1997.

Basic Foods and Functions

The major classes of nutrients are water, carbohydrates, fats, proteins, vitamins, and minerals. Each has an important place in our diet (also called "food plan"), and overall health status depends on the correct amounts and proportions of these classes.

We tend to ignore *water* as a special nutrient, yet even a few days without water is dangerous and can lead to death. This is not the case for other nutrients, which we can do without for considerable periods of time and still survive. Water is obtained from solid food as well as from beverages. Some solid foods, such as potatoes, peas, and lettuce, are 75% to 96% water by weight. It is very important to replace water as it is lost during physical activity to provide the water needed for sweat production. Failure to do so increases the chance of heat injury (see chapter 20). The amount of water stored in the body also varies with the type of diet consumed. Carbohydrates require water for storage in the body; for example, 2.7 lb of water are needed for every pound of carbohydrate stored in the liver and muscles. When an individual begins a low-carbohydrate diet, the body's store of carbohydrate decreases quickly over the next

day or two, and the water stored with the carbohydrate is also lost. This helps to explain why people often experience such a rapid loss of body weight (but not fat loss) with such a diet. Keep in mind that there must be a negative caloric balance of 3500 kcal to lose 1 lb of adipose tissue, a goal that few persons can achieve in one day. These rapid weight loss diets simply cause loss of body water that must—and eventually will—be replaced. Remember, it is the size of the negative caloric balance that is important in weight loss, not the type of diet. Given the dietary goals already mentioned, carbohydrates are the last thing a person should decrease in his or her diet to reduce body fat.

Carbohydrates are a primary source of energy in the diet, containing about 4 kcal per gram. The average American consumes too little carbohydrate relative to the goal of 55% to 60% of total calories. Carbohydrates include both foods that are digestible and can be used for energy (starches and sugars) and those that contain indigestible fiber. Sugars are found in jams, soft drinks, and milk, while starches are found in cereals, breads, and vegetables.

To achieve the dietary goal of a reduction in refined and processed sugars and an increase in complex carbohydrates and fiber, Americans should decrease consumption of soft drinks, cakes, cookies, and other foods containing sugar, and increase intake of whole-grain breads, cereals, fruits, vegetables, and beans. This increase in complex carbohydrates, and therefore caloric intake, is compensated for by a decrease in fat intake.

Fats are a primary source of energy, containing more than twice as many calories per gram (9 kcal) as carbohydrates. Fats can be either liquid (vegetable oils) or solid (lard) at room temperature. Liquid fats are made up of molecules containing few hydrogen atoms, making them "unsaturated" fats, while solid fats are composed mostly of molecules that are filled with hydrogen atoms, making them "saturated" fats. Though there is no difference in the number of kcal per gram for liquid or solid fats, there are major differences between the two in terms of good health. Consumption of large amounts of dietary fats is associated with higher rates of heart disease, with saturated fats identified as a major problem. It should be no surprise, then, that the dietary goals include a reduction in total fat consumption (to 30% or less), and an additional cutback in saturated fats (to less than 10%). This is also true for cholesterol, present in animal fat, which should not exceed 300 mg per day. To accomplish these goals, program participants should do the following:

- Eat more lean meat, fish, poultry, and dry beans and peas as sources of protein
- Use skim or low-fat milk and milk products
- Limit consumption of eggs and organ meats
- Limit intake of fats and oils, especially those high in saturated fats such as butter, lard, shortening, and foods containing palm and coconut oils
- Broil, bake, or boil rather than fry and trim fat off meats

Protein provides the same number of calories per gram as carbohydrate, 4 kcal. Protein, however, is not a primary energy source. Protein is an important nutrient because it contains the amino acids necessary for tissue growth, development, and repair. High-quality protein is found in eggs, meat, fish, milk, poultry, cheese, and soybeans. Grains, vegetables, seeds, and nuts provide lower-quality protein, and more of this is required per day compared to the higher quality protein. The protein requirement for an adult is only 0.8 g per kilogram (g·kg^{-1}) of body weight, so a 154-lb (70-kg) person needs only 56 g, or about 2 oz, per day. A rapidly growing baby requires 2.2 g·kg^{-1}. About 12% of the average American's diet is protein, which is sufficient to meet this standard. The Senate Committee's dietary goals recommend no change in this quantity, but suggest that to keep the intake of fat at a lower level, Americans should eat more fish, poultry, and low-fat dairy products rather than red meat and regular milk products.

Vitamins are special nutrients required in very small amounts, but essential for normal body function. They are classified as *fat-soluble* or *water-soluble* based on whether they dissolve in lipids (fats) or in water. Fat-soluble vitamins include A, D, E, and K. Because of their solubility, they can be stored in the body and are not needed every day, since you can "catch up" on other days. A potential problem with fat-soluble vitamins is that if you take in too much of them over a long period of time, you can actu-

ally develop hypervitaminosis, a toxicity condition that can lead to nervous disorders, gastrointestinal problems, and damage to liver and kidneys.

Water-soluble vitamins, which include the B vitamins, C, folic acid, pantothenic acid, and biotin, are much less likely to induce hypervitaminosis, since the body excretes any excess in the urine. However, high levels of water-soluble vitamins can have toxic effects and should also be avoided. Table 6.1 summarizes these vitamins, their functions, and their food sources.

What about taking vitamin supplements? An individual can meet the daily requirements for all vitamins by eating a varied diet containing the various food groups (discussed later in this chapter), and therefore vitamin supplements generally are unnecessary. However, someone who wants to be sure of getting all the vitamins can generally take a single multivitamin every other day without causing problems. You should nonetheless strive to focus participants' attention on eating a balanced diet to meet these needs in the long run, rather than depending on a supplement. Remember, by eating a balanced diet, people also fulfill their protein and mineral requirements.

Minerals are chemical elements that, like vitamins, are needed in small amounts for normal health. Minerals are divided into two classes: major minerals and trace minerals. Major minerals include calcium for bones, potassium and sodium for nerve and muscle function, and magnesium that is needed for many of the body's enzymes to function. Trace minerals include iron for hemoglobin that transports oxygen in the blood, iodine for the hormone thyroxine that keeps our metabolic rate at the right level, and zinc, selenium, copper, and others needed for the proper functioning of certain enzymes.

An individual can achieve the daily requirements for most of these minerals by eating a varied and balanced diet. However, there is concern that most women do not take in sufficient amounts of iron and calcium, which can lead to anemia (reduced iron stores) and osteoporosis (thinning of the bones). Anemia is a condition in which the red blood cells have a reduced ability to transport oxygen, and the participant's attention should be directed toward eating foods rich in iron, such as red meat, eggs, spinach, and lima

Table 6.1 Vitamins and Their Functions

Vitamin	Function	Sources	Daily adult requirement[a] Men	Women
Thiamin (B-1)	Functions as part of a coenzyme to aid utilization of energy	Whole grains, nuts, lean pork	1.5 mg[b]	1.1 mg
Riboflavin (B-2)	Involved in energy metabolism as part of a coenzyme	Milk, yogurt, cheese	1.7 mg	1.3 mg
Niacin	Facilitates energy production in cells	Lean meat, fish, poultry, grains	19.0 mg	15.0 mg
Vitamin B-6	Absorbs and metabolizes protein; aids in red blood cell formation	Lean meat, vegetables, whole grains	2.0 mg	1.6 mg
Pantothenic acid	Aids in metabolism of carbohydrate, fat, and protein	Whole-grain cereals, bread, dark green vegetables	4-7 mg	4-7 mg
Folic acid	Functions as coenzyme in synthesis of nucleic acids and protein	Green vegetables, beans, whole-wheat products	200 µg[b]	180 µg
Vitamin B-12	Involved in synthesis of nucleic acids, red blood cell formation	Only in animal foods, not plant foods	2 µg	2 µg
Biotin	Coenzyme in synthesis of fatty acids and glycogen formation	Egg yolk, dark green vegetables	30-100 µg	30-100 µg
C	Intracellular maintenance of bone, capillaries, and teeth	Citrus fruits, green peppers, tomatoes	60 mg	60 mg
A	Functions in visual processes; formation and maintenance of skin and mucous membranes	Carrots, sweet potatoes, margarine, butter, liver	1000 µg	800 µg[c]
D	Aids in growth and formation of bones and teeth; promotes calcium absorption	Eggs, tuna, liver, fortified milk	5 µg	5 µg
E	Protects polyunsaturated fats; prevents cell membrane damage	Vegetable oils, whole-grain cereal and bread, green leafy vegetables	10 mg	8 mg
K	Important in blood clotting	Green leafy vegetables, peas, potatoes	80 µg	65 µg

[a]Values are for adults 25 to 50 years of age. The requirements vary for children and pregnant or lactating women. See the appendix.

[b]mg = milligram, µg = microgram, IU = international unit.

[c]µg vitamin A requirements are expressed in microgram of Retinol equivalents.

Reprinted from Howley and Franks 1997.

and navy beans. Osteoporosis is related to hip fractures in the elderly. It is currently believed that one should achieve a high bone mass by the early adult years to have some protection against osteoporosis in the later years. Bone mass is related to the intake of calcium and participation in physical activity. The recommended calcium intake was adjusted upward to deal with this problem. Those 11 to 24 years of age should consume 1200 to 1500 mg per day. Women from 25 to 50 years old and men from 25 to 65 years old should consume 1000 mg every day (instead of the standard recommendation of 800 mg). Postmenopausal women not taking estrogen should consume 1500 mg per day; those on estrogen need take in only 1000 mg daily. Table 6.2 summarizes the minerals and their functions.

Recommended Dietary Allowances

The National Research Council of the National Academy of Sciences has established standards of nutrient intake that are consistent with the requirements of healthy people. These standards are called the Recommended Dietary Allowances (RDA), and are listed in the appendix on pages 215-218. They differ for infants, children, and adults, including pregnant and lactating women. Although one can evaluate the adequacy of a regular diet against these values, each requirement does not have to be met on a daily basis. The participant's diet needs to be evaluated over a period of several days to see if, on average, it provides enough of these nutrients.

The RDA values are based on a substantial amount of research. We do not have as much information about some other vitamins and minerals; however, a range of values given as "estimated safe and adequate daily dietary intakes" for these nutrients is presented in the appendix. Is it possible to design a diet to meet these RDA standards?

Meeting the Dietary Goals and the RDA

A good diet allows an individual to achieve the RDA for protein, minerals, and vitamins, while emphasizing carbohydrates and minimizing

fats. Over the years a variety of food plans have been suggested as models to follow to meet RDA standards, such as the Basic Four Food Group Plan. The model currently recommended by the U.S. Department of Agriculture is the Food Guide Pyramid: A Guide to Daily Food Choices. The Food Guide Pyramid, figure 6.2, lists five food groups:

- Breads, cereals, rice, and pasta
- Fruit
- Vegetable
- Milk, yogurt, and cheese
- Meat, poultry, fish, dry beans, eggs, and nuts

The base of the Food Guide Pyramid emphasizes carbohydrates (with 6 to 11 servings), and the top of the pyramid recommends limiting use of fats, oils, sweets, and alcohol. The latter items contribute little of nutrient value to the diet, while increasing the caloric content. Table 6.3 shows sample foods and serving sizes and the recommended number of servings for three levels of caloric intake. Choosing the lowest fat options within each food group will keep fat intake well below the 30% goal mentioned previously.

Evaluation of Dietary Intake

We have just presented the standards of good nutrition and a plan that can be used to meet those standards. But how do you know whether participants have met those standards or are taking in the proper number of calories needed to maintain or lose weight? The first step is to have individuals complete a dietary history that will help them get a sense of how food fits into their lives. Have them answer the questions in table 6.4.

This fill-in-the-blank review should give participants an idea of how their dietary habits compare to the recommendations mentioned earlier that aim to reduce fat intake and increase consumption of complex carbohydrates. Further, by focusing attention on cooking habits, likes and dislikes, consumption of snacks, and the circumstances surrounding eating, the participants may now be ready to take a look at how to control their caloric intake.

Table 6.2 Minerals and Their Functions

Mineral	Function	Sources	Daily adult requirement[a]	
			Men	**Women**
		Major minerals		
Calcium	Bones, teeth, blood clotting, nerve and muscle function	Milk, sardines, dark green vegetables, nuts	800 mg[b]	800 mg
Chloride	Nerve and muscle function, water balance (with sodium)	Table salt	750 mg	750 mg[c]
Magnesium	Bone growth; nerve, muscle, and enzyme function	Nuts, seafood, whole grains, leafy green vegetables	350 mg	280 mg
Phosphorus	Bone, teeth, energy transfer	Meats, poultry, seafood, eggs, milk, beans	800 mg	800 mg
Potassium	Nerve and muscle function	Fresh vegetables, bananas, citrus fruits, milk, meats, fish	2000 mg	2000 mg[c]
Sodium	Nerve and muscle function, water balance	Table salt	500 mg	500 mg[c]
		Trace minerals		
Chromium	Glucose metabolism	Meats, liver, whole grains, dried beans	.05-.2 mg	.05-.2 mg
Copper	Enzyme function, energy production	Meats, seafood, nuts, grains	1.5-3 mg	1.5-3 mg
Fluoride	Bone and teeth growth	Drinking water, fish, milk	1.5-4 mg	1.5-4 mg
Iodine	Thyroid hormone formation	Iodized salt, seafood	150 μg[b]	150 μg
Iron	O_2 transport in red blood cells; enzyme function	Red meat, liver, eggs, beans, leafy vegetables, shellfish	10 mg	15 mg
Manganese	Enzyme function	Whole grains, nuts, fruits, vegetables	2.5-5 mg	2.5-5 mg
Molybdenum	Energy metabolism in cells	Whole grains, organ meats, peas, beans	.075-.25 mg	.075-.25 mg
Selenium	Works with vitamin E	Meat, fish, whole grains, eggs	70 μg	55 μg
Zinc	Part of enzymes, growth	Meat, shellfish, yeast, whole grains	15 mg	12 mg

[a]Values are for adults 25 to 50 years of age. The requirements vary for children and pregnant or lactating women. See the appendix.

[b]mg = milligram, μg = microgram.

[c]Minimum requirements for healthy people. See the appendix.

Reprinted from Franks and Howley 1989.

Reprinted from Franks and Howley 1989.

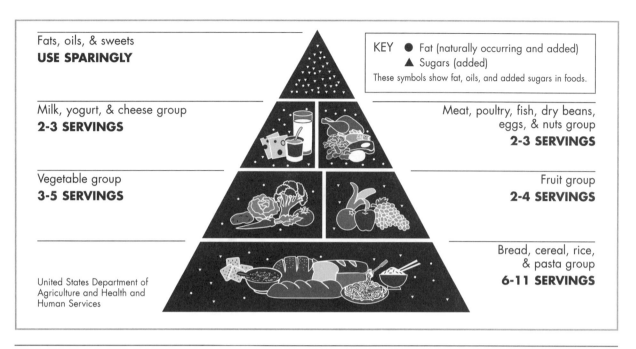

Figure 6.2 The Food Guide Pyramid.

Table 6.3	Food Guide Pyramid: Food Groups, Sample Foods, and Daily Servings			
Food group	**Sample foods and serving size**	**Servings for 3 levels of daily caloric intake (kcal/day)**		
		1,600	**2,200**	**2,800**
Breads	1 slice of bread 1 oz ready-to-eat cereal 1/2 c of cooked cereal, rice, or pasta	6	9	11
Vegetable	1 c of raw leafy vegetables 1/2 c of other vegetables 1/4 c of vegetable juice	3	4	5
Fruit	1 medium apple 1/2 c of chopped, cooked, or canned fruit 1/4 c of fruit juice	2	3	4
Milk	1 c of milk or yogurt 1-1/2 oz of natural cheese 2 oz of processed cheese	2-3	2-3	2-3
Meat	2-3 oz of cooked lean meat, poultry, or fish (1/2 cup cooked beans or 1 egg counts as 1 oz of lean meat)	2-3 servings equal to 5 oz of lean meat	2-3 servings equal to 6 oz of lean meat	2-3 servings equal to 7 oz of lean meat

Source: U.S. Department of Agriculture.

Table 6.4 Eating Context

Instructions: Complete each question.

- How many times a day do you eat? _____

- Do you enjoy eating? _____

- Do you eat when you are hungry or according to a time schedule? _____

- What times do you eat meals? _____ Snacks? _____

- What foods do you eat most often? _____

- What are your favorite snacks? _____

- What are some of your least favorite foods? _____

- How long does it take you to eat a meal? _____

- Do you eat more or less than other people? _____

- Are you on a diet? _____ What kind? _____

- Do you use vitamin and mineral supplements? _____

- How much solid fat (butter, margarine, lard) do you use? _____ Oils? _____

- Do you add salt to your food while cooking? _____ At the table? _____

- Do you use low-fat or regular dairy products? _____

- How many times a week do you eat meat? _____ Poultry? _____ Fish? _____

- Do you primarily fry, bake, broil, or boil your meats? _____

- How long has your weight been what it is now? _____

- When you eat at home, who does the cooking? _____

- How often do you eat out? _____ For what meals? _____

Note. From *Fitness Leader's Handbook* (2nd ed.) by B.D. Franks and E.T. Howley, 1998, Champaign, IL: Human Kinetics. This form may be copied by the fitness leader for distribution to participants.

Table 6.5 provides a means of listing foods eaten at different times of the day. Participants should fill out this dietary record over a period of at least three days, including a Saturday or Sunday. In this way, the participant can obtain a reasonable estimate of his or her average dietary intake.

The focus in table 6.5 is not only on the foods eaten, but also on the eating pattern. For example, if participants always find themselves eating snacks in an easy chair watching television, there may be an association between the eating of the snack and the comfort of the TV room. To change unhealthy habits, including dietary ones, you may first have to help the person change the circumstances associated with the habit. Restricting all eating to the kitchen may help change eating habits. Additional details on how to help persons change habits are presented in chapter 15.

The information collected in table 6.5 can be used to determine if an individual is meeting the recommendations in the Food Guide Pyramid. Table 6.6 provides space for an individual to organize the foods consumed over a 3-day period according to the food groups. This provides good information about which groups

Table 6.5	Suggested Dietary Record Format							
	Time	**Food**	**Amount**	**Calories**	**Where are you?**	**Who is with you?**	**What are you doing?**	**How do you feel?**
DAY 1								
Breakfast								
Snack								
Lunch								
Snack								
Dinner								
Snack								
DAY 2								
Breakfast								
Snack								
Lunch								
Snack								
Dinner								
Snack								
DAY 3								
Breakfast								
Snack								
Lunch								
Snack								
Dinner								
Snack								

Note. From *Fitness Leader's Handbook* (2nd ed.) by B.D. Franks and E.T. Howley, 1998, Champaign, IL: Human Kinetics. This form may be copied by the fitness leader for distribution to participants.

Adapted from Katch and McArdle 1977.

are underrepresented and which are overrepresented. By carefully selecting foods, a person will come close to meeting the goals of the Food Guide Pyramid and may also alter caloric intake. Remember, the plan should emphasize variety and low-fat meats and dairy products.

Weight Loss Methods to Avoid

We have tried to present some basic, sound information relating diet to health and weight control. There is no question about the interest in this topic—just look at all the dieting books

Table 6.6	**Three-Day Record for Food Guide Pyramid**

Instructions:

1. By referring to your record of food intake, determine for each day the actual number of servings you had in each food group and record this in the appropriate box below. If you ate no servings in a food group, record a zero.

2. Total the number of servings in each food group for the 3 days and calculate an average for the 3 days.

Food groups	Recommended daily servings	1st day	2nd day	3rd day	Average
1. Bread, cereal, rice, pasta	6-11				
2. Fruit	2-4				
3. Vegetable	3-5				
4. Milk, yogurt, cheese	2-3				
5. Meat, poultry, fish, dry beans, eggs, and nuts	2-3				
6. Fats, oils, sweets	use sparingly				

and programs for sale in every community. Unfortunately, but not surprisingly, some books and programs provide incorrect and potentially dangerous information regarding diet, exercise, and weight loss. The purpose of this section is to discuss fads and gimmicks sold under the pretense that they will help a person achieve a weight loss goal.

A sound weight reduction plan creates a caloric imbalance of about 500 to 1000 kcal per day through modifications in diet and exercise. This adjustment will cause a fat loss of about 1 or 2 lb per week, and focus attention on exercise and eating behaviors. We cannot overemphasize the need to make *small and systematic changes* in diet and activity levels to cause the weight loss and to maintain the new weight when the goal is achieved. In the process, the fitness participant will learn how to plan meals better to meet the dietary goals and RDA standards. Table 6.7 is a checklist that you can use to help individuals make decisions about the different weight loss diets.

There are products and diets available that "guarantee" weight loss on the way to producing a more beautiful person. The vast majority of people who lose weight using these gim-

micks regain it within a year because they have not adjusted the factors involved in the energy balance equation: energy expenditure and caloric intake. In addition, they have not paid attention to changing lifestyle behaviors that are related to patterns of eating and exercise.

There is no lack of fad diets and commercial enterprises that promise an incredible weight loss in a short period of time. As we mentioned earlier, vendors want to make money with their offerings, and you should help people be wary of exaggerated claims. The saying "If it's too good to be true, it probably is" is a good way to approach weight loss diets and gimmicks. You can help educate participants as to the more common gimmicks used to "lose" weight:

• **Diuretics.** These drugs cause sodium, potassium, and water loss from the body. The weight change that occurs as a result is therefore unrelated to body fatness.

• **Laxatives.** These medications are usually used to loosen fecal matter in the large intestine and promote bowel movements. People who use laxatives for weight loss are under the assumption that if laxatives speed things along the intestinal track, some food will not be

Table 6.7	Weight Loss Diet Evaluation Checklist

The following checklist can be used to evaluate weight loss diets. A *No* answer to any of the questions indicates an inadequate weight reduction plan. Does your diet

	Yes	No
1. aim for a weight loss of 1-2 lb per week?	❑	❑
2. provide at least 1,200 kcal per day?	❑	❑
3. recommend a regular endurance exercise program?	❑	❑
4. provide a balance of foods from all four food groups?	❑	❑
5. provide for variety to prevent boredom?	❑	❑
6. establish eating and exercise habits that can be maintained the rest of your life?	❑	❑
7. conform to your personal lifestyle?	❑	❑
8. work without pills, drugs, or other gadgets?	❑	❑

absorbed into the body. This is not true. Laxatives have little effect on absorption but instead cause the loss of important minerals and water from the body.

• **"Sauna" suits.** These suits are made of materials impermeable to sweat, which must be evaporated from the surface of the skin to cool the body during exercise. Because evaporation does not occur when these suits are worn, the body sweats more in an attempt to cool itself. This results in a loss of water weight that will (and must) be replaced as soon as possible. These suits do not "burn" calories away. Sitting in a sauna room has the same effect on water weight.

• **Elastic belts.** These belts are made to be worn around the waist and allegedly "melt" fat away, causing changes in waist size. As it turns out, waist size does decrease because the tissues are compressed; within a few hours, however, the tissues return to their normal size and the effect disappears.

• **Vibrators or massagers.** These devices promise to break up fat in localized areas, cause "spot reduction," and speed weight loss. Spot reduction is a dream that can't come true because weight is lost from the body in a pattern opposite to the way it went on. If the fat went to the hips first and the face last, it will come from the face first and the hips last when body fat is lost. These machines may be enjoyable to use, but they do not increase energy expenditure, which is necessary for weight loss.

Summary

The recommended diet (or food plan) includes a balanced food intake with 55% to 60% of calories coming from carbohydrates, no more than 30% from fats (less than 10% from saturated fats), and 10% to 15% from proteins. Help fitness participants increase complex carbohydrates and reduce fats in their diets. Specific recommendations include decreasing consumption of soft drinks, cakes, cookies, and other high-sugar foods; increasing intake of whole-grain breads, cereals, fruits, vegetables, and beans; and using low-fat milk, less and leaner meat, and fish, poultry, and dry beans and peas as sources of low-fat protein. Encourage individuals to limit eggs and organ meats as well as fats and oils, especially those high in saturated fats (e.g., butter, lard, and palm and coconut oils). This chapter has provided examples of foods in each group in the Food Guide Pyramid. Finally, some cautions concerning weightloss gimmicks were presented.

Chapter 7
Desired Aerobic Fitness

Aerobic Fitness
Tests of Cardiorespiratory Fitness

Cardiorespiratory fitness (CRF), also called cardiovascular or aerobic fitness, is a good measure of the heart's ability to pump oxygen-rich blood to the muscles. Although there are technical differences in terms using cardio (heart), vascular (blood vessels), respiratory (lungs and ventilation), and aerobic (working with oxygen), they all reflect various aspects of this component of fitness. The person with a healthy heart can pump great volumes of blood with each beat and has a high level of CRF.

Measures of Cardiorespiratory Function

Cardiorespiratory fitness values are expressed in the following ways: liters of oxygen used by the body per minute ($L \cdot min^{-1}$), milliliters of oxygen used per kilogram of body weight per minute ($ml \cdot kg^{-1} \cdot min^{-1}$), and METs. One MET describes the amount of oxygen used by the body at rest and is equal to 3.5 $ml \cdot kg^{-1} \cdot min^{-1}$. If you can use 35 $ml \cdot kg^{-1} \cdot min^{-1}$ of oxygen during maximal exercise, your CRF is 10 METs ($35 \cdot 3.5^{-1} = 10$). Aerobic training programs increase the heart's ability to pump blood, so it is no surprise that CRF increases as a result of such programs.

Historically, measurements of heart rate (HR), blood pressure (BP), and the electrocardiogram (ECG) taken at rest were used to evaluate CRF. Static pulmonary function tests (such as vital capacity) were used to characterize respiratory function. It became clear, however, that measurements made at rest told little about the way a person's cardiorespiratory system responds during work. We now use a graded exercise test (GXT) to evaluate the HR, BP, ECG, ventilation, and oxygen uptake responses during work.

Results from these tests form the basis for exercise recommendations, and they allow fitness professionals and participants to evaluate positive or negative changes in CRF resulting from physical conditioning, aging, illness, or inactivity. Given what we know about the effect of childhood obesity and inactivity on adult health status, there is good reason to include CRF evaluation throughout life, from early childhood to old age. These test scores can point out where the individual stands relative to others and, more importantly, will alert the individual to subtle changes in lifestyle that may compromise positive health.

Choices in Fitness Testing and Activities

Choosing an appropriate test takes several factors into account. People differ in age, fitness level, known health problems, and risks of CHD. Financial considerations determine the amount of time that can be devoted to each individual and the type of work tasks available. Physical fitness testing and activities are well integrated into a fitness program. When people come to the same fitness center over a period of time, they should experience a logical sequence for fitness testing and activities (table 7.1 and figure 7.1). When people come in for fitness testing but will not continue their involvement with the fitness center, then all the tests (with the possible exception of a

maximal test) are usually a part of the same testing protocol.

Other sections of this book discuss elements of the testing sequence. Chapter 4 dealt with screening. The person to be tested needs to understand clearly all the procedures, potential risks, and benefits; that the data will be confidential; and that he or she can terminate any test at any time. (You will find a sample testing consent form in chapter 21.) Chapter 3 dealt with procedures for determining current health status. Advise follow-up testing for those with symptoms of health problems as their histories may warrant a referral to other professionals.

Typical resting tests include a 12-lead ECG, BP, and blood chemistry profile. A physician's evaluation of the ECG may discover abnormalities requiring further medical attention. People with extreme BP or blood chemistry values should also be referred to their personal physician. If the resting tests reflect normal values, and there are no contraindications for testing (see table 7.2), then you can administer a submaximal test.

The submaximal test provides HR and BP responses to different intensities of work from light work up to a predetermined point (usually 85% of predicted maximum HR). You can use a bench, cycle ergometer, or treadmill for this test. Once again, if the person has unusual

Table 7.1	Sequence of Testing and Activity Prescription
Step	**Test or activity**
1	Informed consent
2	Health history
3	Screening
4	Resting CRF, body composition, and psychological tests
5	Submaximal CRF
6	Tests for low-back function
7	Begin light activity program here
8	Tests for muscular strength and endurance
9	Maximal CRF
10	Revise activity program; include games and sports here
11	Periodic retest (and activity revision)

Reprinted from Howley and Franks 1997.

responses to the submaximal test, you should refer him for further medical tests. If the results appear normal, then begin an activity program at an intensity lower than that reached on the test (e.g., if the participant reaches 85% of maxi- mal HR on the test, start the fitness program at 70%). After the participant has become accustomed to regular exercise and appears to be adjusting to fitness activities, you can administer a maximal test.

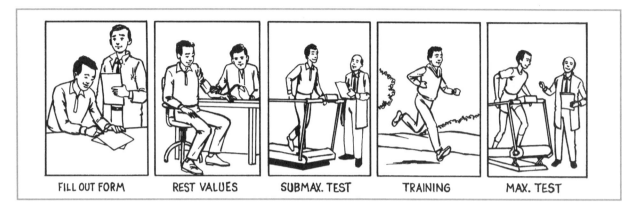

FILL OUT FORM   REST VALUES   SUBMAX. TEST   TRAINING   MAX. TEST

Figure 7.1 Sequence of testing.

Table 7.2 Contraindications to Exercise Testing	
Absolute contraindications:	**Relative contraindications:**
1. A recent significant change in the resting ECG suggesting infarction or other acute cardiac event	1. Resting diastolic blood pressure > 115 mmHg or resting systolic blood pressure > 200 mmHg
2. Recent complicated myocardial infarction (unless patient is stable and pain-free)	2. Moderate valvular heart disease
3. Unstable angina	3. Known electrolyte abnormalities (hypokalemia, hypomagnesemia)
4. Uncontrolled ventricular arrhythmia	4. Fixed-rate pacemaker (rarely used)
5. Uncontrolled atrial arrhythmia that compromises cardiac function	5. Frequent or complex ventricular ectopy
6. Third-degree AV heart block without pacemaker	6. Ventricular aneurysm
7. Acute congestive heart failure	7. Uncontrolled metabolic disease (e.g., diabetes, thyrotoxicosis, or myxedema)
8. Severe aortic stenosis	8. Chronic infectious disease (e.g., mononucleosis, hepatitis, AIDS)
9. Suspected or known dissecting aneurysm	9. Neuromuscular, musculoskeletal, or rheumatoid disorders that are exacerbated by exercise
10. Active or suspected myocarditis or pericarditis	10. Advanced or complicated pregnancy
11. Thrombophlebitis or intracardiac thrombi	
12. Recent systemic or pulmonary embolus	
13. Acute infections	
14. Significant emotional distress (psychosis)	

Reprinted from American College of Sports Medicine 1971.

Maximal aerobic power, also called maximal oxygen uptake, describes the greatest rate at which the human body (primarily muscle) can utilize oxygen. The term also describes the upper limit of the cardiorespiratory system's ability to deliver oxygen-rich blood to those muscles. Maximal aerobic power thus is not only a good index of cardiorespiratory fitness but also a good predictor of performance capability in aerobic events such as distance running, cycling, cross-country skiing, and swimming (see chapter 16 for more information on maximal oxygen uptake).

Basically, two types of maximal tests are used to estimate CRF—laboratory tests that measure physiological responses (e.g., oxygen uptake) to increasing levels of work and unmonitored endurance performance tests (such as time to exhaustion on a treadmill or time on a mile run). *Health standards* for endurance runs and maximal oxygen uptake are listed in table 7.3.

You can use the results of the CRF test to revise the activity program. After the participants achieve a minimum level of fitness, they can include a wider variety of activities (games and sports) in their fitness program. Finally, you should retest them periodically to determine their progress and to revise the program in areas where the gains are not as great as desired.

Graded Exercise Testing

Many fitness programs use a graded exercise test (GXT) to evaluate CRF. You can administer these multilevel tests using a bench, cycle ergometer, or treadmill (see figure 7.2).

Bench stepping is very economical. You can use it for both submaximal and maximal testing. Disadvantages include the number of stages that can be feasibly included for any one bench height and individual fitness level, and the difficulty of taking certain measurements during the test (such as BP) compared to the cycle ergometer or treadmill.

The *cycle ergometer* is less expensive than a treadmill. Additional measurements are easy to obtain since the upper body is essentially stationary during the test. One difference between the cycle ergometer and the other task forms normally used is that body weight is supported by the seat. This may be viewed as either an advantage or a disadvantage, depending on the purpose of the test. One of the major disadvantages of using the cycle ergometer for maximal tests with noncycling individuals is that local muscle fatigue is often a limiting factor. In addition, when a small person does the same work rate on the cycle ergometer as a large person, the smaller individual is operating at a higher MET level.

A particular testing protocol on the *treadmill* is very reproducible. A person must keep up with the set pace, whereas one may go too slow or too fast on either the bench or the cycle. Its major disadvantage is cost—it is the most expensive type of exercise testing equipment.

All equipment must be calibrated (checked with known standards). The speed and grade of the treadmill, resistance scale on the cycle ergometer, timing devices, gas analysis, and other equipment should all be calibrated at specific intervals (see figure 7.3). Manuals for the equipment normally include detailed instruc-

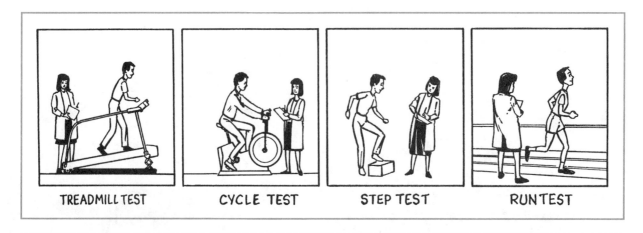

TREADMILL TEST   CYCLE TEST   STEP TEST   RUN TEST

Figure 7.2 Analyzing cardiorespiratory function.

	$\dot{V}O_2max$ ml·kg⁻¹·min⁻¹		1.5-min run (min:s)		12-min run (mi)	
Age[a]	**Female[b]**	**Male**	**Female**	**Male**	**Female**	**Male**
Good						
15-30	>40	>45	<12	<10	>1.5	>1.7
35-50	>35	>40	<13:30	<11:30	>1.4	>1.5
55-70	>30	>35	<16	<14	>1.2	>1.3
Adequate for most activities						
15-30	35	40	13:30	11:50	1.4	1.5
35-50	30	35	15	13	1.3	1.4
55-70	25	30	17:30	15:30	1.1	1.3
Borderline						
15-30	30	35	15	13	1.3	1.4
35-50	25	30	16:30	14:30	1.2	1.3
55-70	20	25	19	17	1.0	1.2
Needs extra work on CRF						
15-30	<25	<30	>17	>15	<1.2	<1.3
35-50	<20	<25	>18:30	>16:30	<1.1	<1.2
55-70	<15	<20	>21	>19	<0.9	<1.0

Table 7.3 Standards for Maximal Oxygen Uptake and Endurance Runs

Note. These standards are for fitness programs. People wanting to do well in endurance performance need higher levels. For those at the *Good* level, emphasize maintaining this level the rest of their lives. For those in the lower levels, emphasize setting and reaching realistic goals.

[a]CRF declines with age.

[b]Women have lower standards because they have a larger amount of essential fat.

Reprinted from Howley and Franks 1986.

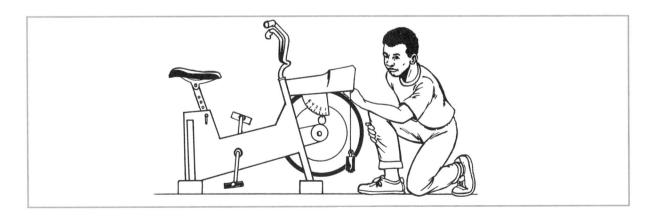

Figure 7.3 Calibrate your equipment.

tions for calibration. Do not assume that any dial setting or meter is accurate. In addition, you must carefully monitor and adjust the work rates (grade and speed on a treadmill, load and revolutions per minute on a cycle, or stepping rate on a bench) throughout a test.

Variables

The variables commonly measured during resting and submaximal tests include HR, BP, and rating of perceived exertion (RPE). Maximal testing often measures maximal oxygen uptake ($\dot{V}O_2$max) and the final stage achieved on a GXT.

Heart Rate. Heart rate is often used as a fitness indicator at rest and during a standard submaximal work task. During an ECG recording, the HR can be taken from the ECG strip (divide 1500 by the number of millimeters between the peaks of two QRS complexes). Heart rate watches can measure HR throughout a test and are quite accurate. You can also take the HR by using a stethoscope with the microphone placed on the chest or by palpating an artery at the wrist or neck. Exercise leaders should use their fingers (not thumb), preferably using the participant's wrist. If monitoring HR at the neck, be sure not to apply too much pressure. Doing so could trigger a reflex that causes the HR to slow down.

Maximal HR is useful for determining the target HR for fitness workouts, but it is not a good fitness indicator as it changes very little with training. The HR at rest or during steady-state exercise should be taken for 30 s for higher reliability. However, when taking HR after exercise, it should be taken at exactly the same time after work (e.g., 5 s after stopping the work) and taken for 10 or 15 s, because the HR is changing so rapidly. The 10- or 15-s rate is multiplied by 6 or 4, respectively, to calculate beats·min[-1].

Blood Pressure. Systolic blood pressure (SBP) and diastolic blood pressure (DBP) are often determined at rest as well as during and after work. You must use a proper-sized cuff and a sensitive stethoscope to obtain accurate values at rest and during work. At rest, the person should place both feet flat on the floor and assume a relaxed position with the arm supported. The cuff should be wrapped securely around the arm. The stethoscope should be below, not under, the cuff. Place the stethoscope where you can most easily hear the sound—often toward the inside of the arm. During exercise the first and fifth Korotkoff sounds (the first sound heard and when sound changes tune) are used for SBP and DBP, respectively. If SBP fails to increase or if DBP increases excessively (>115 mmHg) with increased work, then you should stop the test.

Rating of Perceived Exertion. Borg (1970) introduced the *rating of perceived exertion* (RPE) based on a scale from 6 to 20 (roughly based on resting to maximal heart rate—60 to 200 beats·min[-1]). Table 7.4 contains this scale. You can use this scale with a GXT both to provide useful information during the test as the participant approaches exhaustion and as a reference point for exercise recommendations. (*Note.* To understand the scale and its administration, all users should read Borg, G. 1998. *Borg's Perceived Exertion and Pain Scales.* Champaign, IL: Human Kinetics.)

You should give the participant the following instructions when using the RPE scale (ACSM, 1995, p. 77):

> During the exercise test we want you to pay close attention to how hard you feel the exercise work rate is. This feeling should reflect your total amount of exertion and fatigue, combining all sensations and feelings of physical stress, effort, and fatigue. Don't concern yourself with any one factor such as leg pain, shortness of breath, or exercise intensity, but try to concentrate on your total inner feeling of exertion. Try not to underestimate or overestimate your feeling of exertion; be as accurate as you can.

Pretest Instructions

Because the resting and submaximal exercise HR, BP, and RPE values are influenced by a variety of factors, you must take care to minimize these or at least to minimize the variation in each from one testing period to the next. These factors include, but are not limited to the following:

- The temperature and relative humidity of the testing room
- Number of hours of sleep
- Emotional state
- Hydration state
- Medication
- Time of day
- Time elapsed since the last meal, cigarette smoking, caffeine, and exercise

Paying attention to these factors increases the likelihood that changes in HR, BP, or RPE from one test to the next are a result of changes in physical activity habits. Table 7.5 is a sample pretest instruction sheet.

Termination of the GXT

You should use a series of "end points" to stop a GXT when testing apparently healthy adults (see table 7.6).

Table 7.4	Rating of Perceived Exertion Scales		
Original rating scale	**CR10 scale**		
6 No exertion at all	0	Nothing at all	"No P"
7	0.3		
8 Extremely light	0.5	Extremely weak	Just noticeable
9 Very light	1	Very weak	
10	1.5		
11 Light	2	Weak	Light
12	2.5		
13 Somewhat hard	3	Moderate	
14	4		
15 Hard (heavy)	5	Strong	Heavy
16	6		
17 Very hard	7	Very strong	
18	8		
	9		
19 Extremely hard	10	**Extremely strong "Max P"**	
20 Maximal exertion	11		
	●	Absolute maximum	Highest possible

Borg RPE Scale © Gunnar Borg, 1970, 1985, 1994, 1998

Borg CR10 scale © Gunnar Borg, 1981, 1982, 1998

Table 7.5	Pretest Instructions for a Fitness Test

Name: _____ Test date: _____ Time:_____

Report to:_____

Instructions: Please observe the following:

1. Wear running shoes, shorts, and loose-fitting shirt
2. No food, drink (except water), tobacco, or medication for 3 hr prior to test
3. Minimal physical activity on day of test

Cancellation: If you cannot keep this appointment, please call _____ or _____

Table 7.6	General Indications for Stopping a GXT in Apparently Healthy Adults*

1. Onset of angina or angina-like symptoms
2. Significant drop (20 mmHg) in systolic blood pressure or a failure of the systolic blood pressure to rise with an increase in exercise intensity
3. Excessive rise in blood pressure: systolic pressure >260 mmHg or diastolic pressure >115 mmHg
4. Signs of poor perfusion: light-headedness, confusion, ataxia, pallor, cyanosis, nausea, or cold and clammy skin
5. Failure of heart rate to increase with increased exercise intensity
6. Noticeable change in heart rhythm
7. Subject requests to stop
8. Physical or verbal manifestations of severe fatigue
9. Failure of the testing equipment

*Assumes that testing is nondiagnostic and is being performed without direct physician involvement or electrocardiographic monitoring.

Reprinted from American College of Sports Medicine 1995.

Submaximal and Maximal Tests

Graded exercise testing has been used to evaluate CRF in fitness programs for healthy populations and in the clinical assessment of ischemic heart disease. Exercise is used to place a "load" on the heart to determine the cardiovascular response and see if ischemic changes occur in the electrocardiogram (ECG). In this condition, an inadequate blood flow to the heart muscle can cause changes in the ECG. There has been some controversy concerning whether to use submaximal or maximal tests to evaluate ECG changes. Based on thousands of exercise stress tests conducted over the past 3 decades, one should generally use a maximal exercise test to determine the presence of ischemic heart disease. Though submaximal exercise tests are not as effective in identifying disease conditions, they do represent an appropriate means of evaluating cardiorespiratory fitness prior to and following exercise programs.

When the same fitness center is responsible for both the testing and the program, we recommend that you follow the sequence of testing and activity outlined in table 7.1. The main objection to maximal tests is the stress they put on someone who has been inactive. Although the risk of injury during a maximal GXT is very small when accompanied by adequate screening and qualified testing personnel, the discomfort some people may experience in going to the maximum without prior conditioning may discourage participation in a fitness program. Objections to submaximal tests include the fact that they point out fewer abnormal responses to exercise, and estimating one's maximal level from submaximal data is not always accurate. In a fitness program for apparently healthy persons, you can overcome these objections to both maximal and submaximal tests by administering the submaximal test early in the fitness program and waiting until the participant has been involved in a regular exercise program to administer the maximal test.

Any of the GXT protocols can be used for submaximal or maximal testing—the only difference is the criteria for stopping the test. Stop either test if you observe any of the abnormal responses listed previously. In the absence of abnormal responses, the submaximal test is usually terminated when the person reaches a certain HR (often 85% of maximal HR), while the maximal test continues to voluntary exhaustion.

Maximal Testing Protocol. No one protocol is appropriate for all types of people. We recommend that the time, starting points, and increments between stages vary with the type of person. Young, active individuals, normal sedentary individuals, and individuals of questionable health status should start at 6, 4, and 2 METs, respectively. The same three groups would increase 2 to 3, 1 to 2, and 0.5 to 1 METs, respectively, during stages of the test. The duration of each stage can vary from one to three minutes, depending on the health status of the individual and the need to achieve near steady-state responses at each stage. Table 7.7 illustrates how you may use these criteria for a bench, cycle, or treadmill test.

The following testing protocols are examples of tests that can be used for different populations. You can use the first protocol in table 7.8 with deconditioned subjects by starting at a very low MET level, with slow walking, and increasing one MET per 3-min stage. The Balke Standard protocol can be used for "typical" inactive adults by starting at a higher MET level and progressing at 1 MET per 2-min stage. More active or younger people can use the Bruce protocol, which starts at a moderate MET level and goes up 2 to 3 METs per 3-min stage. Unfortunately, some testing centers attempt to use the same testing protocol for everyone, which results in an initial stage that is either too high or too low and increments in work at each stage that are either too little or too much for the individual being tested.

Table 7.7 Testing Protocol for Different Groups

		Bench		Cycle		Treadmill	
Stage	METs	Height (cm)	Steps·min⁻¹	Work rate (kpm·min⁻¹)	RPM	Speed (km·hr⁻¹)	Grade (%)
Individuals with questionable health							
1	2	0	24	0	50	3.2	0
2	3	16	12	150	50	4.8	0
3	4	16	18	300	50	4.8	2.5
4	5	16	24	450	50	4.8	5.0
5	6	16	30	600	50	4.8	7.5
"Normal" sedentary individuals							
1	4	16	18	360	60	4.8	2.5
2	6	16	30	540	60	4.8	7.5
3	7-8	36	18-24	720-900	60	4.8-5.5	10.0
4	9	36	27	900-1080	60	5.5	12.0
5	10-11	36	30-33	1080-1260	60	9.7	0-1.75
Young active individuals							
1	6	16	30	630	70	4.8	7.5
2	9	36	27	1060	70	5.5	12.0
3	12	36	36	1270	70	9.7	3.5
4	15	50	33	1900	70	11.3	7.0
5	17	50	39	2110	70	11.3	11.0

Reprinted from Chung 1979.

Table 7.8	Treadmill Protocols for Various Categories			
Stage	**METs**	**Speed (km·hr⁻¹)**	**Grade (%)**	**Time (min)**
For deconditioned people[a]				
1	2.5	3.2	0	3
2	3.5	3.2	3.5	3
3	4.5	3.2	7	3
4	5.4	3.2	10.5	3
5	6.4	3.2	14	3
6	7.3	3.2	17.5	3
7	8.5	4.8	12.5	3
8	9.5	4.8	15	3
9	10.5	4.8	17.5	3
For normal inactive people[b]				
1	4.3	4.8	2.5	3
2	5.4	4.8	5	3
3	6.4	4.8	7.5	3
4	7.4	4.8	10	3
5	8.5	4.8	12.5	3
6	9.5	4.8	15	3
7	10.5	4.8	17.5	3
8	11.6	4.8	20	3
9	12.6	4.8	22.5	3
10	13.6	4.8	25	3
For young active people[c]				
1	5	2.7	10	3
2	7	4	12	3
3	9.5	5.4	14	3
4	13	6.7	16	3
5	16	8	18	3

[a]Adapted from Naughton and Haider 1973.

[b] Based on data from Balke 1970.

[c] Adapted from Bruce 1972.

Submaximal Exercise Test Protocol. You can use any graded exercise test protocol for submaximal or maximal testing. Fitness centers typically use a submaximal GXT to estimate a participant's $\dot{V}O_2$max or simply to show changes in selected fitness variables that have resulted from an exer-cise program. Changes in HR, BP, and RPE as a result of an exercise conditioning program make the submaximal test a good mechanism for show-ing improvements in cardiorespiratory function.

The initial stage and rate of progression of the GXT should be selected on the basis of the criteria mentioned earlier. In the following example, the Balke Standard protocol (3 mph, 2.5% grade increase every 2 min) was used with HR monitored in the last 30 s of each stage. The test was terminated at 85% of age-adjusted maximal HR. Maximal aerobic power was estimated by extrapolating the HR response to the subject's estimated maximal HR (220 – age). Figure 7.4 presents the results of this test with a graph showing the HR response at each work rate. Note that the HR response is somewhat "flat" between the 0% and 5% grade. This finding is not uncommon and may be due to the subject's initial excitement or to the fact that stroke volume changes are accounting for the changes in cardiac output at these low work rates (see chapter 16). The HR response is normally quite linear between 110 beats·min^{-1} and the subject's 85% of maximal HR cutoff; that is, HR increases proportionally to work rate.

To estimate $\dot{V}O_2$max, draw a line through the HR points from 7.5% grade to the final work rate. The line is extended (extrapolated) to the subject's estimated maximal heart rate (220 – subject's age; in this example, 220 – 37 = 183

beats·min^{-1}). Drop a vertical line from the last point to the baseline to estimate the subject's maximal aerobic power, which in this case is 11.8 METs or 41.3 ml·kg^{-1}·min^{-1}.

Administration of Graded Exercise Test (GXT). The fitness leader needs to complete several tasks before administering a GXT:

• Calibrate equipment.

• Check supplies and data forms.

• Select the appropriate test protocol for the participant.

• Obtain informed consent.

• Provide instruction in the task, including the cool-down procedure.

• Have the participant practice the task, if needed.

• Check to see that the participant followed the pretest instructions.

Many fitness programs use the YMCA submaximal cycle ergometer test to evaluate cardiorespiratory fitness (see figure 7.5). Table 7.9 on page 73 describes the steps in giving a submaximal cycle ergometer test.

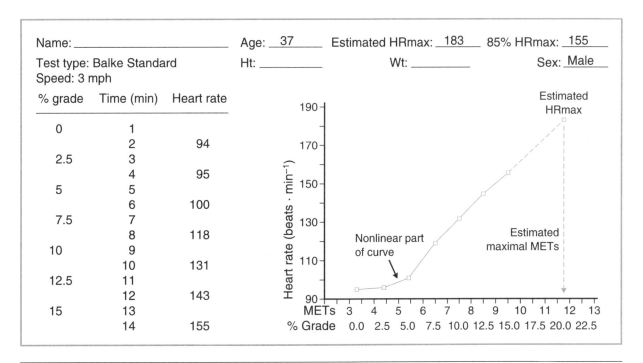

Figure 7.4 Maximal aerobic power estimated by measuring the heart rate response to a submaximal graded exercise test (GXT) on a treadmill.

Reprinted from Howley and Franks 1997.

To assess the participant's progress, you should administer a second test after several weeks of conditioning and compare the results with those of the initial test. Using the same testing protocol, the participant should be able to do the same work with a lower HR and RPE, indicating improved fitness.

You can also use the test results to estimate the participant's maximal oxygen uptake. Figure 7.6 on page 74 illustrates this procedure. Plot the heart rates above 110 (in this case the HRs at stages 3 and 4), and draw a line between them. Extend (extrapolate) this line from these heart rates to the estimated maximal HR (170 in this case), and draw a vertical line from the intersection of the line of best fit and the maximal HR to the baseline. The point where this intersected vertical line touches the baseline is the estimated maximal oxygen uptake (in this case, 1.77 L·min⁻¹).

On the treadmill and the bench, oxygen uptake is measured in METs because the work rate is proportional to the subject's body weight. On the cycle ergometer, however, body weight is supported, and the work is dependent on the speed and resistance of the flywheel. Thus, the oxygen uptake is measured in L·min⁻¹. You can convert maximal oxygen uptake from L·min⁻¹ to METs by following the steps listed in table 7.10.

You can evaluate the participant's estimated maximal oxygen uptake using the standards in

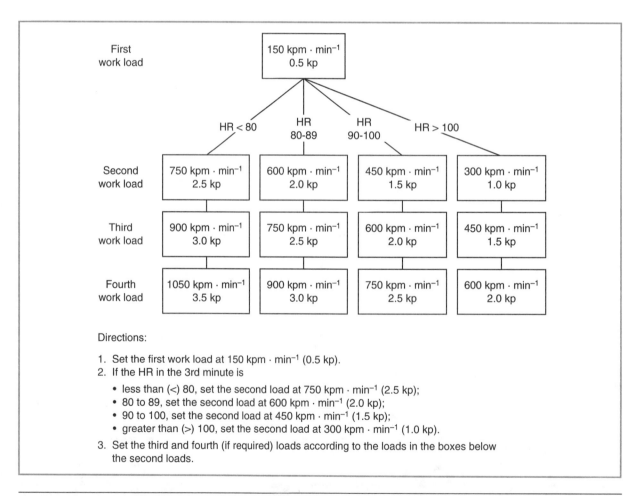

Figure 7.5 Guide for setting power units (work loads) for men and women on a YMCA cycle ergometer test, using the Y's *Way to Physical Fitness* protocol.

Reprinted from *Y's Way to Physical Fitness* with permission of the YMCA of the USA, 101 N. Wacker Drive, Chicago, IL 60606.

Table 7.9	Administration of Submaximal Cycle Ergometer Test

1   Complete pretest items.

2   Select test protocol (see figure 7.5).

3   Estimate participant's max HR (220 – age = beats·min^{-1}).

4   Determine 85% of participant's max HR (max HR x .85 = 85% max HR).

5   Review procedure with participant.

6   Set and record seat height (leg to be slightly bent at knee when foot is at bottom of pedaling stroke).

7   Start metronome (set at 100 beats·min^{-1} so that one foot is at bottom of pedaling stroke on each beat, resulting in 50 complete rpm).

8   Have participant begin pedaling in rhythm with metronome.

9   As soon as correct pace is achieved, set resistance according to protocol chosen (see figure 7.5).

10   Start timer for beginning of 3-min stage.

11   Check resistance setting (it may drift) and observe participant for signs or symptoms that require terminating the test.

12   At 1:30 into the stage, take and record blood pressure.

13   At 2:30, take and record heart rate either from ECG or manually from 2:30-2:45.

14   At 2:50, get and record participant's rating of perceived exertion (RPE).

15   At 2:55, ask participant, "How are you doing?"

16   At 3:00, if HR is less than 85% of max HR, blood pressure is responding normally, and participant is all right, increase resistance to the next stage.

17   Repeat steps 10 through 16 until participant reaches 85% of max HR or there is another reason to stop the test. Go back to stage 1 (for cool-down) and repeat steps 10 through 15, stopping at 3:00 in the cool-down stage.

18   Talk with participant and check out any problems.

Table 7.10	Conversion of Maximal Oxygen Uptake From Liters per Minute to METs

1.   Multiply L·min^{-1} by 1000 to get ml·min^{-1}
   1.77 L·min^{-1} x 1000 ml = 1770 ml·min^{-1}

2.   Divide ml·min^{-1} by kg of body weight.
   1770 ml·min^{-1} ÷ 78 kg = 22.7 ml·kg^{-1} x min^{-1}

3.   Divide ml·kg^{-1} · min^{-1} by 3.5 ml·kg^{-1}·min^{-1}.
   22.7 ml·kg^{-1} · min^{-1} ÷ 3.5 ml·kg^{-1}·min^{-1} = 6.5 METs

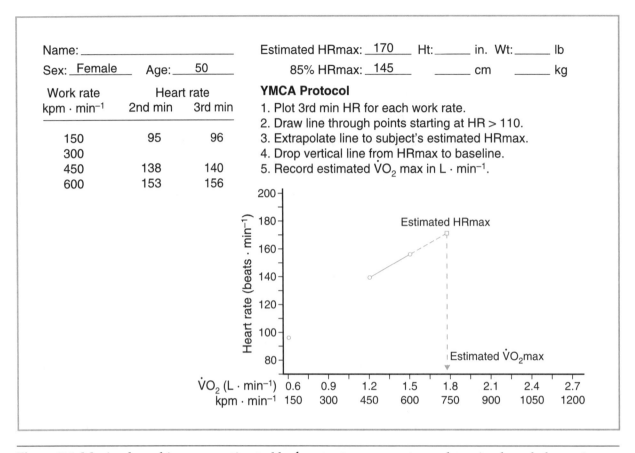

Name: _____   Estimated HRmax: __170__ Ht: _____ in. Wt: _____ lb

Sex: __Female__   Age: ___50___   85% HRmax: __145__   _____ cm   _____ kg

Work rate	Heart rate	
kpm · min⁻¹	2nd min	3rd min
150	95	96
300		
450	138	140
600	153	156

YMCA Protocol
1. Plot 3rd min HR for each work rate.
2. Draw line through points starting at HR > 110.
3. Extrapolate line to subject's estimated HRmax.
4. Drop vertical line from HRmax to baseline.
5. Record estimated $\dot{V}O_2$ max in L · min⁻¹.

Figure 7.6 Maximal aerobic power estimated by heart rate response to a submaximal graded exercise test on a cycle ergometer.

Reprinted from *Y's Way to Physical Fitness* with permission of the YMCA of the USA, 101 N. Wacker Drive, Chicago, IL 60606.

table 7.3. The results show that this participant's cardiorespiratory fitness is at a low level, and you should strongly encourage her to begin an exercise program.

Field Tests

You can also estimate CRF with a variety of field tests. They are called "field tests" because they require very little equipment, can be done just about anywhere, and use the simple activities of walking and running.

Because these tests involve running or walking as fast as possible over a set distance, they are not recommended at the start of an exercise program. Instead, we recommend beginning with the graduated walking or jogging programs outlined in chapters 12 and 13 before taking these tests. The graduated nature of the fitness program allows participants to start at a low, safe level of activity and gradually improve. It is then appropriate to administer a walk or run test to evaluate fitness status.

Field tests rely on the observation that the heart must pump great volumes of oxygen to the muscles for a person to be able to walk or run at high speeds over long distances. Therefore, the average speed maintained in these walk and run tests gives an estimate of CRF. The higher the CRF score, the greater the capacity of the heart to transport oxygen. Endurance runs of a set distance for time or a set time for distance provide information about a person's cardiorespiratory endurance, as long as the distance is 1 mile or more. Some advantages of the endurance run are that it is a natural activity and it allows a large number of individuals to be tested in a short period of time. The disadvantages are that it is difficult to monitor physiological responses, other factors (e.g., motivation) affect the outcome, and endurance running cannot be used for graded or submaximal testing.

Walk Test. You can also estimate CRF in adults, especially older adults, using a 1-mi-walk test. Table 7.11 outlines administration of the test.

Use table 7.12 to predict the participant's CRF based on the time of the walk and the postexercise heart rate. To use table 7.12, find the section of the table that pertains to the individual's sex and age, then read across the top until you find the time (to the nearest minute) it took to walk a mile. Look down that column until it intersects with the person's postexercise heart rate (listed in the far left column). The number where the mile time and postexercise heart rate meet is the participant's CRF value in terms of oxygen used per kilogram of body weight per minute ($ml \cdot kg^{-1} \cdot min^{-1}$). You can evaluate cardiorespiratory fitness by comparing this estimate with the standards presented in table 7.12. For example, a 25-year-old man who walks the mile in 20 min and has a postexercise heart rate of 140 beats·min⁻¹ has an estimated maximal oxygen uptake of 29.2 $ml \cdot kg^{-1} \cdot min^{-1}$. His maximal oxygen uptake is "borderline," indicating a need for improvement.

Jog-Run Test. One of the most common CRF fields is the 12-min or 1.5-mi run popularized by Dr. Kenneth Cooper. This test is very much like

Table 7.11 Steps to Administer the Mile-Walk Test

Step	Activity

Before test day

1. Arrange to have the following elements at the test site:
   - A person to start and read the time from a stopwatch
   - A partner with a watch (with a second hand) for each walker (perhaps with a sheet to mark off laps)
   - A stopwatch for the timer (with a spare ready)
   - A score sheet or scorecard
2. Explain the purpose of the test (i.e., to determine how fast they can walk a mile, which reflects the endurance of their cardiovascular system).
3. Select and mark off (if needed) a level area for the walk.
4. Explain to people being tested that they are to walk the mile in the fastest time possible. Only walking is allowed, and the goal is to cover the distance as fast as possible.

Test day

1. Have participants warm up with stretching and slow walking.
2. Have several people walk at the same time.
3. Explain the procedure again.
4. The timer says, "Ready, go," and starts the stopwatch.
5. Each individual has a partner with a watch with a second hand.
6. The partner counts the laps and tells the individual at the end of each lap how many more lap(s) to walk.
7. The timer calls out the minutes and seconds as each person finishes the mile walk.
8. The partner listens for the time when his or her walker finishes the mile and records it (to the nearest second) immediately on a scorecard.
9. The walker takes a 10-s HR immediately after the end of the mile walk while the partner times.

					Min·mi⁻¹						

Table 7.12 Estimated Maximal Oxygen Uptake $(ml·kg^{-1}·min^{-1})$ for Men and Women, 20-69 Years Old

HR	10	11	12	13	14	15	16	17	18	19	20
Men (20-29)											
120	65.0	61.7	58.4	55.2	51.9	48.6	45.4	42.1	38.9	35.6	32.3
130	63.4	60.1	56.9	53.6	50.3	47.1	43.8	40.6	37.3	34.0	30.8
140	61.8	58.6	55.3	52.0	48.8	45.5	42.2	39.0	35.7	32.5	29.2
150	60.3	57.0	53.7	50.5	47.2	43.9	40.7	37.4	34.2	30.9	27.6
160	58.7	55.4	52.2	48.9	45.6	42.4	39.1	35.9	32.6	29.3	26.1
170	57.1	53.9	50.6	47.3	44.1	40.8	37.6	34.3	31.0	27.8	24.5
180	55.6	52.3	49.0	45.8	42.5	39.3	36.0	32.7	29.5	26.2	22.9
190	54.0	50.7	47.5	44.2	41.0	37.7	34.4	31.2	27.9	24.6	21.4
200	52.4	49.2	45.9	42.7	39.4	36.1	32.9	29.6	26.3	23.1	19.8
Women (20-29)											
120	62.1	58.9	55.6	52.3	49.1	45.8	42.5	39.3	36.0	32.7	29.5
130	60.6	57.3	54.0	50.8	47.5	44.2	41.0	37.7	34.4	31.2	27.9
140	59.0	55.7	52.5	49.2	45.9	42.7	39.4	36.1	32.9	29.6	26.3
150	57.4	54.2	50.9	47.6	44.4	41.1	37.8	34.6	31.3	28.0	24.8
160	55.9	52.6	49.3	46.7	42.8	39.5	36.3	33.0	29.7	26.5	23.2
170	54.3	51.0	47.8	44.5	41.2	38.0	34.7	31.4	28.2	24.9	21.6
180	52.7	49.5	46.2	42.9	39.7	36.4	33.1	29.9	26.6	23.3	20.1
190	51.2	47.9	44.6	41.4	38.1	34.8	31.6	28.3	25.0	21.8	18.5
200	49.6	46.3	43.1	39.8	36.5	33.3	30.0	26.7	23.5	20.2	16.9
Men (30-39)											
120	61.1	57.8	54.6	51.3	48.0	44.8	41.5	38.2	35.0	31.7	28.4
130	59.5	56.3	53.0	49.7	46.5	43.2	39.9	36.7	33.4	30.1	26.9
140	58.0	54.7	51.4	48.2	44.9	41.6	38.4	35.1	31.8	28.6	25.3
150	56.4	53.1	49.9	46.6	43.3	40.1	36.8	33.5	30.3	27.0	23.8
160	54.8	51.6	48.3	45.0	41.8	38.5	35.2	32.0	28.7	25.5	22.2
170	53.3	50.0	46.7	43.5	40.2	36.9	33.7	30.4	27.1	23.9	20.6
180	51.7	48.4	45.2	41.9	38.6	35.4	32.1	28.8	25.6	22.3	19.1
190	50.1	46.9	43.6	40.3	37.1	33.8	30.5	27.3	24.0	20.8	17.5
Women (30-39)											
120	58.2	55.0	51.7	48.4	45.2	41.9	38.7	35.4	32.1	28.9	25.6
130	56.7	53.4	50.1	46.9	43.6	40.4	37.1	33.8	30.6	27.3	24.0
140	55.1	51.8	48.6	45.3	42.1	38.8	35.5	32.3	29.0	24.7	22.5
150	53.5	50.3	47.0	43.8	40.5	37.2	34.0	30.7	27.4	24.2	20.9
160	52.0	48.7	45.4	42.2	38.9	35.7	32.4	29.1	25.9	22.6	19.3
170	50.4	47.1	43.9	40.6	37.4	34.1	30.8	27.6	24.3	21.0	17.8
180	48.8	45.6	42.3	39.1	35.8	32.5	29.3	26.0	22.7	19.5	16.2
190	47.3	44.0	40.8	37.5	34.2	31.0	27.7	24.4	21.2	17.9	14.6

					Min·mi⁻¹						
HR	**10**	**11**	**12**	**13**	**14**	**15**	**16**	**17**	**18**	**19**	**20**
				Men (40-49)							
120	57.2	54.0	50.7	47.4	44.2	40.9	37.6	34.4	31.1	27.8	24.6
130	55.7	52.4	49.1	45.9	42.6	39.3	36.1	32.8	29.5	26.3	23.0
140	54.1	50.8	47.6	44.3	41.0	37.8	34.5	31.2	28.0	24.7	21.4
150	52.5	49.3	46.0	42.7	39.5	36.2	32.9	29.7	26.4	23.1	19.9
160	51.0	47.7	44.4	41.2	37.9	34.6	31.4	28.1	24.8	21.6	18.3
170	49.4	46.1	42.9	39.6	36.3	33.1	29.8	26.5	23.3	20.0	16.7
180	47.8	44.6	41.3	38.0	34.8	31.5	28.2	25.0	21.7	18.4	15.2
				Women (40-49)							
120	54.4	51.1	47.8	44.6	41.3	38.0	34.8	31.5	28.2	25.0	21.7
130	52.8	49.5	46.3	43.0	39.7	36.5	33.2	29.9	26.7	23.4	20.1
140	51.2	48.0	44.7	41.4	38.2	34.9	31.6	28.4	25.1	21.8	18.6
150	49.7	46.4	43.1	39.9	36.6	33.3	30.1	26.8	23.5	20.3	17.0
160	48.1	44.8	41.6	38.3	35.0	31.8	28.5	25.2	22.0	18.7	15.5
170	46.5	43.3	40.0	36.7	33.5	30.2	26.9	23.7	20.4	17.2	13.9
				Men (50-59)							
120	53.3	50.0	46.8	43.5	40.3	37.0	33.7	30.5	27.2	23.9	20.7
130	51.7	48.5	45.2	42.0	38.7	35.4	32.2	28.9	25.6	22.4	19.1
140	50.2	46.9	43.7	40.4	37.1	33.9	30.6	27.3	24.1	20.8	17.5
150	48.6	45.4	42.1	38.8	35.6	32.3	29.0	25.8	22.5	19.2	16.0
160	47.1	43.8	40.5	37.3	34.0	30.7	27.5	24.2	20.9	17.7	14.4
170	45.5	42.2	39.0	35.7	32.4	29.2	25.9	22.6	19.4	16.1	12.8
				Women (50-59)							
120	50.5	47.2	43.9	40.7	37.4	34.1	30.9	27.6	24.3	21.1	17.8
130	48.9	45.6	42.4	39.1	35.8	32.6	29.3	26.0	22.8	19.5	16.2
140	47.3	44.1	40.8	37.5	34.3	31.0	27.7	24.5	21.2	17.9	14.7
150	45.8	42.5	39.2	36.0	32.7	29.4	26.2	22.9	19.6	16.4	13.1
160	44.2	40.9	37.7	34.4	31.1	27.9	24.6	21.3	18.1	14.8	11.5
170	42.6	39.4	36.1	32.8	29.6	26.3	23.0	19.8	16.5	13.2	10.0
				Men (60-69)							
120	49.4	46.2	42.9	39.6	36.4	33.1	29.8	26.6	23.3	20.0	16.8
130	47.9	44.6	41.3	38.1	34.8	31.5	28.3	25.0	21.7	18.5	15.2
140	46.3	43.0	39.8	36.5	33.2	30.0	26.7	23.4	20.2	16.9	13.6
150	44.7	41.5	38.2	34.9	31.7	28.4	25.1	21.9	18.6	15.3	12.1
160	43.2	39.9	36.6	33.4	30.1	26.8	23.6	20.3	17.0	13.8	10.5

(continued)

				Min·mi⁻¹							
HR	**10**	**11**	**12**	**13**	**14**	**15**	**16**	**17**	**18**	**19**	**20**
				Women (60-69)							
120	46.6	43.3	40.0	36.8	33.5	30.2	27.0	23.7	20.5	17.2	13.9
130	45.0	41.7	38.5	35.2	31.9	28.7	25.4	22.2	18.9	15.6	12.4
140	43.4	40.2	36.9	33.6	30.4	27.1	23.8	20.6	17.3	14.1	10.8
150	41.9	38.6	35.3	32.1	28.8	25.5	22.3	19.0	15.8	12.5	9.2
160	40.3	37.0	33.8	30.5	27.2	24.0	20.7	17.5	14.2	10.9	7.7

Table 7.12 *(cont'd)*

Note. Calculations assume 170 lb for men and 125 lb for women. For each 15 lb beyond these values, subtract 1 ml·kg⁻¹·min⁻¹.

Reprinted from Howley and Franks 1997.

the walk test just described: The participant jogs or runs as fast as possible for 12 min or for 1.5 mi. Average running speed depends on the ability of the heart and lungs to transport oxygen to the working muscles. This test makes use of this observation, and the CRF score depends on the speed maintained over the distance. Find a measured track and have the participant run as far as possible in 12 min or run 1.5 mile for time. Table 7.3 lists the values for CRF as *good, adequate, borderline,* and *needs extra work.* The table takes age and gender into consideration. For example, a 40-year-old woman who runs 1.5 mile in 14 min 15 s (14:15) rates between *adequate* and *good.* This time of 14:15 corresponds to a CRF value of about 35 to 40 ml·kg⁻¹·min⁻¹. We recommend that you encourage participants to try to achieve and maintain the *good* value for their age and gender. If they are not at that level, help them plan to make small and systematic progress toward the goal using the walking and jogging programs in chapter 13.

Administration of an Endurance Run. Many youth fitness programs use a 1-mi run. Table 7.13 lists the steps to follow before the test day as well as the procedures for conducting the test.

Activity Recommendations for Cardiorespiratory Fitness

Chapter 12 includes the recommendations for physical activity based on the individual's current activity level and desired health, fitness, and performance goals. Chapter 13 describes a variety of activities participants can use to improve and maintain cardiorespiratory fitness.

Summary

This chapter provided several ways you can evaluate the cardiorespiratory fitness levels of your fitness participants. You can use a walking test and measure heart rate to estimate maximal aerobic power. This chapter described the use of heart rate, blood pressure, and perceived exertion in a graded exercise test. You should emphasize to fitness participants that resting, submaximal tests, and a beginning conditioning program should precede all-out field tests. Do *not* administer a running test to determine cardiorespiratory fitness level until after participants have successfully completed a beginning fitness program.

Table 7.13	Steps to Administer the 1-Mile Run
Step	**Activity**

Before test day

1. Arrange to have the following elements at the test site:
   - A person to start and read the time from a stopwatch
   - A partner for each runner (perhaps with a sheet to mark off laps)
   - A stopwatch for the tester (with a spare ready)
   - A scoresheet or scorecard
2. Explain the purpose of the test (i.e., to determine how fast participants can run a mile, which reflects the endurance of their cardiovascular system).
3. Do *not* administer the test until participants have had several fitness sessions, including some with running.
4. Have participants practice running at a set submaximal pace for one lap, then two, and so on, several times prior to test day.
5. Select and mark off (if needed) a level area for the run.
6. Explain to people being tested that they are to run the mile in the fastest time possible. Walking is allowed, but the goal is to cover the distance as fast as possible.

Test day

1. Have participants warm up with stretching, walking, and slow jogging.
2. Have several people run at the same time.
3. Explain the procedure again.
4. The timer says, "Ready, go," and starts the stopwatch.
5. Each individual has a partner with a watch with a second hand.
6. The partner counts the laps and tells the individual at the end of each lap how many more lap(s) to run.
7. The timer calls out the minutes and seconds as the runner finishes the mile run.
8. The partner listens for the time when the runner finishes the mile and records it (to the nearest second) immediately on a scorecard.
9. The runners continue to walk one lap after finishing the run.

Reprinted from Howley and Franks 1997.

Chapter 8
Muscular Strength and Endurance

Muscular Strength
Muscular Endurance
Improvement of Strength and Endurance

Athletes who exercise at high performance levels distinguish muscular strength from muscular endurance and, indeed, need to separate these two characteristics. In fitness programming, you can combine the two concepts, because you want to help participants achieve desired levels of both. Muscular strength describes the *maximum force* that can be generated by a muscle. A person with a great deal of strength can lift very heavy weights. Strength depends on the size of the muscle and the person's ability to "recruit" available muscle fibers, which is related to the individual's level of arousal. In contrast, muscular endurance describes the ability of a muscle to make repeated contractions against a *less-than-maximal load*. An individual who can lift a weight many times before experiencing fatigue has a high level of muscular endurance.

For many years, health-related fitness programs focused on participation in aerobic exercise to improve cardiorespiratory fitness and to expend calories as a part of a weight maintenance goal. Today's fitness programs should broaden this focus to include exercises to improve muscular strength and endurance to help do the following:

• Reduce the chance of osteoporosis

• Maintain muscle mass

• Reduce the chance of low-back pain

• Reduce the effort required to do the activities of daily living

• Improve one's self-concept (confidence)

Osteoporosis, a thinning of the bone that is related to fractures in the elderly, is a growing problem in our society because the "baby boomer" generation is entering its sixth decade. Osteoporosis is related to the reduction in estrogen that occurs at menopause, inadequate calcium intake (see chapter 6), and inadequate exercise and strength. The downward force associated with exercise in the standing position (weight-bearing activities such as walking or jogging) and the lateral forces exerted by muscle contractions help retain bone mass. Maintaining muscle mass also maintains the resting metabolic rate, the largest portion of our total daily energy expenditure. This helps prevent weight gain that occurs with age (see chapter 5). Inadequate abdominal muscle strength and endurance makes it more difficult to maintain the pelvis in its proper orientation, resulting in an exaggeration of the "curves" of the low back and subsequent back pain. Adequate muscular strength and endurance makes the usual daily activities less strenuous and reduces the stress that might be transferred to weaker tissues when an individual can't lift a load properly. Lastly, individuals who are strong feel better about themselves. This alone justifies including muscular strength and endurance exercises as a regular part of your participants' workouts. *Fitness Facts* will provide participants with information on measurement, principles, and training programs for muscular strength and endurance.

Measuring Muscular Strength

Strength can be measured with static (isometric) and dynamic tests. You can measure isometric strength with instruments such as the *grip dynamometer*, which measures the force of your grip, or the *cable tensiometer*, which can measure the strength of most muscle groups. In an isometric contraction, the muscle does not shorten ("isometric" means "constant length"), even though the person is exerting maximal force. Isometric strength varies depending on the angle of the joint, and it does not provide a measure of strength throughout the normal range of motion. This type of test is especially helpful for individuals who need strength at one set position.

One measure of dynamic strength uses a special "isokinetic" machine that controls the speed at which you move a joint through its range of motion. One of the subject's limbs, such as the lower leg, is attached to a lever arm that controls how fast the limb moves. When a muscle contracts with as much force as possible to move the limb, sensors in the machine monitor the force

throughout the range of motion while allowing the limb to move at a selected speed. These machines are expensive and can usually be found in physical therapy and athletic training facilities.

In contrast to measurements made using isokinetic machines, dynamic strength is usually measured as the heaviest weight lifted through a normal range of motion. You may measure dynamic strength using "free weights" (barbells and dumbbells) or machines. Free weights provide a constant resistance during the particular lift (since the weight doesn't change), but the muscles will exert varying degrees of effort while lifting the weight through that joint's range of motion. In contrast, machines such as the Nautilus brand alter the actual resistance on the muscle as the participant moves through the range of motion. These machines attempt to match the resistance to the muscle's capacity to generate force at the different joint angles. For this reason you will see strength training programs divided into "dynamic constant resistance (free weights) programs," and "dynamic variable resistance (machine) programs." Although some suggest that one form of training is better than the other for performance, either program can create adequate muscular strength and endurance from a health-related standpoint, as long as the program exercises a variety of muscle groups in an appropriate manner. Figure 8.1 shows two subjects doing an arm curl test to measure the strength of the arm flexors (biceps); one is using a barbell (free weight) and the other, a machine.

The greatest weight the subject can lift once in good form through a joint's range of motion is called the one-repetition maximum or 1-RM, and is a measure of maximal muscle strength. To test someone's 1-RM, have the participant lift a weight (starting with one you think he or she can lift), then gradually add more weight. Have the participant lift each new load only once until you find a weight the individual cannot lift. The last weight lifted in good form is the 1-RM. Some measure the 3-RM or 5-RM because it doesn't require individuals to go to their limit.

Measuring Muscular Endurance

We typically measure muscular endurance by counting the number of lifts a person can do with a fixed weight. This is sometimes called absolute

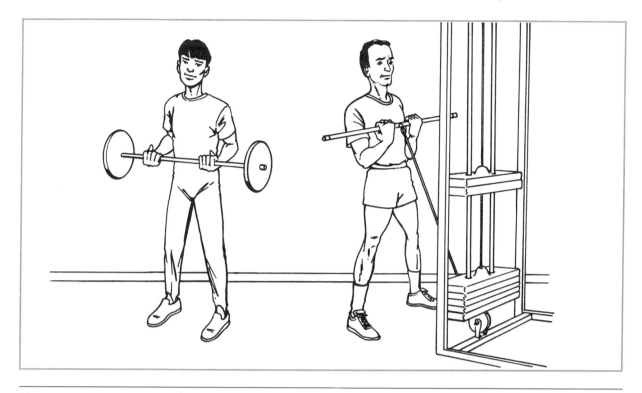

Figure 8.1 Dynamic strength testing.

muscular endurance, as the weight that is lifted is a fixed (absolute) quantity. You can use this approach to show the participant's progress over time. For example, a person might have been able to do only 5 arm curls with a 25-lb weight prior to a training program, but might have increased that number to 20 after the program.

Another approach is to measure relative muscular endurance, which shows how many times a weight that is a certain percent (e.g., 70%) of the 1-RM can be lifted. Because the 1-RM (maximal strength) will change during a training program, this approach allows you to show the participant how muscular endurance changes as strength increases. For example, at the beginning of a training program the participant's 1-RM might be 60 lb for an arm curl, and the person might lift 42 lb (70% of 60 lb) 10 times. At the end of the training program you determine the new 1-RM, which might be 80 lb, and you see how many times the participant can lift 56 lb (70% of 80 lb). If muscular strength increases faster than muscular endurance, then the number of repetitions at the new 70% of 1-RM will be less than 10. If strength and endurance improve at the same rate, the number of repetitions will be 10. If endurance increases more

than strength, the number of repetitions will be greater than 10.

Another way to test arm and shoulder strength and endurance is to use the modified pull-up (see figure 8.4 later in this chapter). Since the participants' feet support part of their weight, this test is more appropriate for many fitness participants than a standard pull-up requiring them to lift their full weight. You can easily build a modified pull-up stand for a fitness program (see figure 8.6 at the end of this chapter). You can also use the 90° push-up as a test of arm and shoulder strength and endurance (see figure 8.8).

Basis for Improving Muscular Strength and Endurance

Help the participant understand the principles of overload and specificity that apply to training programs for muscular strength and endurance. The overload principle states that to make improvements, a muscle must lift a heavier weight than that to which it is accustomed. As the muscle adapts to that new, heavier load, the participant must overload the muscle again to gain additional strength (see figure 2.2).

The principle of specificity states that the type of adaptation that occurs is related to the type of exercise used. It is best illustrated by comparisons between gains in muscular strength and gains in muscular endurance. If a person lifts heavy weights the *primary* change is an increase in the *size* of the muscle cells, a process called *hypertrophy*. This increase in muscle size is associated with the increase in muscle strength. On the other hand, if a person does many repetitions with lighter weights (such as 50% of 1-RM), the *primary* changes in the muscle are found in the energy-producing parts, called mitochondria, and in the number of capillaries that bring oxygen to the muscle cell. Muscle size does not increase very much with endurance exercise. Though the effects of training are specific to the type of exercise performed, there is some overlap in the areas of strength and endurance—a person cannot completely isolate one from the other.

Strength increases over the course of a training program, but hypertropy doesn't occur until later (more than 10 weeks) in the program. The strength gain early in the program comes primarily from neural changes related to coordination of the major muscle groups and the ability to recruit more muscle fibers. Men typically experience more hypertrophy than women as a result of a long-term training program. This is primarily because men have more testosterone, a hormone that has more anabolic (tissue building) properties than estrogen.

Activities for Improving Muscular Strength and Endurance

Progressive resistance exercise (PRE) generally describes a method to progressively and systematically overload a muscle group. A PRE program specifies both the weight (load) lifted and the maximum number of repetitions the load is lifted (RM). The term "set" describes the number of repetitions done before a rest period. For example, you may want to have the participant do two sets of a 10-RM routine, choosing a weight (guidelines described shortly) that can be lifted a maximum of 10 times (10 RM), and then do the following:

1. Lift the weight 10 times
2. Rest
3. Lift the weight 10 times
4. Rest

For gains in muscular *strength*, have the participant follow a 4- to 8-RM routine (choose a weight that the participant can lift a maximum of 4 to 8 times), and do two to three sets. When the participant can lift the weight more than 8 times in each of three sets, increase the weight (the overload principle). This progressively increases the load against which the participant's muscle must work.

For gains in muscular *endurance*, have the participant do two to three sets of a 15- to 30-RM routine. High repetitions with lighter weights result in specific muscular-endurance adaptations. Participants should do weight training, like aerobic exercise, on an every-other-day basis.

Two general guidelines can help determine the amount of *weight* to use in weight training:

1. For exercises with the arms, start the PRE program with a weight equal to 1/4 to 1/3 of body weight. For example, if the participant weighs 180 lb, start with 45 (1/4 of 180) to 60 (1/3 of 180) lb.

2. For exercises with the legs, start the PRE program with a weight equal to 1/2 to 2/3 of body weight. For example, if the individual weighs 180 lb, start with 90 (1/2 of 180) to 120 (2/3 of 180) lb.

Table 8.1 provides a summary of starting weights for people of different body weights. Remember, in helping a participant choose a starting point, it is better to do too little rather than too much.

You can use the following selected weight-training activities to increase muscular strength and endurance (see figures 8.2, a-f). Similar exercises can be done using machine weights (e.g., Nautilus). To maximize safety you should direct the participant to do the following:

- Warm up before exercise and cool down after exercise
- Use a "spotter" for free-weight workouts to prevent being trapped under a weight (such as the bench press)
- Use collars on plate-loading equipment such as dumbbells

- Perform the lift with the correct form and controlled speed
- Breathe normally during a lift; breathe out when weight is lifted and in when weight is lowered
- Don't "bounce" weights off the body; use a lighter weight

- Be in a stable and controlled position prior to the lift
- Always select a load that is within his or her capacity to lift

As you work with participants, observe any problems with equipment that can be a safety hazard and report it at once.

Table 8.1	Starting Weights (in Pounds) for Weight Training for Arms and Legs	
Body weight (lb)	**Arms**	**Legs**
100	25-33	50-67
120	30-40	60-80
140	35-46	70-93
160	40-53	80-107
180	45-60	90-120
200	50-66	100-133

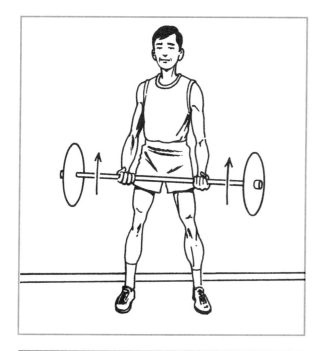

Figure 8.2a *Arm curl.* With arms extended, hold the barbell with an underhand grip. While keeping the elbows close to the sides, flex the forearms and raise the barbell to the chest; lower to the starting position. Suggested beginning load: 1/4 to 1/3 of body weight.

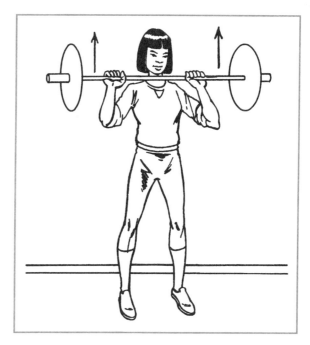

Figure 8.2b *Overhead press.* Hold the barbell at chest level with an overhand grip. Push the bar straight up to full extension and then lower to the starting position. Do not hyperextend the back. Suggested beginning load: 1/4 to 1/3 of body weight.

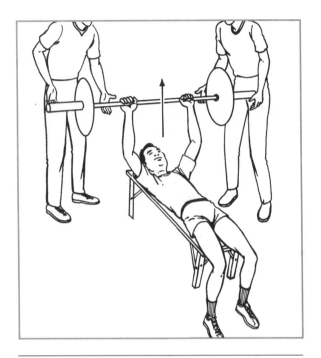

Figure 8.2c *Bench press.* Hold barbell above chest with hands slightly wider than shoulder width. Lower barbell to chest and push back to starting position. Suggested starting load: 1/4 to 1/3 of body weight.

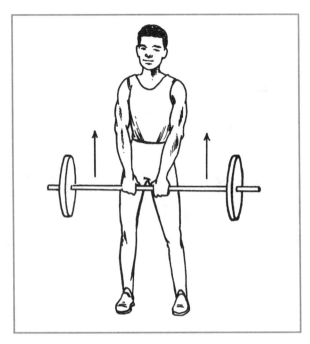

Figure 8.2d *Upright rowing.* Hold barbell with an overhand grip with hands 1-2 in. apart. Keep elbows above the bar while raising it to shoulder position. Suggested beginning load: 1/4 to 1/3 of body weight.

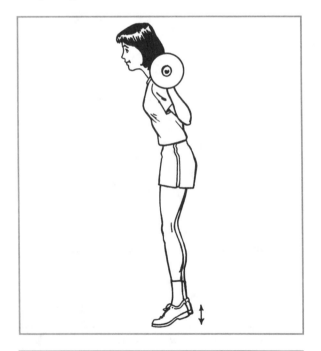

Figure 8.2e *Heel lifts.* With barbell behind shoulder at the back of the neck, raise upward on toes and then slowly return the heels to the floor. Suggested beginning load: 1/2 to 2/3 of body weight.

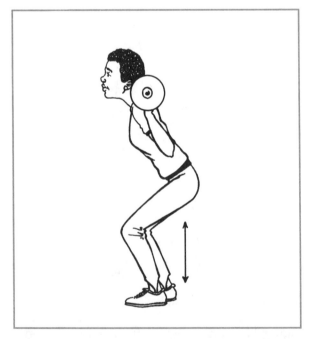

Figure 8.2f *Half-squats.* With barbell behind shoulders at the back of the neck, gradually lower body to a semi-squat position. Keep back straight. Suggested beginning load: 1/2 to 2/3 of body weight.

Muscular Strength and Endurance Without Weights

Generally, if your fitness program includes running, cycling, or dancing, you are providing enough stimulus to maintain an adequate level of muscular strength and endurance in the leg muscles. These activities do little for the muscular strength and endurance of the arms, shoulders, or trunk, however. One of the most common ways to increase the muscular strength and endurance of these muscle groups is to have participants do exercises in which the participant's own body acts as the weight or resistance against which she works. The following activities focus on developing strength and endurance in the arms and shoulders.

Figure 8.3 shows three forms of push-ups that vary in difficulty and can be done anywhere: the push-away, the bent-knee push-up, and the regular push-up. Start with the push-away for a participant on the low end of the strength and endurance scale. When she can comfortably do three sets of 10 in one workout, she progresses to the bent-knee push-up, start-

ing with two sets of 5 and increasing the number until two sets of 10 can be done in a single workout. Then she can shift to the regular push-up, doing two sets of 5 and gradually working up to two sets of 10. When this goal has been achieved, have her continue to do the two sets of 10 or more in each workout. If you use the push-up for a test, we recommend that you select the 90° push-up (see figure 8.8), in which the individual only comes down to the point where the elbow makes a 90° angle.

Figure 8.4 shows two types of pull-ups that can be used to improve strength and endurance. The standard pull-up is harder to do because the participant must lift his entire body weight. You will often find fitness participants who are unable to do a single pull-up. In contrast, body weight is partially supported in the modified pull-up, making it easier to do. The individual lies on his back with his chest under the bar and his arms extended. Place the bar 1 in above the fingertips and put the rubber band three notches below the bar. The participant grasps the bar and pulls his body up (only his heels continue to touch the ground) until his chin is above the rubber band, then releases back to the starting position and repeats. Start with 2 or 3 modified

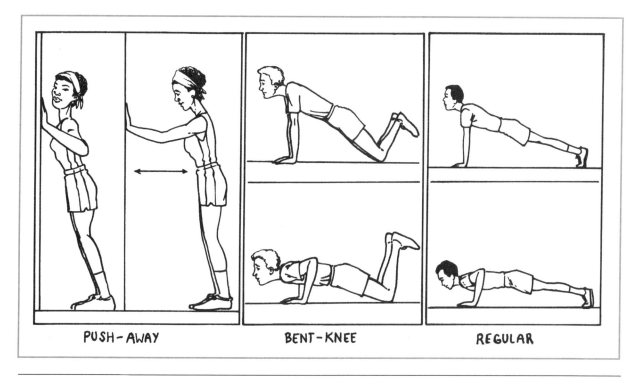

PUSH-AWAY   BENT-KNEE   REGULAR

Figure 8.3 Different types of push-ups.

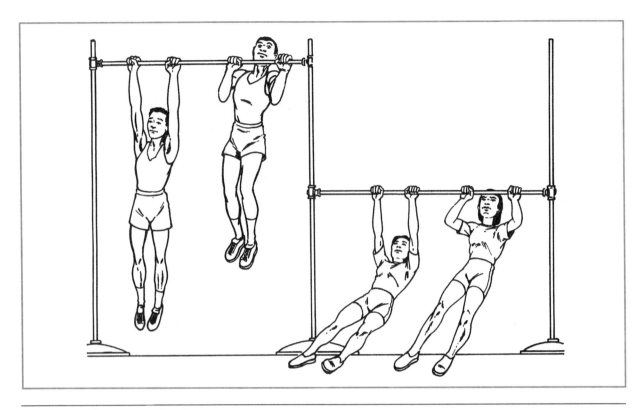

Figure 8.4 Two types of pull-ups.

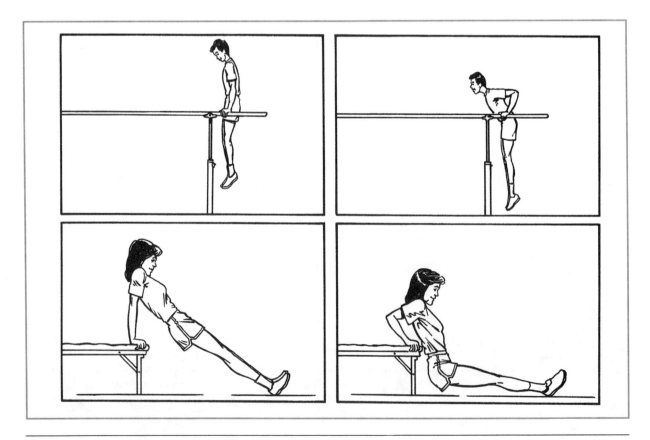

Figure 8.5 Two versions of the dip.

pull-ups, adding some when able and gradually working up to 25 to 35. Figure 8.6 shows specifications for building the modified pull-up stand, and figure 8.7 shows the completed apparatus.

Another exercise that can be used to strengthen the upper body is the "dip," shown in figure 8.5. The weight-supported version is the easier of the two versions shown in this figure.

Summary

Muscular strength is a measure of the maximal force a muscle can generate. Muscular endurance is a measure of the muscle's ability to repeatedly lift a less-than-maximal load. In training programs for strength gains, choose a weight that can be lifted 4 to 8 times and do two to three sets. For endurance, have the participant choose a weight that can be lifted 15 to 30 times and do two to three sets. The starting weight for arm exercises is 1/4 to 1/3 of body weight; for leg exercises, 1/2 to 2/3 of body weight. It is better to do too little rather than too much. Use simple push-ups, pull-ups, and dips to promote strength and endurance of the upper body.

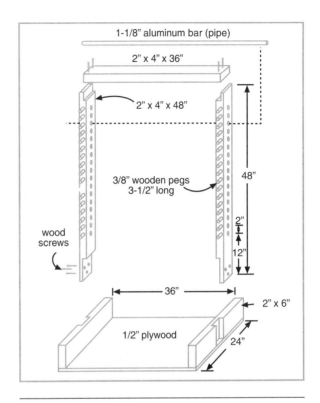

Figure 8.6 Modified pull-up stand specifications.

This figure is reprinted with permission from the *Journal of Physical Education, Recreation & Dance* 68 (9), 1987, 98-102. *JOPERD* is a publication of the American Alliance for Health, Physical Education, Recreation and Dance, 1900 Association Drive, Reston, VA 20191.

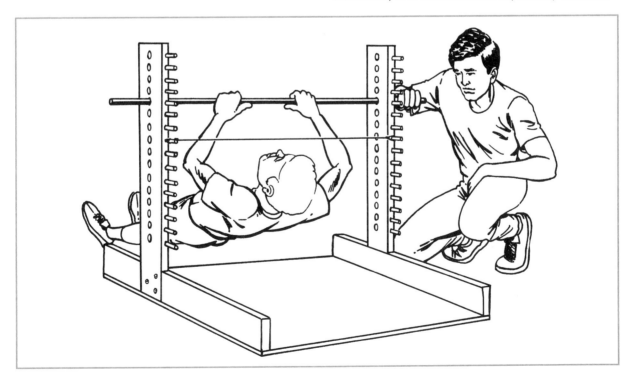

Figure 8.7 Using the pull-up stand.

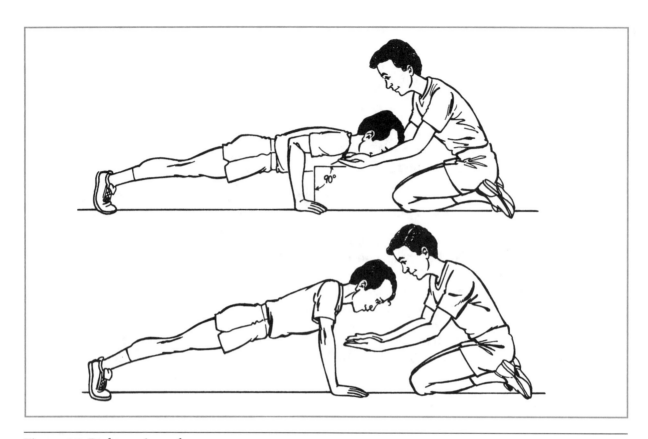

Figure 8.8 Right angle push-ups.
Reprinted from President's Council on Physical Fitness 1997.

Chapter 9
Flexibility

Improving Flexibility

Flexibility measures how well a joint moves through its normal range of motion. The fitness leader must help participants maintain the flexibility of each joint so that they can complete normal, everyday tasks without undue strain. Poor flexibility can be related to medical problems, with low back pain being one example (see chapter 10).

Flexibility, like any trait, is limited by genetic endowment. Regular use of the joints is necessary to develop and maintain that endowment. For example, when a cast is removed from an individual who had a broken bone at the elbow joint, that person's initial attempts to move the joint through its normal range of motion are usually painful and not very successful. While the arm is immobilized in the cast, fibrous connective tissue, or "adhesions," begin to cling to the tendons, ligaments, and bones in the joint, reducing its range of motion. In addition, because the cast holds the arm at a fixed angle,

the upper arm muscles and tendons become shortened and do not allow the arm to straighten when the cast is removed. Flexibility, then, is affected by both the condition of the connective tissues at the joint and the ability of the muscle to stretch. Including stretching exercises in your program can help participants maintain a normal range of motion by maintaining the proper length of the muscle-tendon unit and reducing the development of inappropriate connective tissues at the joint.

Improving Flexibility

Each fitness workout should include specific stretching exercises as a regular part of the warm-up. These stretching exercises, along with other warm-up activities, help prepare the joints for the more strenuous dynamic activity to come by releasing fluids that lubricate the joint and by increasing the size of the joint's soft cartilage that absorbs the shock of impact associated with normal physical activity. In addition, stretching exercises help make the transition from the resting state to the exercise state a little easier.

The principles of training mentioned in the previous chapter, overload and specificity, also apply to stretching and flexibility. If you want the participants to improve their flexibility, have them stretch to the point of some tension (overload). The principle of specificity also applies, as improvements in flexibility are limited to the muscles and joints involved in the stretching exercises.

There are two major types of stretching exercises: static and dynamic. In static stretching, you slowly stretch a muscle group, hold the stretch at the point of *mild* tension, and then relax. The static stretching technique successfully accomplishes flexibility goals with little chance of causing problems. Dynamic stretching involves active movements, but if it becomes "bouncy" with too much momentum it becomes a *ballistic* stretch. A ballistic stretch may cause an individual to exceed a joint's range of motion, causing injury to the connective tissue. Ballistic stretching may also be counterproductive for stretching the muscle. When a muscle is suddenly lengthened, as happens in bouncing, the muscle responds with a reflex contraction. This is the opposite of the intended effect of stretching exercises. Nonetheless, dynamic activity has its place as part of a warm-up. The participants should do the same type of movements they will perform for the workout at a lower intensity as part of the warm-up.

Participants need to do a variety of stretching exercises to maintain the function of as many joints as possible. The recommended stretching exercises start at the neck and proceed downward. Have participants do each slowly, holding each for 10 to 30 s and repeating each two or three times. You can also have the participants do controlled dynamic movements to get the body ready for more strenuous activity.

Should you do static stretching before or after warming up? The argument for warming up indicates that muscles and other tissues are easier to stretch when they are warm. The connective tissues of the muscle-tendon unit have both "elastic" and "plastic" properties. The elastic property allows the tissue to return to its normal length following stretching; the plastic property is what establishes its normal length when at rest. The stretching routine is aimed at changing the plastic property, so that the joint can move through its normal range of motion. It is easier to lengthen the connective tissues while minimizing tissue damage if the muscle-tendon unit is already warm. The contrasting argument suggests that muscles are normally "warm," and light warm-up activities don't increase that very much. We recommend that you have the participants do some light stretching activities at the beginning of an exercise session and a more thorough program of stretching during the cooldown when body temperature is elevated and greater flexibility gains can be made.

Stretching Exercises

These directions are for the participant. The fitness leader should emphasize the following:

1. Stretches are held to the point of mild tension, not pain.

2. Breathe normally during each stretching exercise. Do not hold your breath.

3. Do each exercise slowly.

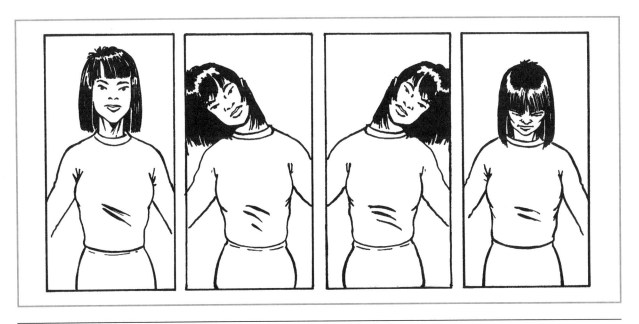

Figure 9.1 *Stretches for the neck.* While sitting or standing with your head in its normal upright position, slowly tilt it to the right until you feel tension on the left side of your neck. Hold that tension for 10 to 30 s and then slowly return your head to the upright position. Repeat to the left side, and then toward the front. Always return to the upright position before moving on.

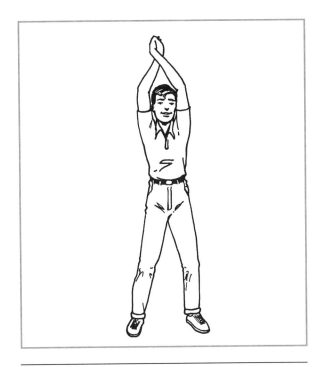

Figure 9.2 *Reach to the sky.* Stand with your feet shoulder-width apart. Raise both arms overhead so that your hands are intertwined, palms facing. Hold for 10 to 30 s and relax.

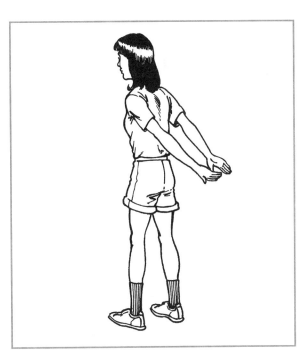

Figure 9.3 *Reach back.* Stand with your feet shoulder-width apart and hold your arms out to the sides with your thumbs pointing down. Slowly move both arms back until you feel tension. Hold for 10 to 30 s and relax.

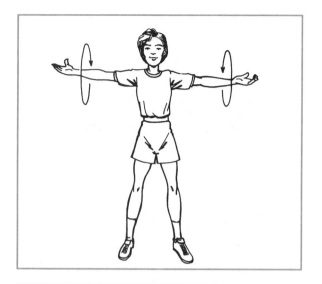

Figure 9.4 *Arm circles*. Stand with your feet shoulder-width apart and hold your arms straight out to the side with your hands facing up. Start moving your arms slowly in small circles and gradually make larger and larger circles. Come back to the starting position and reverse the direction of your arm swinging.

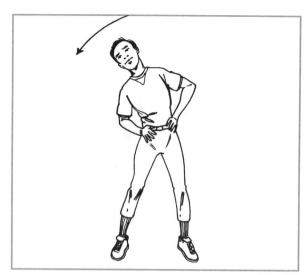

Figure 9.5 *Side bend*. Stand with your feet shoulder-width apart and place your hands on your waist. Slowly bend to the right side until you feel slight tension. Hold for 10 to 30 s and relax. Repeat to the left side.

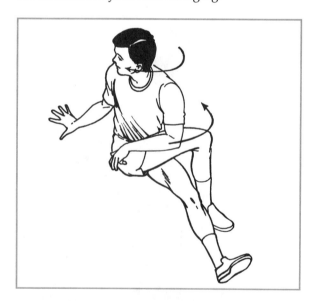

Figure 9.6 *Sit-and-twist*. Sit on a mat with your left leg straight in front of you. Bend your right leg and cross it over your left leg so that your right foot is alongside your left knee. Bring your left elbow across your body and place it on the outside of your right thigh near the knee. Slowly twist your body as you look over your right shoulder. Your left elbow should be exerting pressure against your right thigh. Hold the stretch for 10 to 30 s, relax, and repeat with the other side.

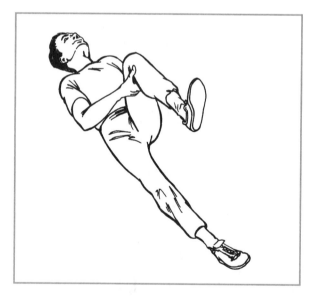

Figure 9.7 *Trunk flexion exercise*. Lie on your back on a mat with your legs straight. Bend your left knee and bring it up toward your chest. Grasp the underside of your thigh and *slowly* pull your thigh to your chest. Hold for 10 to 30 s. Release, and repeat with the right leg.

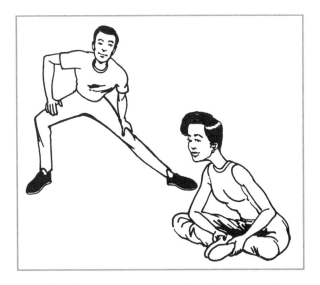

Figure 9.8 *Groin stretch*. Sit on a mat with your knees bent. Put the soles of your feet (or shoes) together and hold onto your ankles. Place your elbows on the inner side of your knees and *slowly* apply downward pressure until you feel tension. Hold for 10 to 30 s and repeat.

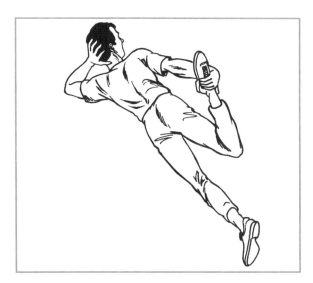

Figure 9.9 *Lying quad stretch*. Lie on your stomach and grasp your right ankle with your right hand. Slowly bring it up until you feel tension on the front side of the thigh. Hold for 10 to 30 s, then repeat with the left leg.

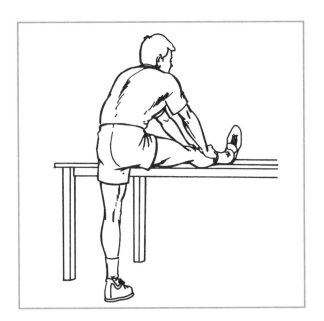

Figure 9.10 *Hamstring stretch*. While standing, raise your right foot onto a table, bench, or chair so that your leg is almost parallel to the floor. Slowly move your hands along your right leg toward your ankle until you feel tension on the underside of the thigh. Hold the tension for 10 to 30 s and relax. Repeat for the other leg. Chapter 10 lists other hamstring stretches.

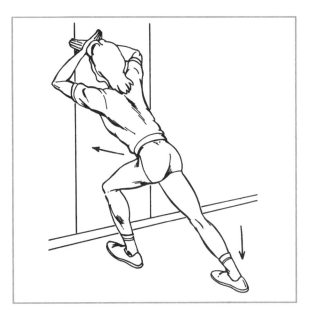

Figure 9.11 *Achilles stretch*. Stand facing a wall with your left foot close to the wall and your left knee bent. With your right leg straight, slowly lean toward the wall, *keeping your right heel flat on the ground*. Hold for 10 to 30 s and relax. Repeat with the left leg.

Summary

Flexibility measures how well a joint can move through its normal range of motion. Flexibility is limited by both the connective tissues at the joint and the muscles that are responsible for moving the joint. Stretching exercises increase a joint's flexibility by acting on both types of tissue; flexibility decreases when those specific exercises are not done on a regular basis. This chapter includes specific exercises for different areas of the body. Help fitness participants do these stretching exercises as a regular part of warming up and cooling down.

Chapter 10
Preventing Low-Back Problems

Causes and Prevention
Special Activities
Tests

Low-back pain is one of the most common complaints among adults in the United States. Low-back problems account for more lost person-hours than any other type of occupational injury and are the most frequent cause of activity limitations in individuals in the U.S. under age 45.

Anatomy of the Low-Back Area

Figure 10.1 shows that the lower part of the spinal column (lumbar region) is balanced on top of the pelvis. Consequently, anything that affects the orientation of the pelvis (such as tipping it too far forward) causes changes in the shape of the curve (the lordotic curve) formed by the lumbar vertebrae. Increasing the lordotic curve places additional stress on the vertebrae in this region and may injure the disc between the vertebrae as well as the connective and muscle tissues supporting the vertebrae. Stretching

of the abdominal muscles as seen in pregnancy and abdominal obesity causes a forward pelvic tilt and increases the risk of low-back pain. In contrast, strengthening the abdominals stabilizes the pelvis and helps to maintain a normal lordotic curve.

Other muscles can affect the orientation of the pelvis. If the quadriceps femoris is too strong and too short, the pelvis will tip forward. If the hamstrings are too short, then normal forward motion of the pelvis (when bending forward) is limited and the load is transferred to the tissues of the low back. Finally, the iliopsoas is connected to the lumbar vertebrae and runs across the pelvis. When this muscle contracts, it pulls the lumbar curve forward, increasing the chance of low-back pain.

It should be no surprise that exercise programs aimed at reducing the risk of low-back problems focus attention on the proper strength and flexibility of the muscles and connective tissues associated with pelvic function.

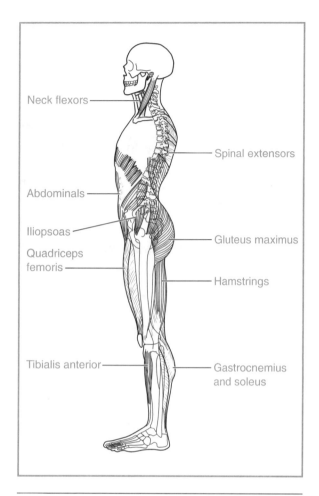

Figure 10.1 Side view of the muscles, spinal column, and pelvis.

Adapted from Howley and Franks 1997.

Causes and Prevention of Low-Back Pain

Low-back problems have many causes, including structural abnormalities, some diseases, accidents, inappropriate lifting, poor posture, lack of proper warm-up prior to vigorous activity, lack of abdominal strength and endurance, lack of flexibility in the back and legs, and inability to cope with stress. A very small percentage of low-back problems are caused by anatomical problems, such as having a deformed spine or one leg longer than the other. These conditions may be altered by some structural device or may require surgery.

Some diseases, such as arthritis or tuberculosis of the spine, are directly related to the back, and obviously can cause back problems. Other

diseases seemingly unrelated to the back can also result in back pain, including kidney or gall bladder disease, peptic ulcers, a tipped uterus, or ovarian infection.

Many physical ailments, including low-back problems, result from accidents. These problems often require long hours of rehabilitation to help the affected person return to a normal lifestyle.

People often injure their backs trying to lift objects that are too heavy or by using poor lifting techniques. Fitness leaders can help participants learn to lift properly (see figure 10.2). You should emphasize that individuals should avoid lifting objects that are too heavy for their strength, use their leg muscles by bending their knees and keeping their backs straight, and keep the object close to the center of their bodies while lifting and carrying.

Low-back pain is rarely caused by a single movement, but comes from "repetitive microtrauma" from an individual doing the same type of improper movement or maintaining an improper posture over a long period of time. The key, then, is to minimize the risk of low-back pain by doing tasks (such as lifting) properly, following guidelines for appropriate postures, warming up prior to strenuous exercise, doing exercises to maintain flexibility and strength, and dealing effectively with stress.

Posture

Because people spend the majority of their time sleeping, sitting, or standing, you should provide guidelines for good posture in these positions. While sitting and lying, avoid extremes in posture; a slight rounding of the back and shoulders is healthy. Take care not to overdo the slouched position. Healthy practices include some mild extension (keeping the head and shoulders back) and using small pillows to maintain the small curve in the lower back. Tell participants to avoid rigid positions (military "attention") and extreme hyperextension (head and shoulders back as far as they can go). Sleeping either face down or on the back with legs straight tends to increase the curve in the lower back and may be a cause of low-back pain or discomfort in some individuals. Sleeping on the side or back with hips and knees bent appears to be comfortable and appropriate for most

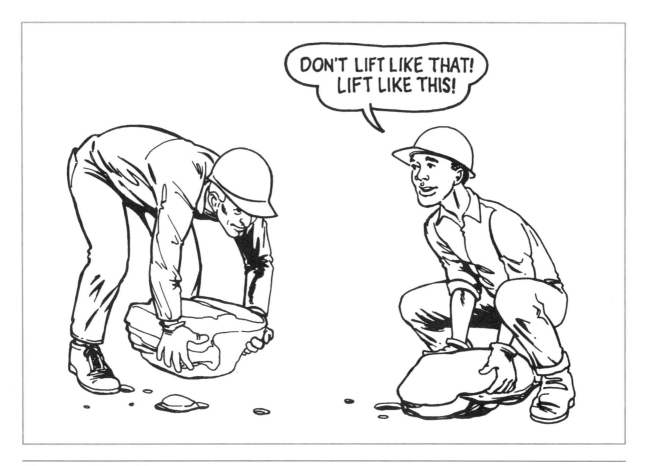

Figure 10.2 Proper lifting.

individuals. The type of mattress can also be a factor; for example, a posture that results in discomfort on a firm mattress may not cause a problem on a water bed.

Standing for long periods of time may cause fatigue in the supporting muscles of the trunk. Whenever possible, an individual should avoid prolonged standing. Bending the knees slightly while standing and shifting weight with one foot slightly elevated during extended standing help prevent back problems.

Warm-Up

Warming up properly can help prevent low-back problems in two ways. The fitness leader should use stretching and strengthening exercises for the midtrunk area (abdominal, back, upper legs) described in chapters 8 and 9 on a regular basis as part of warming up to develop the strength, endurance, and flexibility needed to help prevent low-back problems. One fre-

quent low-back problem is a strain resulting from sudden or forceful bending or twisting while playing a game (e.g., racquetball). Warming up the muscles to be used in the activity prior to a game can help prevent this type of muscle strain.

Abdominal Strength and Endurance

Muscular deficiencies, including lack of abdominal strength, are important considerations in preventing and relieving low-back pain. Abdominal muscles play a major role in preventing an excessive forward tilt of the pelvis, and strong abdominal muscles support the trunk in postures that otherwise could cause back problems. When a person is leaning, strong abdominal muscle contractions can decrease the stress placed on the spine.

To strengthen the abdominal region, participants should do exercises to improve the function of both the rectus abdominis and the external and internal obliques. The latter muscles help to stabilize the pelvis and protect the low back in times of increased loading (lifting). In the "crunch" (figure 10.3), instruct the participant first to flatten the low-back area to the mat and then to lift up no more than 30° from the floor; at that point the work of the rectus abdominis is done. A full sit-up calls the iliopsoas into play and could increase the risk of low-back problems. The "oblique curl" (figure 10.4) involves the internal and external obliques. Both of these exercises can incorporate a 5-s isometric hold in the "up" position. The minimum goal is 10 to 15 repetitions per set in two to three sets.

Flexibility

Chapter 9 dealt with total body flexibility. Poor flexibility in the low back and upper legs can cause low-back problems. The muscles that move the hips in different directions are associated with low-back pain. Either lack of flexibility or lack of strength and endurance in this region can result in back problems. You can help participants deal with this problem with static stretching. This involves slowly lengthening the muscle or muscles to a point of slight discomfort, then holding for 10 to 30 seconds, with one or two repetitions. Have the participants use each of the exercises in chapter 9. Remember, progressively increasing the range of motion results in improved flexibility.

Most low-back stretches involve flexion of the back (moving forward). Most people should also include some extension (moving backward) and slight hyperextension. The participant should seek medical advice if a back problem or pain is experienced with hyperextension. When performing hyperextension (see figure 10.5), the participant should *not* push backward as far as possible.

The fitness leader can have participants do hamstring stretching exercises while sitting or lying (see figures 10.6 and 10.7).

Coping With Stress

Although inability to cope with stress will not itself cause back problems for those who have healthy backs, it does cause problems in those already at risk for back problems. See chapter 11 for suggestions on coping with stress.

Evaluating Progress

We recommend tests for muscular strength, endurance, and flexibility in the midtrunk area for low-back function. One way to use the tests is to administer them periodically and record the participants' scores to monitor their progress.

Because abdominal strength and endurance play an important role in the prevention of low-back pain, we recommend a modified curl-up test. A low score on this test may indicate a high risk for low-back problems. Table 10.1 and figure 10.8 describe this test.

Fitness instructors also commonly use the sit-and-reach test. Unmodified versions of this test were believed to provide a good measure of both

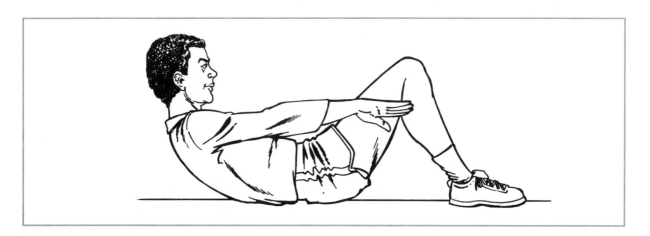

Figure 10.3 Crunch (partial) curl.
Reprinted from Howley and Franks 1997.

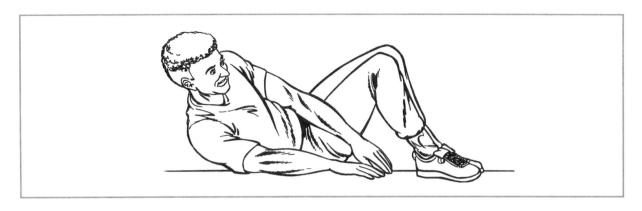

Figure 10.4 Oblique (diagonal) curl.
Reprinted from Howley and Franks 1997.

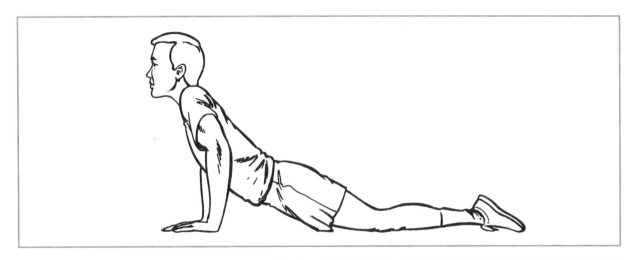

Figure 10.5 Back hyperextension exercise.

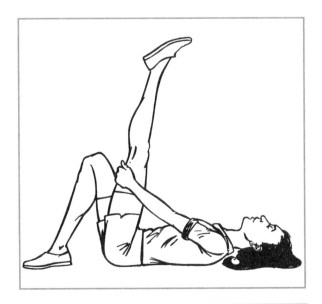

Figure 10.6 Hamstring stretch.

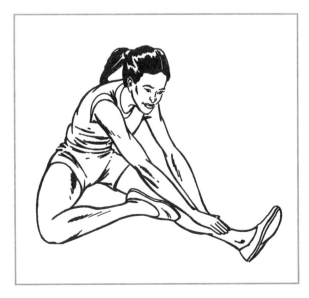

Figure 10.7 Modified hurdler's stretch.

Table 10.1	Administration of Curl-Ups

Needed for curl-ups

1. Flat surface with mat
2. Someone to explain purpose of test
3. Partner for each individual
4. Scoresheet or card

Step	Activity
1.	Explain the purpose of the test (i.e., to determine the endurance of the abdominal muscles to help prevent low back problems).
2.	Several persons can do this at the same time.
3.	Each individual lies on back with knees at about 150° angle, arms extended with fingers on legs.
4.	Partner is behind individual with hands cupped under head.
5.	Individual slowly curls up until fingertips touch knees, then back down (about one curl every 3 s).
6.	Partner counts number of curls (i.e., fingertips to knees and head back to partner's hands).
7.	The individual does as many as possible without stopping, up to a maximum of 35.
8.	Number of curl-ups is recorded on scoresheet or card.

Note. See chapter 17 for curl-up standards.

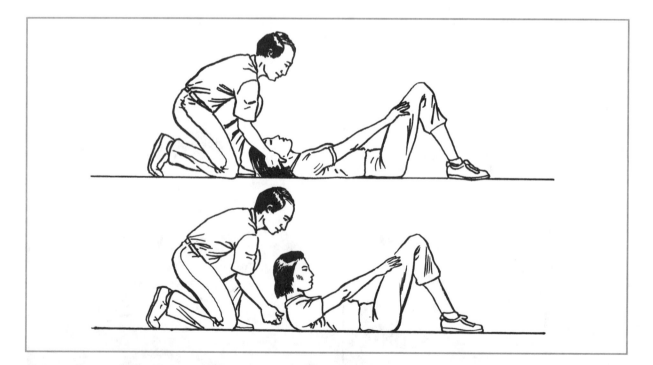

Figure 10.8 Modified curl-up test.
Reprinted from Howley and Franks 1997.

the flexibility of the hamstrings and the low-back area. Some questions have been raised about measuring low-back flexibility and about test design (planter flexion affects the score, and the test did not allow for differences in arm-to-leg or leg-to-trunk length). The current modifications of the sit-and-reach test include doing the test one leg at a time, to reduce the stress on the low back and to obtain information about each leg independently; allowing the foot to flex past the plane of the box against which the foot rests; and making a pretest measure with the subject's back against a wall to see how far she can reach, and subtracting this figure from the maximum distance reached. The following test incorporates the first two modifications (figure 10.9).

Attach a meter stick to the top of the box, with the 9-in (23-cm) mark located above the junction of the feet and the box (see figure 10.10). Instruct the individual being evaluated to slowly reach forward as far as possible (see table 10.2).

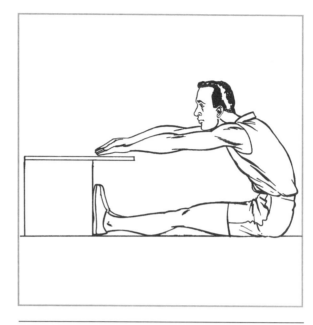

Figure 10.9 Sit-and-reach test of flexibility.
Reprinted from Howley and Franks 1997.

Table 10.2	Administration of the Sit-and-Reach Test

Pretest

- Area for warm-up
- Box (see figure 10.10)
- Administrator
- Scoresheet or card

Test

1. Explain the purpose of the test (i.e., to determine flexibility of the back of the legs to help prevent low-back problems).
2. Persons should *warm up* with static stretches prior to this test.
3. Individual sits with *shoes off*, one leg is straight with the foot flat against box end board; the other leg is bent with foot near the knee of the extended leg (see figure 10.9).
4. Place one hand on top of the other and extend arms forward.
5. Test administrator keeps the knee from bending by placing hands lightly on the extended leg above the knee.
6. Reach forward slowly as far as possible four times.
7. Hold the maximum reach on the fourth try for 1 s.
8. Scorer reads the point that the longest finger on both hands reached the fourth time that was held for at least 1 s.
9. Record the distance to the nearest 1/2 in. or cm.
10. Repeat steps 3 to 9 for other leg.

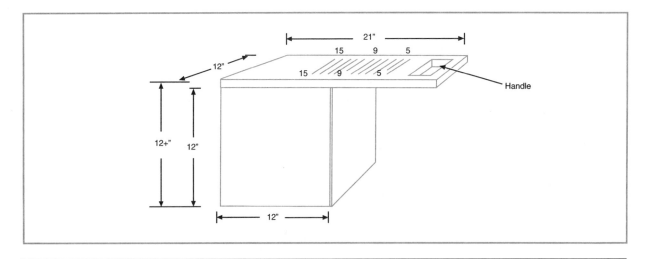

Figure 10.10 Sit-and-reach box specifications.
Reprinted from the American Alliance for Health, Physical Education, Recreation and Dance (1980).

The fitness leader should emphasize flexibility and strengthening exercises for the low-back area. Have the participants do a variety of exercises during each workout, but test flexibility and abdominal endurance only during regular testing periods.

Summary

Low-back problems are caused by a number of factors, including structural abnormalities, disease, accidents, poor posture or lifting mechanics, lack of proper warm-up prior to exercise, and lack of flexibility and muscular strength and endurance in the mid-trunk area. Participants can prevent many of these problems by using appropriate lifting techniques and good posture; warming up before exercise; increasing midtrunk strength, endurance, and flexibility; and learning to cope with stress. Use the suggestions in this chapter for teaching participants proper lifting and posture. Help your fitness participants lower their risk of future low-back problems by including midtrunk flexibility and strength and endurance activities as part of the fitness program and by encouraging participants to do these exercises at least every other day.

Chapter 11
Coping With Stress

Relationship to Health
Physical Activity and Reduced Stress
Coping With Stressors

Physical fitness components include cardiovascular function, relative leanness, and low-back function. Physical fitness also assumes sufficient levels of flexibility and muscular strength and endurance to be able to do daily tasks efficiently.

Though we acknowledge our inability to separate the mental, physical, psychological, social, and spiritual aspects of life, this book emphasizes physical fitness. This chapter deals with an area that bridges the psychological and physiological aspects of fitness.

Healthy people can relax and disregard irrelevant stimuli during quiet times; they can also work and play with vigor and enthusiasm. Physical conditioning enhances both relaxation and vitality. One of the keys to living a healthy life is balancing relaxation and arousal. People who are always relaxed and easygoing don't accomplish very much. But people who have a "get-it-done" attitude toward all aspects of life at all times exhibit coronary-prone behavior.

This chapter discusses a balance between relaxation and arousal by describing the relationships among physical activity, stress, and health.

Stress Continuums

Stress is related to personality—a person's perception of a stimulus or situation determines to a large extent how stressful it is. There are no uniform definitions of stress terms. For our purposes, we define a *stressor* as any stimulus or condition related to an activity that causes physiological arousal beyond what is necessary to accomplish the activity. This excessive arousal is called *stress*.

There are three major components of stress. A complete description of a stressful event includes the amount by which the stress response exceeded the functional demand, how pleasant it is to the individual, and whether it causes development or deterioration.

Functional—Severe Stress

An individual's physiological response to stress at any one time lies on a continuum from what is essential to provide the energy for that task at one end of the continuum to an extreme physiological response beyond what is needed at the other end. Table 11.1 illustrates how typical resting and submaximal heart rates include not only the heart rate needed to provide energy for the body but also increased heart rate (stress) due to chronic stressors (such as excess fat) and acute stressors (such as agitated emotional state).

Enjoyable—Unpleasant

Another aspect of stress is how enjoyable the individual perceives the stressor to be. Attending an exciting concert and taking an examination to qualify for a position may provoke similar stress responses. Most people, however, would perceive the concert as more enjoyable.

Development—Deterioration

The third aspect of stress is what happens to the individual as a result of the stressful experience.

This is, of course, the main criterion for determining whether the stressful event was positive or negative. Positive stressors result in a healthier, stronger person. Negative stressors lead to a weaker individual.

This end result of stress is somewhat independent of the other two aspects of stress. For example, on the one hand, a very stressful event (one that causes a large stress response beyond what is essential) can result in an individual's inspiration to achieve great things, or it may destroy initiative. On the other hand, conditions that cause little stress response may lead to steady development or can gradually wear down a desire to excel. In addition, people can grow and develop from stressors that are pleasant (positive reinforcement) as well as those that are unpleasant (a deadline to finish a project). Either pleasant or unpleasant stressors may tempt people to escape from confronting important areas of their lives. Therefore, be cautious in identifying a specific stressor as healthy or unhealthy based solely on the degree of physiological and psychological stress response or how pleasant the individual found the situation. Instead, determine whether the experience has led toward higher levels of mental, social, or physical health or not.

Table 11.1 Stress Components of Heart Rate

Component of heart rate	Heart rate, beats/min		
	Sitting	Climbing stairs	Running
HR needed to do task	30	50	100
Additional HR due to chronic stressors			
Poor aerobic fitness	+15	+20	+40
Excess fat	+5	+15	+20
Additional HR due to acute stressors			
Not relaxed	+10	+5	0
Emotional state	+15	+10	0
Total heart rate	75	100	160

Note. This HR model shows the contribution of the heart rate necessary to perform various tasks and the additional HR response caused by chronic and acute stressors. The actual HR values will vary with the individual depending on body size, fitness level, and type and severity of stressors.

Reprinted from Howley and Franks 1997.

Relationship Between Stress and Health

Stress is important to both positive and negative aspects of health. No discussion of the highest quality of life possible or of serious health problems is complete without including consideration of stress.

Positive Stress

We often think of stress as a primarily negative influence on our lives, but it has many positive features. Involvement with many stimuli and stressors provides interesting aspects to a full life. Absence of any stress at all results in a bland existence. It is difficult to imagine people developing, learning, growing, and striving toward their optimal potential without encountering stress. One feature of the good life is involvement in special emotional experiences that are remembered forever. These peak moments were probably stressful.

Negative Stress

Stress is also a factor in any discussion of our society's health problems. Stress is a risk factor for many major health problems, including coronary heart disease, hypertension, cancer, ulcers, low-back pain, and headaches. Although inability to cope with stress is probably insufficient to cause any of these problems without predisposition, stress does seem to exacerbate them. So for some people, stress results in a heart attack (see figure 11.1); for others, hypertension, ulcers, low-back pain, or headaches. Two aspects of an inability to cope are our perceptions of and reactions to stress. All of us have found ourselves getting upset (stressed) over something that normally would not bother us because of stress in another area of our lives. Although whether we can make a positive transfer of an adaptation to one stressor to other stressors is open to debate, there is little doubt that *negative* transfers from an inability to cope in one area lead to problems coping with other areas of life.

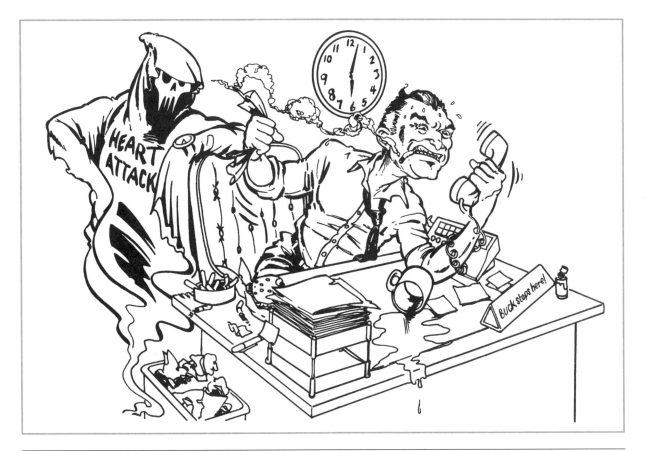

Figure 11.1 Negative aspects of stress.

Physical Activity and Stress Reduction

Many writers have justified exercise programs partly on the basis that they reduce stress. Although the claims have often exceeded the evidence, there is a basis for the relationship between stress reduction and acute (immediate) and chronic (long-range) exercise.

Acute Activity

Three primary factors cause single bouts of exercise to reduce stress: distraction, control, and social interaction.

Exercise (like many other activities) can serve as a temporary distraction from stressors. It is often helpful to step away from a problem, then come back to it later. This technique is healthy, as long as exercise doesn't become an escape from the problem.

One of the primary concepts in a person's ability to cope with stressors is the perception of personal control. For example, increased practice resulting in improved skills reduces stress when playing a game around others. Postcardiac exercise programs often reduce participants' fears that any exertion at all will cause another heart attack.

Another way acute exercise may reduce stress is by providing a time to have either more or less interaction with others. Stress reduction can result when the exercise session provides a time to be alone for people who experience daily stress from constant contact with other people (e.g., the working parent who must spend almost every waking moment in the presence of others, such as children, spouse, employees, employer, and colleagues, all demanding time and attention). That person can use a walk/jog program as a time to be alone with her or his own thoughts. At the other extreme is the person who has little contact with other people during the typical day and for whom loneliness is a potential stressor. Doing activities and having time to talk with other people in an exercise program can aid that person. The HFI should be aware of the needs of individuals in terms of the amount of social interaction during the exercise session.

Chronic Activity

The long-term effects of a regular exercise program also help reduce stress. Increased cardiorespiratory function and decreased body fat cause you to be less stressed throughout the day. With increased fitness levels, physical activity itself becomes less of a stressor. For example, many studies have shown that as a person becomes fit, he or she can do the same amount of external work with lower heart rate, blood pressure, and adrenaline. Thus the functional response to the work (the energy necessary to accomplish the task) remains the same, but the stress response is reduced. Some authorities believe, with some evidence, that adaptation to physical activity provides a basis for better adaptation to other stressors. Others believe, also with some evidence, that adaptation is specific to different stimuli and stressors. The transfer from adaptation to exercise to adaptation to other stressors apparently occurs with some participants, but not everyone.

Motivation

As a fitness leader, you are concerned with motivation for exercise at two levels. First, how can you get people to *begin* a fitness program? The public has been educated to acknowledge, in general, the need for healthy behaviors; most people will agree that they should exercise on a regular basis. There must be, however, convenient programs available that provide personal contact with concerned exercise professionals to complement information about the healthy life. Second, you must consider what will make fitness participants continue physical activity as a part of their lifestyles. Individual attention, realistic goals with periodic testing, options for group participation, involvement of spouse or important others, contracts, and programs that minimize injury all seem to help people adhere to fitness programs. Whether motivating a person to begin or to continue activity, fitness has to achieve priority status in life (like eating and sleeping). Any effort to increase motivation must have that end in sight. Therefore, external, or extrinsic, rewards are only a temporary means to change behavior; maintaining behavior over the long-term requires internal, or intrinsic, motivation.

A positive addiction to exercise can take place as the participants achieve the almost universal perception of "feeling good" as a result of appropriate physical activities. One of the main purposes of a fitness program is to help individuals progress safely to the fitness level at which they become "addicted," at which they look forward to the regular workout. As with all healthy behaviors, however, it is possible to take an exercise addiction to the extreme. Instead of regarding exercise as a healthy part of life, some people become obsessed and overemphasize its importance, spending time exercising that should be spent on other parts of their lives.

One of the key elements in achieving a balance between arousal and relaxation is appreciation of the balance of work and play. The hard-driving, time-conscious, impatient person (often called "Type A") has difficulty taking time just to play and enjoy an activity that is not directly related to productivity; the easy-going person (often called "Type B") has corresponding difficulty in getting down to business and

completing a task. Likewise, fitness leaders who try to pattern their fitness programs after military or athletic models often have a goal orientation without the play. Other leaders who do not discriminate about their selection of activities as long as everyone is having a good time may achieve playfulness without fitness gains. The good fitness program achieves a balance by including activities that provide the necessary fitness components as well as a playful atmosphere in which it is fun to participate.

Coping Methods

People can do many things to maximize the positive aspects of stress while minimizing the negative (see figure 11.2). For instance, simply being exposed to a wide range of experiences helps individuals become better educated and less stressed by new situations. A good fitness program provides a variety of different types of experiences, including cooperative, problem-

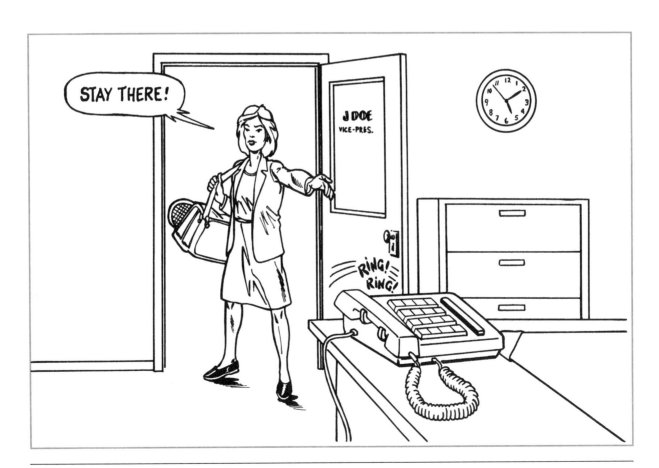

Figure 11.2 Coping with stressors.

solving, competitive, individual, partner, and team activities. This variety enriches the participant by improving fitness as well as the ability to cope with different movement experiences.

Strategies

Fitness leaders should encourage fitness participants to observe the different strategies that seem to enhance coping with potentially stressful situations. Facing the problem, looking at alternatives, talking about it with close friends, seeking professional or technical advice when needed, and stepping back or away from it for a brief time are all behaviors people use in coping with stress. Which ones are better suited for particular situations? Are there some that might help but the participant feels uncomfortable doing? Help participants practice coping behaviors in "easy" settings. In terms of fitness, using a variety of activities in a good program requires different coping strategies.

Developing Optimal Fitness

Developing physical, mental, and social fitness characteristics will cause potential stressors to be less threatening. An individual who can do hard work will not dread physical stressors. A person accustomed to the mental processes that lead to problem solving finds a difficult problem not as stressful. Aspects of social fitness, such as establishing meaningful relationships with other people, can provide a support group that helps a person have positive responses to stressful situations. The fitness leader and fitness class can be conducted in an atmosphere that provides this kind of support group.

Control

Perception of control repeatedly appears as a major element in coping with stress. Therefore, whatever you can do to help participants gain control of their lives will diminish potentially stressful conditions. One of the by-products of exercising, eating nutritious foods, and refraining from using harmful drugs is the feeling of taking responsibility for one's own life. Not only do the healthy behaviors themselves

reduce stress, but the fact that the person has "taken charge" also reduces stress levels. Chapter 15 deals with ways to help people modify behavior. Give attention to whatever things, tasks, and relationships are important to the participant so that he can increase his skills in those areas. Then, an individual who is asked to do something important will experience enhanced self-confidence in being successful. It is also important to recognize unreasonable demands, whether they are self-imposed or imposed by someone else (see figure 11.3). It is essential to good health to be able to point out the problem and work with others (perhaps one's boss or spouse) to try to accomplish common goals in a reasonable way within an appropriate time frame.

Relaxation

Participants can learn techniques to help them relax. Benson and others have demonstrated the benefits of the "relaxation response." One easily used technique, introduced by Edmund Jacobsen, aims at helping individuals recognize the feelings produced by tension. When using this technique, participants should assume a comfortable position with eyes closed. This should be done lying down, but it can be done sitting as well.

Jacobsen's technique calls for participants to tense a specific area of the body, hold for about 20 seconds, then relax; then tense a larger segment, hold, relax, and so forth. During the tension period, tell participants to feel the tension. During the relaxation period, ask the participants if they can feel the tension leave the area. A fitness leader can use the following sequence:

- Right toes
- Left toes
- Right foot
- Left foot
- Right leg below knee
- Left leg below knee
- Right leg below hip
- Left leg below hip
- Both legs below hips
- Abdomen and buttocks
- Right fingers

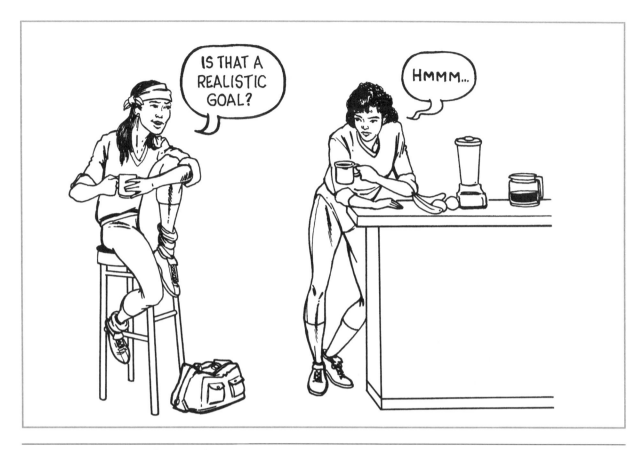

Figure 11.3 Setting realistic goals.

- Left fingers
- Right arm below elbow
- Left arm below elbow
- Right arm below shoulder
- Left arm below shoulder
- Both arms below shoulders
- Chest
- Neck
- Jaw
- Forehead
- Entire head
- Entire body

Extend this last relaxation period, asking the participants to feel tension leaving their bodies and be aware of their slow, deep breathing.

Summary

This chapter helped you understand what stress is and how you can help fitness participants get its positive benefits while reducing its negative aspects. Stress is excessive arousal beyond what is needed to accomplish a task. Small or large amounts of stress may be either enjoyable or unpleasant. Evaluate a stressful event by determining whether it has led to healthy development or deterioration. Ways to maximize the positive elements of stress include exposure to varied stimuli, developing a range of coping abilities, exhibiting healthy behaviors, and gaining as much control over one's life as possible. Finally, this chapter described a method you can use to help participants learn to relax, which is one element of stress management.

PART IV

The Fitness Program

Recommendations for Physical Activity
Fitness Program Components
Energy Cost of Activities
Behavior Modification

Part I provided the basis for fitness programs. Part II dealt with evaluating an individual's health status to determine the appropriate type of fitness program. Part III described the various components of fitness. Part IV of the *Fitness Leader's Handbook* presents the contents of a complete physical fitness program, as well as ways to modify behavior.

Chapter 12 describes how to recommend physical activity for individuals based on recent position statements and reports, such as the *Surgeon General's Report on Physical Activity and Health*. Chapter 13 describes activities that can be used in a well-rounded physical fitness program. Chapter 14 provides methods to determine how many calories a person uses in various activities. Chapter 15 recommends a process for helping participants live healthier lives by adhering to an exercise program and increasing healthful living in other areas of life.

Chapter 12
Recommendations for Physical Activity

Exercise Prescription Based On
Current Activity Status
Health, Fitness, and Performance Goals

Most of the concepts in this chapter have been included in various chapters in the first three parts of the book. This chapter brings them all together in one place to help you recommend appropriate activities for individual fitness participants. This chapter will extend the concept of how to begin a fitness program and progress from one step to the next. Your responsibilities as a fitness leader include providing a continual process of education for participants. In many cases, you must help them not only learn appropriate concepts based on the latest research but also "unlearn" some things they have experienced and been taught in the past. (Having your participants read *Fitness Facts* will help.) One of the most difficult aspects of your educational efforts will be to help participants progress over reasonable periods of time from walking to jogging to playing games and sports. Most participants want to do too much too soon, resulting in unnecessary soreness and

risk of injury that often causes them to drop out of fitness programs.

What physical activity should you recommend? Recommendations for physical activity range from changing TV channels manually without a remote control to running 10 to 15 mi per day to prepare for a marathon. Keep in mind that the public gets advice from official reports from governmental agencies, position statements from professional organizations, and opinions from exercise scientists, physical activity professionals, and sports, entertainment, and journalism figures. Some of the questions raised by these reports, organizations, and professionals include duration, frequency, total amount of work, intensity, type of activity, and whether or not it must be done in one session or can be divided into smaller parts.

Although "how much activity to recommend" is a simple question, there is confusion about its answer both in the research and popular literature.

The confusion comes primarily from failing to consider two factors: the individual's physical activity status and health, fitness, and performance goals. The purpose of this chapter is to describe how you can provide coherent recommendations for physical activity based on research data and expert judgment.

A Brief Historical View

The American College of Sports Medicine (ACSM) has been the major public voice in exercise recommendations for the last 20 years. Its 1978 recommendations have been the most quoted source on this subject. These recommendations (three to five times per week of at least 20 min of vigorous-intensity aerobic activity at 60% to 80% of maximal functional capacity) represented a good summary of the experimental literature on the effects of physical activity on cardiovascular fitness (maximal oxygen uptake). More recent recommendations from ACSM and others expand the earlier statement to include evidence from epidemiological studies on risks of cardiovascular disease, encouraging everyone to engage daily in at least 30 min of moderate-intensity activity. The Surgeon General's report synthesized the research findings concerning physical activity and health, with conclusions similar to the more focused report from the NIH Consensus Conference on Physical Activity and Cardiovascular Health.

Two reasons for the increased interest in physical activity and the modifications of the ACSM recommendations are the evidence that sedentary individuals can reduce their risk of cardiovascular disease with less activity than called for in the original ACSM recommendations, and the rather small percentage of people in the United States who are active at the level suggested by the original ACSM guidelines. In the U.S. adult population, about 15% engage in activities recommended by the original ACSM statement, 22% engage daily in 30 min of moderate-intensity activity, and 24% are completely sedentary, leaving 39% who engage in some activity (but less than the minimum recommended).

Despite these official statements and reports, which have received wide recognition in the media, there is still confusion about how to determine what activity should be recommended, how intense it should be, how often, and how long.

Activity Recommendations

You can harmonize all the various research studies and position statements by using the step-wise model described in table 12.1. You can universally recommend certain activities. Recommending other activities depends on the current activity level of the individual. After a person includes a modest level of physical activity in her lifestyle, recommendations for additional activity largely depend on her specific health, fitness, or performance goals. Table 12.1 summarizes this model for recommending physical activity.

Activities for Everyone

In order to promote general health and well-being and the ability to handle routine tasks, there are common activities recommended for everyone. Each person can increase activity as part of his lifestyle.

This recommendation is based on using common sense to find ways to increase activity in an individual's routines at home, work, and during leisure time. Suggested activities include walking rather than riding when possible; climbing stairs rather than taking the elevator or escalator; parking farther away from the store or office for a short walk to and from the car; and getting off the bus or train one stop earlier for a short walk to the office, store, or home. Daily activities should emphasize weight-bearing activities (such as walking) to use more energy and enhance bone health. People should also include a daily routine of static stretching and abdominal endurance aimed at preventing low-back problems.

For Sedentary Individuals

Sedentary individuals are those who currently do no regular physical activity or who can't walk for 30 min continuously without discomfort or pain (individuals who are unable to walk can substitute moving in a wheelchair, swimming, or the like). They should find ways to include activity in their daily routine as well as engage in 30 min of moderate-intensity activity daily. These activities might include walking, yard work, cycling, slow dancing, and low-impact exercise to music. The activity can be

Table 12.1	Model for Physical Activity Recommendations

• Activities recommended for every one
• Activities for sedentary individuals
• Activities for moderately-active individuals interested in
  • Health
  • Cardiovascular
  • Bone
  • Low back
  • Psychological
	• Physical fitness
	  • Aerobic fitness
	  • Relative leanness
	  • Muscular strength and endurance
	  • Flexibility
	• Activities for vigorously active individuals interested in
	  • Performance
	  • Sport
	  • Physical task(s)

broken into two to four segments; for example, one person might take two 10-min exercise breaks during the work day, another exercise break in the morning or at night during the week and taking a 30-min walk on weekend days. Weight-bearing activities should be included, emphasizing simply being active, without concern about the intensity level.

For Moderately Active Individuals

Moderately active individuals are those who currently engage in 30 min of activity daily, or who can walk 30 min continuously without pain or discomfort, but can't jog 3 mi (or walk 6 mi fast, cycle 12 mi, or swim 3/4 mi) continuously at target heart rate without discomfort and undue fatigue. These individuals should continue to include activity in their normal routine, and engage in 30 min of moderate-intensity activities every day.

At this point, your recommendations should depend upon the individual's health and fitness goals. Chapter 1 illustrated the different levels of health, fitness, and performance. This chapter will describe how you can recommend different activities for specific health, fitness, and performance goals.

Table 12.2 includes recommended activities for common health and fitness goals. Important health goals include cardiovascular, bone, low back, and psychological health. Health-related

physical fitness includes aerobic fitness, relative leanness, muscular strength and endurance, and flexibility.

Cardiovascular Health and Aerobic Fitness. Those individuals who want to prevent cardiovascular and other diseases and to promote general health should emphasize including activity as part of the daily routine and doing 30 min of moderate-intensity activity daily. Evidence shows that this type of activity will reduce the risk of cardiovascular disease. There is some additional benefit from longer duration or more vigorous activity. The goal of improving aerobic fitness (see chapter 7) is related to the health goal for cardiovascular health and performance goals involving endurance activities.

To increase aerobic fitness, the participant should schedule at least 20 min of vigorous-intensity activity (preceded and followed by 5 to 10 min of moderate-intensity activity) 3 or 4 days each week. These activities can include fast walking, jogging, cycling, fast dancing, low- to moderate-impact exercise to music, and swimming. Heart rate during these activities should be 70% to 85% of maximal heart rate (see chapter 2). She must warm up and cool down for 5 to 10 min prior to and following the vigorous-intensity workout. She can include low-back exercises (see chapter 10) as part of the warm-up or cool-down. The aerobic activities will, over time, increase maximal oxygen uptake, make current submaximal tasks less stressful, and reduce resting and submaximal

Table 12.2 Physical Activity for Health Goals

Health goal	Recommended activities
Cardiovascular	Accumulate 30 min of daily, moderate-intensity activity Include longer duration and (or) higher intensity
Bone	Weight-bearing activities Resistance exercises
Low back	Static stretching in midtrunk and thigh regions Abdominal curl-ups
Psychological	Enjoyable activities and atmosphere

Note. These activities should be considered **after** an individual is already doing those activities recommended for everyone. These activities should be done *in addition to* activities recommended for sedentary individuals.

heart rate. These activities will further reduce the risk of cardiovascular disease and provide the basis for a number of endurance-type sports and activities.

Relative Leanness. The amount of fat related to the total body weight is a key element for both health and fitness (see chapter 5). Recommendations for relative leanness include both nutrition and activity. For those with too little fat, increase caloric intake, especially carbohydrates, and begin resistance exercises. You should consider having such people evaluated for possible eating disorders.

People with too much fat should reduce their total caloric intake and the proportion of fat in their diet. You should encourage them to include activity as part of their routines, engage in at least 30 min of moderate-intensity activity daily, and either continue the moderate-intensity activity for longer duration or include vigorous-intensity activities such as those recommended for aerobic fitness. Emphasize activities that use energy (calories). You should also recommend resistance exercise to increase the active fat-free mass, thereby increasing the number of calories burned throughout the day. Resistance activities to maintain muscle mass are important for individuals who are restricting their caloric intake, and you should emphasize activities designed to improve muscular strength and endurance (see chapter 8).

Bone Health and Muscular Strength and Endurance. Emphasize weight-bearing activities and resistance exercise for healthy bones. Although elite performers need to distinguish between strength (one contraction) and endurance (repeated contractions), a fitness perspective considers strength and endurance together (see chapter 8). Individuals need modest levels of strength and endurance to be able to function in normal routines that include lifting, moving, and carrying. One or two sets, 10 to 15 repetitions each, of resistance exercise for each muscle group, two or three times per week, will improve or maintain muscular strength and endurance.

Low-Back Health, Flexibility, and Abdominal Endurance. For a healthy low back (see chapter 10), we recommend daily static stretching in the midtrunk area, two or three repetitions, holding each for 10 to 30 s, and 15 to 30 abdominal curl-ups (slow, without feet held). The flexibility fitness goal includes the ability to move all joints through their complete range of motion without pain, which is important for daily tasks (see chapter 9).

Psychological Health and Fitness. Psychological well-being is a major part of one's overall health and fitness. Feeling good, a positive outlook on life, and the ability to capture the positive aspects of stress while minimizing its negative side effects are all components of psychological health. There is increasing evidence that an active lifestyle is associated with improved psychological well-being. While we cannot precisely define specific activity recommendations for psychological health at this time, it seems logical that the emphasis for psychological health should be on selecting enjoyable activities and creating or finding an appropriate workout environment. Each individual's desired activities and atmosphere will vary. For example, many people enjoy the social interaction of being part of a group jogging, playing games, or exercising to music, while others look forward to that time to be alone with their own thoughts. Relaxation techniques can also be helpful with psychological well-being.

Other Elements of Health. Physical activity may help prevent or minimize many other health problems we have not listed. More research is needed before definitive exercise prescriptions can be made for each specific potential health problem. In general, the activities recommended for cardiovascular health are appropriate for a variety of health concerns.

Although the emphases for health goals are on including more activity as part of one's routine and accumulating 30 min of daily activity, there is some additional benefit in more activity. It appears that either doing more activity (longer duration) or activities that are more intense can create additional health benefits. The nature of the additional activities can often be determined by looking at specific physical fitness goals.

For Vigorously Active Individuals

Individuals who can run 3 mi continuously (or walk fast 6 mi, cycle 12 mi, or swim 3/4 mi) at target HR, three or four times per week without discomfort or pain can, if interested, now engage in a variety of sport and performance activities. Some individuals have specific performance goals. They may want to be better tennis players or run a 10K race in a certain time. Table 12.3 lists recommended activities for achieving performance goals.

These individuals should continue to include activity as part of their life, engage in 30 min daily of moderate-intensity activity, and include vigorous-intensity activity at target HR those weeks when not engaging in sport or performance activities. Performance activities include a wide range, such as soccer, basketball, racquet-

ball, badminton, high-impact exercise to music, and road races. It is impossible to make general recommendations for performance. Different performance sports or tasks need additional fitness levels, as well as developing the skills and strategies of the game. For example, running, cycling, or swimming races demand high levels of aerobic fitness in that mode of activity, specific form to increase efficiency of movement, and strategy and mental readiness for the event. Racquetball requires aerobic and anaerobic energy, court agility and coordination, different types of strokes (e.g., serve, kill, lob, hitting after the ball rebounds from the wall), plus strategy and mental readiness for the match. Being a fire fighter requires ability to respond quickly to emergencies, anaerobic capacity in smoke-filled air, muscular endurance for carrying heavy loads up and down ladders or stairs, and so on. All activities require energy sources, but each activity has its own mix of aerobic and anaerobic tasks. Interval training that mimics the energy demands of the performance is one important aspect of training. The point is that each performance has its own need for the underlying fitness levels and specific skills.

Quality of Life

Perhaps everyone's overall goal is to be able to participate in and enjoy life fully. For most individuals, this will include several health, fitness, and performance goals. Thus, it seems logical to start with the health goals, then progress to the fitness goals, finally adding performance goals for those interested. In this way, the fitness program can enhance the overall quality of each participant's life.

Finally

We have presented two factors to consider in exercise prescription: current activity status and health, fitness, and performance goals. We believe your initial recommendations for activity should be based on each individual's activity status, getting him involved in routine activities and daily moderate-intensity activities. Then, after he is engaging in daily activities on a regular basis without any problems of discomfort or

Table 12.3	Physical Fitness Goals and Recommended Activities

Physical fitness goals	Recommended activities
Aerobic fitness	20-40 min vigorous-intensity activity, 3-5 days per week
Relative leanness	
Too little fat	Eat more calories, especially carbohydrates
	Resistance exercise
Too much fat	Reduce calories, especially fat
	Increase duration of aerobic activities
	Include resistance exercise
Muscular strength and endurance	Resistance exercise 1-2 sets, 10-15 reps, each muscle group
Flexibility	Static stretching, 10-30 s, 2-3 times, each joint

Note. These activities should be considered only **after** an individual is doing the activities in table 12.2. These activities should be done *in addition to* table 12.2 activities.

fatigue, he might consider the health and fitness goals for which he desires improvement. After he has included the daily and fitness activities as part of his lifestyle, he might consider a variety of performance goals that are of interest.

To return to the original question: What activity should you recommend? You can answer that question consistent with the research data and recommendations of experts by considering the individual's current activity status and her health, fitness, and performance goals. The answer includes these steps:

Essential for Everyone

1. Include more activity in routine aspects of one's lifestyle.
2. Engage in at least 30 min of moderate-intensity daily activity.
3. Include activities aimed at health goals.

Optional

4. Include activities aimed at fitness goals.
5. Include activities aimed at performance goals.

In short, people who adopt an active lifestyle obtain enhanced quality of life.

Summary

Coherent individualized recommendations for physical activity can be consistent with the research data and expert judgment by using the individual's current activity status and the health, fitness, and performance goals in the following sequence:

Activity Status	Recommended Activities
Everyone	Include activity in every-day life.
Sedentary	Engage in 30 min of daily moderate-intensity activities.
Moderately active	Based on health and fitness goals.
Vigorously active	Based on performance goals.

Chapter 13
Fitness Activities

Walking and Jogging
Cycling
Games
Aquatic Activities
Exercising to Music

In this chapter we will provide details on walking, jogging, and cycling programs as well as comment on other fitness activities. You will, of course, want to help fitness participants modify these activities to establish a program that enables them to achieve their fitness goals (see figure 13.1).

Walking, Jogging, and Running

Walking involves keeping one foot in contact with the ground at all times. During jogging or running there is a period of "flight" during which both feet are off the ground. The extra energy required to propel the body off the ground and to absorb the force of impact when landing makes jogging or running a better way to expend calories, but it also increases the chance of injury. It is more difficult to distinguish jogging from running. A world-class runner may "jog" through a warm-up at 7 mph while a person of average fitness may be running all out at the same speed. Jogging usually refers to a submaximal running speed.

Shoes

Specialized walking shoes are now available from major shoe manufacturers catering to the growing market of walking enthusiasts. For most people, however, a comfortable pair of ordinary shoes offering side support is sufficient to start a walking program. Specialized walking shoes may be a reasonable investment for someone who has chosen walking as a primary activity. A good quality pair of jogging-running shoes with the usual cushioning to absorb the shock of impact

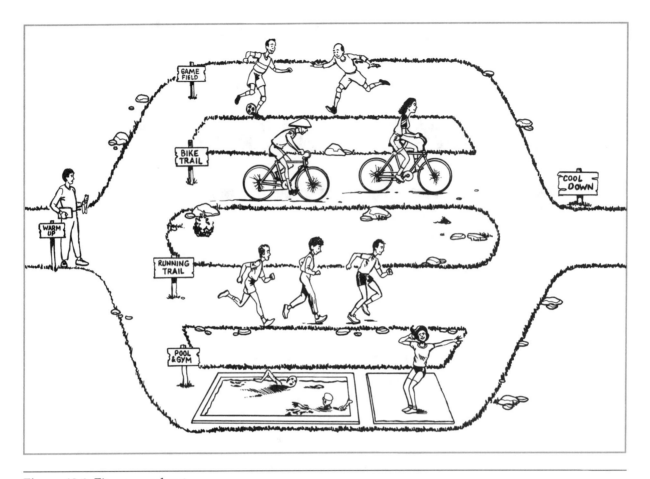

Figure 13.1 Fitness workout.

and the structural support to resist movement of the heel upon landing is also suitable for walking. As participants progress from the walking to the jogging and running phases of a fitness program, encourage them to invest in a pair of good-quality running shoes. We recommend that participants purchase shoes at a store that specializes in athletic shoes, fitting the shoes late in the day (when feet are at their largest) while wearing the same kind of socks they wear during a workout.

Clothes

Emphasize selecting clothes that make the participant feel as comfortable as possible during the exercise session. In addition, bright, easily visible clothing is a wise choice. In hot weather, recommend loose-fitting, light-colored clothing and a hat with a brim for exercise in direct sunlight. Cotton fabrics are best because they help bring sweat to the surface for evaporation and cooling of the body. Alert participants to mis-

leading advertising that suggests that by wearing plastic, nylon, or rubber clothing, they will lose more weight when exercising in warm weather. The weight lost is water weight, not fat weight, and wearing these fabrics can create a potentially dangerous situation by making it more difficult to keep cool.

When exercising outdoors in the cold weather, participants should wear layers of clothing so that they can remove a layer or two as they warm up and begin to sweat. The idea is to not produce too much sweat, which can accelerate heat loss and result in hypothermia (a lowering of the body temperature). Wool and polypropylene fabrics are best because they maintain their insulating qualities even when wet with sweat. You should recommend a hat and gloves or mittens, since a great deal of heat is lost from the head and hands. For those who tend to have cold hands, wearing a pair of polypropylene gloves inside the mittens provides additional comfort. The emphasis should be on comfort—not looks.

Location and Surface

Safety is the first consideration in choosing a workout site. Walking is a good activity, but walking in some urban areas after dark is not healthful (or smart!). Remind participants to consider the traffic flow, lighting, and surface when selecting an exercise area. Low-traffic areas are more relaxing and reduce the chance of an accident. If walking, jogging, or running in the streets, recommend that participants run toward oncoming traffic so they can see what is ahead. Encourage participants to yield to traffic at each intersection and driveway even though they may legally have the right of way. The following poem reinforces this point:

> Here lies the body of Benjamin Bay.
> He died maintaining his right of way.
> He was right—dead right—as he jogged
> along,
> But he's just as dead as if he'd been wrong.

The surface should be relatively smooth. Remind the participants to be aware of cracks, holes, and debris to avoid sprains and strains. The hardness of the surface is not important for those who walk, since the force of impact is relatively low. For those who jog or run, however, the surface can influence their comfort, especially if they have arthritis in their ankles, knees, or hips. A soft surface like grass or a cushioned track will relieve some of the problems. When jogging on grass, however, caution participants to watch for roots and holes. Given the concern for injuries and safety, the area should be well-lighted.

Walking Program

The walking program shown in table 13.1 takes the participant from a very light level of activity to the point of being able to walk 60 min at a brisk pace. The fitness leader should encourage the participants to follow the five rules at the top of the table.

The most important rule for the participants is to not progress to the next stage until they are comfortable at the current stage. Continually encourage them to take their time and enjoy steady progress toward fitness goals. We recommend that they increase the distance walked at a slow speed before increasing the walking speed. We have not stated a particular walking speed, however, because what is comfortable for one person may be too fast for another.

At the end of the walking program, when the participants can walk 3 mi or so at a brisk pace, they are ready to start the jogging program. As mentioned, however, some individuals will prefer to stay at the "brisk walk" stage of the walking program as their most intense activity. Individuals should start slowly and go at a pace that is appropriate for them. This is a good time for the leader to walk with different individuals to see if they have questions and to encourage them to continue their activity.

Jogging Program

Table 13.2 describes a jogging program. Remember, though, that the first rule to follow is to make sure the participant completes the walking program first. In addition, the first five levels of the program emphasize the need to mix walking with jogging to stay at the low end of the THR zone—where the participant perceives the exercise as being easy. This gradual transition will result in less muscle soreness. The fitness leader can suggest that participants who achieve their THR at the same pace jog together.

Running Races

In almost every community there are opportunities to compete in running races—whether 1-mi "fun runs" or social 10K (6.2-mi) runs. For those interested in jogging or running as a primary form of activity, these runs can, and should, be fun. Their focus should be on completing the course comfortably.

Remember, the focus of this book is on helping participants become fit, not on achieving world-class status as runners. The fitness leader should refer those interested in running performance to additional educational material on long-distance running and local or regional running clubs. Those who choose to emphasize competitive running, with a main goal of running faster and faster, should expect more injuries and muscle soreness to accompany their efforts.

Table 13.1	Walking Program

Rules:

1. Start at a level that is comfortable to you.
2. Be aware of new aches or pains.
3. Don't progress to next level if not comfortable.
4. Monitor heart rate and record it.
5. It would be healthful to walk at least every other day.

Stage	Duration (min)	Heart rate	Comments
1	15	_____	_____
2	20	_____	_____
3	25	_____	_____
4	30	_____	_____
5	30	_____	_____
6	30	_____	_____
7	35	_____	_____
8	40	_____	_____
9	45	_____	_____
10	45	_____	_____
11	45	_____	_____
12	50	_____	_____
13	55	_____	_____
14	60	_____	_____
15	60	_____	_____
16	60	_____	_____
17	60	_____	_____
18	60	_____	_____
19	60	_____	_____
20	60	_____	_____

Note. From *Fitness Leader's Handbook* (2nd ed.) by B.D. Franks and E.T. Howley, 1998, Champaign, IL: Human Kinetics. This form may be copied by the fitness leader for distribution to participants.

Cycling

A cycling program can use a regular bicycle or one of the many stationary cycle ergometers found in fitness centers. Cycling is a good exercise alternative for people who do not like to jog or run and can also give relief to those who have joint tenderness. Adjust the seat height so that the partici-pant's knee has only a slight bend when each foot is at the bottom of a pedal swing. Table 13.3 shows a cycling program that progresses in much the same way that the walk and jog programs do.

The emphasis at the beginning of the program is on simply riding the equivalent of 1 to 2 mi, three times per week. After that, participants should work at the low end of the THR zone (60%

Table 13.2	Jogging Program

Rules:

1. Complete the walking program before starting this program.
2. Begin each session with stretching and walking.
3. Be aware of new aches and pains.
4. Don't progress to next level if not comfortable.
5. Stay at low end of THR zone; record heart rate for each session.
6. Do program on a work-a-day, rest-a-day basis.

Stage 1 Jog 10 steps, walk 10 steps. Repeat five times and take your heart rate. Stay within THR zone by increasing or decreasing walking phase. Do 20 to 30 min of activity.

Stage 2 Jog 20 steps, walk 10 steps. Repeat five times and take your heart rate. Stay within THR zone by increasing or decreasing walking phase. Do 20 to 30 min of activity.

Stage 3 Jog 30 steps, walk 10 steps. Repeat five times and take your heart rate. Stay within THR zone by increasing or decreasing walking phase. Do 20 to 30 min of activity.

Stage 4 Jog 1 min, walk 10 steps. Repeat three times and take your heart rate. Stay within THR zone by increasing or decreasing walking phase. Do 20 to 30 min of activity.

Stage 5 Jog 2 min, walk 10 steps. Repeat two times and take your heart rate. Stay within THR zone by increasing or decreasing walking phase. Do 30 min of activity.

Stage 6 Jog 1 lap (400 m, or 440 yd) and check heart rate. Adjust pace during run to stay within the THR zone. If heart rate is still too high, go back to the Stage 5 schedule. Do 6 laps with a brief walk between each.

Stage 7 Jog 2 laps and check heart rate. Adjust pace during run to stay within the THR zone. If heart rate is still too high, go back to Stage 6 activity. Do 6 laps with a brief walk between each.

Stage 8 Jog 1 mi and check heart rate. Adjust pace during the run to stay within THR zone. Do 2 mi.

Stage 9 Jog 2-3 mi continuously. Check heart rate at the end to ensure that you were within THR zone.

Note. From *Fitness Leader's Handbook* (2nd ed.) by B.D. Franks and E.T. Howley, 1998, Champaign, IL: Human Kinetics. This form may be copied by the fitness leader for distribution to participants.

of maximal heart rate) until they can comfortably do 15 to 25 min of activity. Have the participants stay within the THR zone as they progress through the program. Individuals should not advance to the next stage until they can easily complete the current stage. The fitness leader can provide films or television for participants to watch as these will make riding the stationary cycles more enjoyable. Suggest that groups of participants who ride at about the same speed to reach their THR zones ride together.

Games

One characteristic of childhood that is often lost in adults is a sense of playfulness. A child doesn't need to justify spending time playing a game simply for the fun of it. Inability to appreciate play for its own sake is an attribute that seems to be present in coronary-prone behavior. Perhaps one way that a good fitness program can benefit people is to provide them with activities that increase both fitness and playfulness. *The*

Table 13.3	Cycling Program			

Rules:

1. Start at a level that is comfortable for you.

2. Use either a regular bicycle or a stationary exercise cycle.

3. If you are starting at Stage 1, simply get used to riding 1 or 2 miles. Don't be concerned about time or reaching the lower end of your target heart rate (THR) zone.

Stage	Distance (mi)	THR (% of max HR)	Time (min)	Frequency (days/week)
1	1-2	—	—	3
2	1-2	60	8-12	3
3	3-5	60	15-25	3
4	6-8	70	25-35	3
5	6-8	70	25-35	4
6	10-15	70	40-60	4
7	10-15	80	35-50	4-5

Note. From *Fitness Leader's Handbook* (2nd ed.) by B.D. Franks and E.T. Howley, 1998, Champaign, IL: Human Kinetics. This form may be copied by the fitness leader for distribution to participants.

New Games Book (1976) offers a number of specific games of varying intensity for different numbers of people. This book presents a playful, fun, and inclusive approach to games.

For the reasons we have mentioned, you can have interested individuals play games in a fitness program. But we do recommend that a person first be able to move through the walking and the jogging programs. This is because those programs emphasize more controlled types of activity at an intensity that will help achieve cardiovascular fitness levels and change body composition to facilitate involvement in games. Indeed, if the participant is not fit enough to play a game, there is a lower chance of having fun and a greater chance of injury.

The first component for games is enjoyment. This means balancing cooperation and competition, continued participation by everyone, and the chance for everyone to be a winner.

A key ingredient for a fitness game is that everyone be included. This may mean modifying normal rules. For example, in a game of tag, if someone is tagged by the person who is "it," the tagged player also becomes "it" and continues to play, rather than sitting down until the game is over.

Many good games are inclusive and fun, but relatively inactive. For example, having children sing a song while performing limb and body movements. These can be used as part of a warmup and cool-down or can be interspersed between vigorous games. The main body of the workout should include games in which all participants are continuously active in the THR range. Once again, you may have to alter rules to ensure this continued vigorous activity. For example, in a game like softball, in which players are inactive during most of the game, a new rule might require all players to shift positions each time another player comes to the plate to bat. In games like soccer, basketball, or ultimate Frisbee, in which a few persons tend to dominate the action, playing with two or three balls (or Frisbees) at the same time increases participation by everyone.

Having small groups solve problems together or cooperate to accomplish fitness tasks can be enjoyable and healthy. For example, have each volleyball team see which one can keep their ball in the air for the longest time (using one ball on each side). As you can see, you can change competitive games to cooperative events by simple rule changes. Once again using volleyball as an example, you can apply the usual rules, but the "score" is changed to the number of times the ball is hit across the net (or the total number of hits counting both sides) before it hits the ground. This is not to say you need to avoid competition, but you should deemphasize winning. Winning's importance should not be used to exclude anyone from participation.

Games of Skill

Most games can become fitness games when played vigorously. Some require certain minimum levels of skill that you can teach as part of the fitness program. Games like badminton, racquet- or paddleball, squash, and tennis all require a certain amount of skill in hitting a ball (or bird) with a racket. Some general guidelines can enhance the fitness qualities of these games, including singles play and matching players of similar ability. Energy expenditure is often a little less than it would be for the same amount of time spent running, but you can use these types of games as a fun part of the fitness program.

Some activities and games require a minimum of special skills, equipment, or facilities. Normal fitness activities can be done in ways that accomplish other goals. For example, creativity can be enhanced by groups of three or four people playing "follow the leader" for warm-up, aerobic, or cool-down activities, changing the leader often so that each person has a chance to lead the group. Trust can be developed by having one person lead a partner whose eyes are closed in warm-up or cool-down activities, communicating solely through the hands. The game of tag is another example of low-organization activity. Some variations of tag include persons touching the spot on their bodies where they were tagged as they try to tag others; a person cannot be tagged while hugging someone (with a time limit for hugs); or a person has to be enclosed, rather than tagged, by the two persons who are "it" holding hands, then the tagged person joins hands with those who are "it" until everyone has been enclosed.

A good example of a low-organization game that can be modified to make it a physical fitness game is musical chairs, in which players walk around chairs—numbering one less than the number of players—until the music stops,

and then each person tries to sit in a chair. The one who doesn't is "out." Two changes can make this a good fitness game. First, players jog, rather than walk, around the chairs, which are arranged in a big circle. Second, as soon as two people are "out," they begin a second circle. As the first circle gets smaller, the second one gets larger (each person who is out in the first circle continues to participate in the second circle—each time the music stops a chair is deleted from the first circle and one added to the second circle). Thus everyone continues to play. Another modification is to change musical chairs from a competitive to a cooperative game. The person who can't find a chair, instead of being put out of the circle or going to another circle, has to sit or stand on a part of a chair or on part of another person on a chair. Continue the game by removing one more chair each time the music stops (or the whistle blows), until everyone has to be supported by one chair. For this modification, make sure you have sturdy chairs, and caution players to be careful.

Fitness Stations

One way of organizing the exercise session is to have different activities at different stations, with the participants rotating to each station or choosing those stations they would like to use. This uses limited space or equipment efficiently while adding variety to the workout.

Special Considerations

Warm-up and cool-down activities are for participants at any fitness level. More vigorous games usually involve high-intensity bursts, stopping, starting, and quickly changing directions. These are not recommended for people at the early stages of a fitness program. You should include some additional stretching and easy movements in different directions as part of the warm-up. Obviously the space, number of people, and available equipment have to be considered in the selection of activities.

The fitness leader must emphasize safety and should change the rules immediately when something is not working. For example, if the person who is "it" is unable to tag anyone, the space can be made smaller or a second "it" can be named. If a few individuals are dominating a team game, then you can introduce a new rule—everyone on the team has to touch the ball before shooting. Another modification of a team game like basketball, soccer, or volleyball is to award points based on how many people touched the ball by the team as part of the scoring play—one point if only one person made contact with the ball, two points for contact by two players, and so on.

In some classes, you will want to have different activities going on simultaneously. For example, if there are only two racquetball courts, then most of the fitness participants will engage in some activity other than racquetball, but four could play each period. Offer a variety of games so that people with different skill levels can participate. When large groups are involved in activities, there should be frequent changes in activities to maintain interest. Finally, in addition to warm-up and cool-down activities, alternate higher- and lower-intensity activities to prevent undue fatigue. Encourage participants to go at their own pace. Target heart rate should be checked periodically to ensure that participants are within their range.

Aquatic Activities

A person doesn't have to play games, run, or cycle to achieve a cardiorespiratory training effect. Swimming is a good alternative. Aquatic activities, however, include more than just swimming. Participants can walk, jog, or run across the pool; hold onto the side of the pool and do flexibility exercises; and play games in the water. Swimming or one of these other activities is a good choice for persons who have chronic orthopedic problems or a recent injury that will not allow them to do their regular workouts. Water supports body weight to relieve the load on ankles, knees, and hips while providing enough resistance to require the expenditure of a large number of calories and achieve THR.

The maximal heart rate is about 13 beats·min⁻¹ lower when immersed in water. This shifts the THR zone back about 10 beats·min⁻¹, since THR depends on the maximal heart rate. Have participants progress from low-intensity to higher-intensity activities in the pool in much the same way you do on land. Flexibility activities include moving the legs forward, backward, and to the side in a gentle and easy motion while holding onto the side of the pool with one hand. You can

also have participants hang onto the side of the pool with both hands, so that the body is floating, and practice kicking patterns that are part of regular swimming.

Those who cannot swim can walk or jog across the pool while doing a swimming stroke. Water offers enough resistance to this movement so that most people can achieve THR. Participants can vary the workout by walking backward or skipping side to side while moving across the pool. Moreover, they can use flotation devices to help them along while swimming; flotation offers a good deal of resistance while providing support. In this way even a nonswimmer can achieve a satisfying workout while "swimming" up and down the pool.

Swimming laps in the pool requires a certain level of skill—a poor swimmer will be exhausted at the end of one or two laps and will be unable to complete the duration of the workout needed to expend the necessary 200 to 300 kcal (remind participants that kcal is what the public usually calls calories). Individuals can learn to swim at any age and, besides the survival value of such a skill, swimming provides a special alternative for the individual who cannot perform other exercise activities due to injury, disease (e.g., arthritis), or situation. The (lower) THR should be checked during the swimming workout in much the same way as during running. The distance the individual has to swim to expend 200 to 300 kcal varies with the stroke used and the swimmer's skill level. A very rough rule of thumb is that a 1-mi swim is equal to about 4 mi of jogging. Begin each workout with a gradual warm-up and finish with a cool-down. Table 13.4 includes a list of steps to follow in a swimming program.

Participants can start this swim program at any of the levels, depending on their skill and current fitness levels. Also, don't hesitate to vary the components to suit the individual participant. For example, a participant might like to jog four widths, swim four widths, and walk two widths, repeating the sequence to achieve 20 to 30 minutes of activity at the THR. Simply remember to have participants take their time in making the transition to longer duration and more intense activities. In addition, you can use many of the ideas mentioned previously for working with groups in the water too, such as playing games and grouping together people who work at similar intensities.

Table 13.4	Swimming Program

Rules:

1. Start at a level that is comfortable for you.

2. Don't progress to next stage if not comfortable with current one.

3. Monitor and record heart rate.

Stage 1 In chest-deep water, walk across the width of the pool four times and see if you are close to THR. Gradually increase the duration of the walk until you can do two 10-min walks at THR.

Stage 2 In chest-deep water, walk across and jog back. Repeat twice and see if you are close to THR. Gradually increase the duration of the jogging until you can complete four 5-min jogs at THR.

Stage 3 In chest-deep water, walk across and swim back (any stroke). Use kickboard or flotation device if needed. Repeat this cycle twice and see if you are at THR. Keep up this pattern of walk-swim to do about 20 to 30 min of activity.

Stage 4 In chest-deep water, jog across and swim back (any stroke); repeat and check THR. Gradually decrease the duration of the jog and increase the duration of the swim until four widths can be completed within the THR zone. Accomplish 20 to 30 min of activity per session.

Stage 5 Slowly swim 25 yards, rest 30 seconds, slowly swim another 25 yards, and check THR. On the basis of the heart rate response change the speed of the swim and (or) the length of the rest period to stay within the THR zone. Gradually increase the number of lengths you can swim (three, then four, and so on) before checking THR.

Stage 6 Increase the duration of continuous swimming until you can accomplish 20 to 30 min without a rest.

Note. From *Fitness Leader's Handbook* (2nd ed.) by B.D. franks and E.T. Howley, 1998, Champaign, IL: Human Kinetics. This form may be copied by the fitness leader for distribution to participants.

Movement to Music

One of the best things to happen to fitness exercises in the past 20 years has been setting them to music. It has provided an exercise opportunity for people who do not like to jog or run. In addition, exercising to music (often called "aerobics") provides one less excuse to those who would skip exercise sessions because it is (pick one) too hot, too cold, raining, and so on.

Music provides a sense of pace and the motivation to keep at it, in contrast to other, more isolated activities such as cycling, jogging on a treadmill, or swimming laps in a pool. The pace can be varied by the tempo of the music, which becomes a distraction from the exercise as one listens to changing rhythms. In addition, musical exercise sessions offer a better balance of activities to achieve fitness goals in flexibility, muscular endurance, and cardiorespiratory endurance. Generally speaking, participants will have no problem reaching their THR during an exercise-to-music session. In fact, individuals may find it easy to reach THR, and you should recommend that they do too little rather than too much of this type of exercise. Emphasize enjoying the session, not competing with others, either in the types of steps used or in continuing when the body is saying "slow down." As we mentioned earlier, the idea of "no pain, no gain" still heard in some health clubs is wrong! "Train, don't strain" is more appropriate and will bring more benefits in the long run.

The reason for doing too little rather than too much is that exercise-to-music programs lead to more than their share of injuries. The routines tend to isolate smaller muscle groups and skeletal structures. In addition, people may start this kind of activity program before they are ready. We recommend that participants achieve a minimum level of fitness (equivalent to jogging 3 mi at THR) before undertaking this kind of activity. Further, we suggest participants alternate this kind of exercise with other activities, like cycling and swimming, that do not put as much stress on the joints.

Fitness centers now offer a wider variety of exercise-to-music classes than they did in the past. This is partly in response to the incidence of injuries in regular-level classes and partly related to the recognized need to offer classes suited to older and more sedentary individuals. It is reasonable to have participants start with beginner and low-impact classes and move up to more advanced classes, including water classes, as their fitness and interest increase.

Summary

We recommend a progression from walking to jogging to games. Participants should be able to walk 3 to 4 mi at a brisk pace before undertaking more strenuous activities. The jogging program begins with walk-jog intervals and gradually increases to continuous jogging. When individuals can jog about 3 mi (or equivalent in cycling [12 mi] or swimming [3/4 mi]), they are ready for fitness activities, including games and exercise to music. Swimming is a good alternative to walking or jogging because it takes a load off the joints. The THR is about 10 beats·min^{-1} lower in swimming than for land activities. Exercise to music provides good motivation and variety in a workout but may also cause more than an average number of injuries. Substituting or alternating with cycle or swim workouts relieves some of the stress on the joints.

Chapter 14
Measuring Energy Expenditure

Methods of Determining Energy Cost
Energy Costs of Various Activities

We have discussed the importance of modifying both diet and exercise for fitness participants to help them achieve weight loss goals and maintain the new weight. You will be helping participants burn 200 to 300 kcal during each exercise session. Though most people are familiar with the caloric values of food, as values are usually printed on food packages and can be found in calorie-counter tables, such is not the case for the caloric costs of physical activity. This chapter provides information you can use to help participants expend the desired number of kcal.

When oxygen is used by the body, energy is produced to contract a muscle, move a nerve impulse, repair a bone, or carry out any number of other cellular functions. Oxygen goes from the lungs to the blood and finally to the tissues where it is used. For each liter of oxygen used, the body produces about 5 kcal. Knowing this,

we can measure the amount of energy produced during the course of a day simply by measuring oxygen consumption. We can then estimate the amount of energy a person uses for different activities and provide an overall estimate of what a person might expend in one day.

When we are sitting at rest, we produce about 1 kcal per hour for every kg (2.2 lb) of body weight. The value of 1 kcal per kilogram per hour (kcal·kg^{-1}·hour^{-1}) is 1 resting metabolic unit or 1 MET. METs have already been used to quantify cardiorespiratory fitness (CRF) in chapter 7. METs are also used in expressing the energy costs of activities; for example, running at 6 mph requires 10 METs, or 10 times the rate of energy expended at rest. Before discussing the energy costs of physical activity, however, we need to focus on the energy associated with sitting at rest—the largest energy-producing task in the lives of most people! Given that we produce about 1 kcal of energy per kilogram of body weight per hour at rest, you can estimate a fitness participant's resting energy expenditure (also called basal metabolic rate, or BMR) by

- multiplying 24 kcal times body weight in kilograms (pounds divided by 2.2) or
- multiplying 11 kcal times body weight in pounds; for example, for a 150-lb person,
  150 lb x 11 kcal·lb^{-1} = 1650 kcal.

This, of course, represents only resting energy expenditure. To obtain an estimate of overall energy expenditure, the participant must add the energy cost of other activities performed on a regular basis. This is done by adding from 400 to 800 kcal, depending on whether the individual is sedentary or very active. So, if our 150-lb person is sedentary, the estimated total energy expenditure is 2050 kcal per day (1650 kcal + 400 kcal). Remember that this is a rough estimate, and like any estimate may be too high or too low for any particular individual. Use it as a guide, but if you find the participant gaining weight while eating just enough food to meet the estimated energy expenditure, decrease your estimate by about 10% and see if the individual can maintain weight on that new estimate. Remember, if caloric intake is reduced to a very low level, the body responds by decreasing its resting metabolic rate to protect its limited energy stores. In such a circumstance the formula we have offered will result in an overestimation of energy expenditure.

Estimate Your Daily Energy Expenditure

1. Determine resting metabolic rate: Multiply 11 by body weight: 11 x ___ lb = ___ kcal

2. Select 400 kcal if sedentary, 600 kcal if moderately active, and 800 kcal if active: ___

3. Daily energy expenditure: Line 1 ___ kcal + Line 2 ___ kcal = ___ kcal

---

Energy Costs of Common Activities

The techniques used to measure energy expenditure at rest have also been used to measure the energy required to do certain activities. This section presents information on the energy required for some of the most common activities associated with physical fitness programs.

Walking

We recommend a walking program for anyone who has not been active for some time. The program provides stages of gradually increasing duration and intensity and may be a lead-in to a jogging or running program. For many people, the walking program may be all they wish or need to do to maintain fitness. Walking has the advantage that it can to be done anywhere, any time, by virtually anyone. Scientists have studied the energy cost of walking indoors using a treadmill, as well as outdoors on a track, beach, or farm. Walking on a beach or across a plowed field requires more energy than walking at the same speed on a flat, firm surface. Because most people exercise on a firm surface, however, we will discuss the energy costs of walking on a smooth surface.

Table 14.1 shows the energy required to walk at different speeds. The values are given in kcal·min^{-1}. Not surprisingly, the energy cost of walking increases with the speed of walking; however, the rate of increase is higher at the higher speeds. For example, when walking speed increases from 2 to 3 mph for a 150-lb person, the energy required increases from 2.8 to 3.7 kcal·min^{-1}. But going from 4 to 5 mph increases the energy required from 5.6 to 9.0 kcal·min^{-1}. As we mentioned earlier, fitness walking can be done by just about anyone. The very sedentary individual can walk at slow speeds and achieve THR while the relatively fit individual can walk at high speeds and reach THR while using more energy.

Jogging and Running

Many people jog and run to achieve their fitness and weight loss goals. The energy requirement of jogging is about twice that of walking at 3 mph but is nearly the same as walking at 5 mph. Table 14.2 shows the energy required to jog or run at

Table 14.1	Energy Costs of Walking (kcal/Minute)						
	Miles per hour						
Body weight (lb)	2.0	2.5	3.0	3.5	4.0	4.5	5.0
110	2.1	2.4	2.8	3.1	4.1	5.2	6.6
120	2.3	2.6	3.0	3.4	4.4	5.6	7.2
130	2.5	2.9	3.2	3.6	4.8	6.1	7.8
140	2.7	3.1	3.5	3.9	5.2	6.6	8.4
150	2.8	3.3	3.7	4.2	5.6	7.0	9.0
160	3.0	3.5	4.0	4.5	5.9	7.5	9.6
170	3.2	3.7	4.2	4.8	6.3	8.0	10.2
180	3.4	4.0	4.5	5.0	6.7	8.4	10.8
190	3.6	4.2	4.7	5.3	7.0	8.9	11.4
200	3.8	4.4	5.0	5.6	7.4	9.4	12.0
210	4.0	4.6	5.2	5.9	7.8	9.9	12.6
220	4.2	4.8	5.5	6.2	8.2	10.3	13.2

Note. Multiply value by the duration of activity to obtain total calories expended.

different speeds. As you can see, the energy requirement increases with increasing speed, but the increase in the energy cost from one speed to the next is similar at slow and fast speeds, about 1.7 kcal·min^{-1} per mph increase in speed for a 150-lb person. This proportional increase in energy cost means that when participants jog 1 mi at 6 mph (10 min per mi) they will finish the mile twice as fast as when jogging at 3 mph, but the energy required per mile is about the same. We will discuss this topic further in the next section.

Caloric Costs of Walking and Running One Mile

In spite of the vast amount of information available regarding the energy costs of walking and running, a good deal of misunderstanding exists. We still hear claims that the energy cost of walking 1 mi is equal to that of running the same distance. Table 14.3 shows the energy cost of walking 1 mi, and table 14.4 shows the energy cost of running 1 mi. Given that energy cost depends on body weight (heavier people require more energy to travel 1 mi than lighter people do), the caloric cost is given for different body weights.

The table contains two numbers for each weight, one expressing the gross cost of the activity and the other expressing the net cost. Gross cost includes the resting metabolic rate (the cost of just sitting around), while net cost subtracts this quantity out. For weight control programs it is important to use the net cost of an activity, as it measures the energy used over and above that of sitting around. When moving at slow to moderate speeds (2 to 3.5 mph), the net cost of walking a mile is about half that of jogging or running a mile. This means that the person who jogs a mile at 3 mph will be working at twice the metabolic rate of someone who walks the same distance, and, of course, heart rate response will be higher as well. Because most people who walk move at these slower speeds, it is important to remember that the energy cost per mile is half that of running. However, if we now look at very high walking speeds (5 mph—1 mi in 12 min), we see that the net energy cost of walking is similar to that of jogging or running. If you try it, you will find that the participant's heart rate response is as high during walking as during running at that speed. If individuals can walk at these high speeds, they can easily reach THR and expend kcal at about the same rate as during running.

Table 14.2 — Energy Costs of Jogging and Running (kcal/Minute)

Body weight (lb)	Miles per hour							
	3.0	4.0	5.0	6.0	7.0	8.0	9.0	10.0
110	4.7	5.9	7.2	8.5	9.8	11.1	12.3	13.6
120	5.1	6.4	7.9	9.3	10.6	12.1	13.4	14.8
130	5.5	7.0	8.6	10.0	11.5	13.1	14.6	16.1
140	5.9	7.5	9.2	10.8	12.4	14.1	15.7	17.3
150	6.4	8.1	9.9	11.6	13.3	15.1	16.8	18.5
160	6.8	8.6	10.5	12.4	14.2	16.1	17.9	19.8
170	7.2	9.1	11.2	13.1	15.1	17.1	19.1	21.0
180	7.6	9.7	11.8	13.9	15.9	18.1	20.2	22.2
190	8.1	10.2	12.5	14.7	16.8	19.1	21.3	23.5
200	8.5	10.8	13.2	15.4	17.7	20.1	22.4	24.7
210	8.9	11.3	13.8	16.2	18.6	21.1	23.5	25.9
220	9.3	11.8	14.5	17.0	19.5	22.2	24.7	27.2

Note. Multiply value by the duration of activity to obtain total calories expended.

Table 14.3 — Gross and Net (Gross/Net) Cost in kcal per Mile for Walking

Body weight (lb)	Miles per hour						
	2.0	2.5	3.0	3.5	4.0	4.5	5.0
110	64/39	58/39	54/39	53/39	60/48	68/57	79/69
120	69/42	63/42	59/42	57/42	66/52	75/63	86/75
130	75/45	68/45	64/45	62/45	71/57	81/68	93/81
140	80/49	73/49	69/49	67/49	77/61	87/73	100/88
150	87/52	79/52	74/52	72/52	82/65	93/78	108/94
160	92/56	84/56	79/56	76/56	88/70	100/84	115/100
170	98/59	90/59	84/59	81/59	93/74	106/89	122/107
180	104/63	95/63	89/63	86/63	99/78	112/94	129/113
190	110/66	100/66	94/66	91/66	104/83	118/99	136/119
200	115/70	105/70	99/70	95/70	110/87	124/104	144/125
210	121/73	111/73	104/73	100/73	115/92	131/110	151/132
220	127/77	116/77	109/77	105/77	121/96	137/115	158/138

Note. Multiply value by the number of miles walked to obtain the total (gross/net) calories expended.

Table 14.4 shows that the net caloric cost of running a mile is independent of speed. It does not matter whether participants jog the mile at 3 mph or run it at 6 mph—the caloric cost is the same. It obviously takes twice as long to run 1 mi at 3 mph than at 6 mph, but again, the net cost is about the same. There is no question that at 6 mph the individual will be expending energy at about twice the rate expended at 3 mph, but since the mile is finished in half the time, the total energy expenditure is about the same. Heart rate response will, of course, be higher during the 6-mph run.

Another point about the costs of walking and running a mile concerns the actual number of kcal expended per mile. A person weighing 154 lb (70 kg) expends about 54 and 107 kcal as a result of walking and running a mile, respectively. If this formerly sedentary person walks 4 mi a day, he expends 216 kcal (4 x 54 kcal) above his resting rate, and when coupled with a reduction in caloric intake of 300 kcal a day, the person will lose about 1 lb of fat per week (500 kcal x 7 days = 3500 kcal). Figure 14.1 shows the relationship between exercise energy expenditure and food energy. You can help the participant think,

before taking that next handful of chips, how many miles it will take to "burn" them off. Indeed, a person should not justify a milkshake by walking only 1 mi. Remember, it is the small, systematic changes made in diet and exercise habits that lead to weight loss and allow participants to maintain the weight when the goal is achieved.

One final comment about the energy costs of walking and running: As weight is lost, the energy the body requires to walk or run 1 mi decreases—there is simply less weight to carry around. This may help explain why some people experience a leveling off of body weight even though they are careful to keep the distance of their walks or runs the same during a weight loss program. Knowing this, you should have participants increase the distance they cover as they lose weight to keep up the same rate of weight loss.

Walking and running are not the only activities used in exercise programs to achieve fitness goals and expend calories. We will now discuss bicycle riding, exercising to music, rope skipping, and swimming. In addition, we'll include a summary table at the end to tie things together.

Table 14.4	Gross and Net (Gross/Net) Cost in kcal/Mile for Jogging and Running							
Body weight (lb)	Miles per hour							
	3.0	4.0	5.0	6.0	7.0	8.0	9.0	10.0
110	93/77	89/77	86/77	84/77	84/77	83/77	82/77	81/77
120	101/83	97/83	94/83	92/83	92/83	90/83	89/83	89/83
130	110/90	105/90	102/90	100/90	99/90	98/90	97/90	96/90
140	118/97	113/97	110/97	108/97	107/97	106/97	104/97	104/97
150	127/104	121/104	118/104	115/104	114/104	113/104	112/104	111/104
160	135/111	129/111	125/111	123/111	122/111	121/111	119/111	119/111
170	144/118	137/118	133/118	131/118	130/118	128/118	127/118	126/118
180	152/125	146/125	141/125	138/125	137/125	136/125	134/125	133/125
190	161/132	154/132	149/132	146/132	145/132	143/132	141/132	141/132
200	169/139	162/139	157/139	154/139	153/139	151/139	149/139	148/139
210	177/146	170/146	165/146	161/146	160/146	158/146	156/146	155/146
220	186/153	178/153	173/153	169/153	168/153	166/153	164/153	163/153

Note. Multiply value by the number of miles walked to obtain the total (gross/net) calories expended.

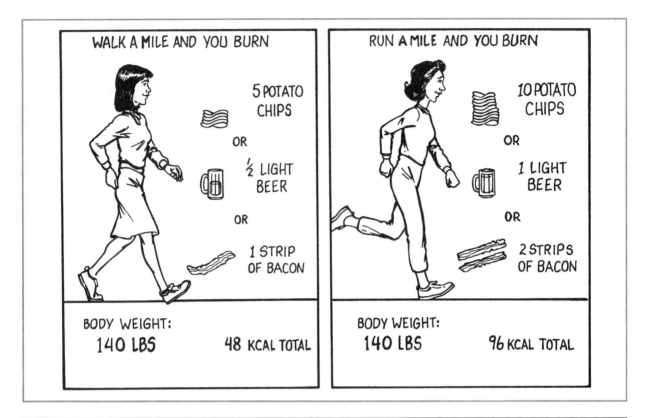

Figure 14.1 Energy intake and expenditure.

Bicycling

Traveling by bicycle is more efficient than walking or running. Consequently, a person has to pedal more miles than he or she would have to walk to expend the same amount of energy. In general, one has to bicycle about 2 to 3 mi to expend the same number of calories as walking 1 mi. As most people can comfortably ride a bike at 6 to 9 mph, they can accomplish the same energy expenditure goal and take no more time than the person who walks at 3 mph.

Exercising to Music

As you know, one of the most popular forms of exercise in fitness facilities is exercising to music. The intensity of the session depends on the type of activities being done—flexibility, muscular endurance, or cardiovascular. In addition, energy expenditure depends on whether a person walks through the exercises or does low-impact, regular, or advanced routines. The energy requirement for exercising to music (table 14.5) ranges from as low as 4 METs

for someone who walks through the session (about the same as walking at 3.5 mph) to as high as 10 METs in an advanced session (about the same as jogging or running at 6 mph). Figure 14.2 indicates that, as in walking and running, there is a clear need to be realistic about just how many calories are expended during this form of activity. If a 132-lb (60-kg) woman works at an average of 5 METs for an entire 40-min session, she will expend 200 kcal, equal to the gross cost of walking 3 mi. Given that she is making gains in cardiovascular fitness, flexibility, and muscular endurance, this is a very reasonable number of calories to expend. Because these exercises involve small muscle groups and require other muscles to stabilize body positions, heart rate response tends to be elevated at any level of energy expenditure.

Rope Skipping

Rope skipping can be done indoors or out, requires little equipment, and can be an effective part of a fitness program for people with high levels of fitness and regular activity. We

Table 14.5	Gross Energy Cost of Exercising to Music (kcal per Minute)		
Body weight (lb)	Low intensity	Moderate intensity	High intensity
110	3.3	5.8	8.3
120	3.6	6.4	9.1
130	3.9	6.9	9.8
140	4.2	7.4	10.6
150	4.5	7.9	11.3
160	4.8	8.5	12.1
170	5.1	9.0	12.8
180	5.4	9.5	13.6
190	5.7	10.1	14.3
200	6.0	10.6	15.1
210	6.3	11.1	15.9
220	6.6	11.7	16.7

Note. Multiply value by duration of activity to obtain total calories expended.

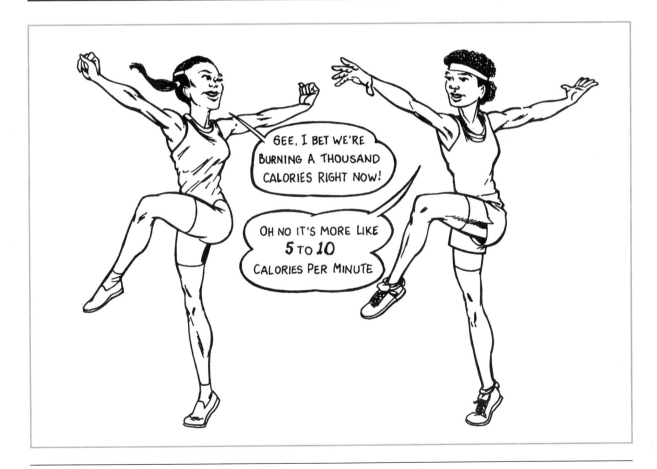

Figure 14.2 Energy cost of exercising to music.

emphasize the latter point because rope skipping places a load primarily on the lower leg, involves smaller muscle groups than walking and running, and causes a disproportionately higher heart rate response. Overdoing this activity, especially at the beginning of a fitness program, is inappropriate. The reason for such concern is the high energy cost of rope skipping (table 14.6), which is 9 METs (with a HR of 150 beats·min⁻¹) in young fit subjects even at very slow skipping rates (60 to 80 turns a minute). Skipping at 120 turns a minute increases the energy cost only to 11 METs. As a result, skipping is not a "graded" activity—even the lowest skipping rate (60 to 80 turns a minute) requires an energy expenditure equal to or higher than the CRF of many formerly sedentary people.

Swimming

Swimming is an excellent activity because it involves the large muscle groups and provides little trauma to joints while expending a relatively large number of calories. However, predicting the caloric cost of swimming is difficult because it depends on the type of stroke used, swimming speed, and the skill of the swimmer.

A poor swimmer must expend greater quantities of energy just to stay afloat or move at a slow pace, while a highly skilled swimmer expends very few calories doing the same thing. As a rule of thumb, the net caloric cost of swimming 1 mi is about four times that of running 1 mi (400 kcal versus 100 kcal). Table 14.7 shows the estimated caloric cost per mile of swimming the forward crawl for men and women. Because of their greater buoyancy associated with higher body fatness, women expend fewer calories per mile than men, independent of skill level. Remember, the maximal HR is about 13 beats·min⁻¹ lower in water than on land. For this reason, THR should be reduced about 10 beats·min⁻¹ from that calculated using the 220 − age formula.

Summary of Energy Costs

We have presented only a few of the most common activities used in activity programs. Table 14.8 provides some details about other activities in which the fitness participants may be involved, either in your fitness program or on their own. The MET level gives some indication of the relative intensity of each activity and should provide some guidance as to whether you should include

Table 14.6	Gross Energy Cost of Rope Skipping (kcal per Minute)		
Body weight (lb)	**Slow skipping**		**Fast skipping**
110	7.5		9.2
120	8.2		10.0
130	8.9		10.9
140	9.5		11.7
150	10.2		12.5
160	10.9		13.4
170	11.6		14.2
180	12.3		15.0
190	13.0		15.9
200	13.6		16.7
210	14.3		17.5
220	15.0		18.4

Note. Multiply value by duration of activity to obtain total calories expended.

Table 14.7 Caloric Cost Per Mile (kcal per Mile) of Swimming the Front Crawl for Men and Women by Skill Level

Skill level	Women	Men
Competitive	180	280
Skilled	260	360
Average	300	440
Unskilled	360	560
Poor	440	720

Note. Multiply value by number of miles to obtain total calories expended.

Adapted from Holmer 1979.

Table 14.8 Summary of Measured Energy Cost of Various Physical Activities

Activity	METs $kcal \cdot kg^{-1} \cdot hr^{-1}$	$kcal \cdot hr^{-1}$ 50 kg/110 lbs	70 kg/154 lbs	90 kg/198 lbs
Archery	3.5	175	245	315
Backpacking (general)	7	350	490	630
Badminton (social)	4.5	225	315	405
Badminton (competitive)	7	350	490	630
Basketball (game)	8	400	560	720
Basketball (general)	6	300	420	540
Billiards	2.5	125	175	225
Bowling	3	150	210	270
Boxing (in ring)	12	600	840	1080
Canoeing (moderate)	7	350	490	630
Canoeing (vigorous)	12	600	840	1080
Cricket	5	250	350	450
Croquet	2.5	125	175	225
Cycling (light)	6	300	420	540
Cycling (moderate)	8	400	560	720
Cycling (vigorous)	10	500	700	900
Dancing (ballroom, slow)	3	150	210	270
Dancing (ballroom, fast)	5.5	275	385	495
Dancing (aerobic)			see table 14.5	
Fencing	6	300	420	540

(continued)

Table 14.8 *(cont'd)*

Activity	METs kcal·kg⁻¹·hr⁻¹	kcal·hr⁻¹		
		50 kg/110 lbs	70 kg/154 lbs	90 kg/198 lbs
Field hockey	8	400	560	720
Fishing (general)	4	200	280	360
Fishing (in waders)	6	300	420	540
Football (touch)	8	400	560	720
Golf (pulling clubs)	5	250	350	450
Golf (carrying clubs)	5.5	275	385	495
Golf (power cart)	3.5	175	245	315
Handball (general)	12	600	840	1080
Hiking	6	300	420	540
Horseback riding (trotting)	6.5	325	455	585
Horseshoe pitching	3	150	210	270
Hunting (general)	5	250	350	450
Jogging		see tables 14.2, 14.4		
Paddle/racquetball, general	6.5	325	455	585
Paddle/racquetball, competitive	10	500	700	900
Rock climbing, ascending	11	550	770	990
Rope jumping		see table 14.6		
Running		see tables 14.2, 14.4		
Sailing (general)	3	150	210	270
Scuba diving (general)	7	350	490	630
Shuffleboard	3	150	210	270
Skating, roller and ice	7	350	490	630
Sledding	7	350	490	630
Snowshoeing	8	400	560	720
Squash	12	600	840	1080
Soccer (general)	7	350	490	630
Soccer (competitive)	10	500	700	900
Swimming		see table 14.7		
Table tennis (general)	7	350	490	630
Tennis (general)	7	350	490	630
Volleyball (general)	3	150	210	270
Walking		see tables 14.1, 14.3		

Note. Values from: Ainsworth, B.E., Haskell, W.L., Leon, A.S., Jacobs, D.S., Jr., Montoye, H.J., Sallis, J.F., and Paffenbarger, R.S., Jr. (1993). Compendium of physical activities: Classification by energy costs of human physical activities. *Medicine and Science in Sports and Exercise.* 25:71-80.

it in your program for specific participants. Remember to select activities consistent with the participant's fitness level and to recommend a duration that will result in the expenditure of an appropriate number of calories. Caloric expenditures are listed for three body weights, indicating an approximate range of energy expenditures associated with each activity.

An Easy Way to Estimate Energy Expenditure

Estimating energy expenditure can be simplified so you can obtain a reasonable figure without having to consult all sorts of tables and figures. The estimate is based on the observation that when working in the THR zone a participant is at about 70% of maximal CRF. For example, a person with a maximal CRF value of 10 METs will be exercising at about 7 METs while in the THR zone. Because 1 MET is equal to 1 kcal·kg^{-1}·hour^{-1}, a person working at 7 METs is working at 7 kcal·kg^{-1}·hour^{-1}. If that person weighs 70 kg (154 lb), it means that 490 kcal are expended per hour in the activity. If the activity lasts only 30 min, then half that, or

245 kcal, is expended. Therefore, by knowing your maximal MET value (CRF value) you can obtain a reasonable estimate of how many kcal you are expending in a workout. Table 14.9 is based on those calculations for a 30-min workout. Locate the participant's estimated CRF on the left and look across the table to the approximate body weight to find the estimated energy expenditure for a 30-min workout at THR.

Summary

This chapter described the caloric costs of a variety of activities. Daily energy expenditure can be determined by multiplying body weight (in lb) by 11 and adding from 400 to 800 kcal based on activity level. At normal speeds, it costs about twice as much energy to run as to walk a set distance. Exercising to music can use as much energy as walking or running depending on the intensity of the exercise. To expend the same amount of energy as it takes to run a set distance, an individual has to cycle about four to six times or swim about one-fourth of that distance.

Table 14.9	**Estimated Energy Expenditure (kcal) for 30 Minutes of Exercise at 70% Cardiorespiratory Fitness Value (CRF) for Persons of Different Body Weights**		
V̇O₂max (kcal·kg⁻¹·hr⁻¹)	**70% CRF (kcal·kg⁻¹·hr⁻¹)**	**Body weight [kg (lb)]**	
		50 (110)	**70 (154)**	**90 (198)**
20	14.0	350	490	630
18	12.6	315	441	567
16	11.2	280	392	504
14	9.8	245	343	441
12	8.4	210	294	378
10	7.0	175	245	315
8	5.6	140	196	252
6	4.2	105	147	189

Adapted from Sharkey 1984.

Chapter 15
Behavior Modification

```
Stages of Behavior Change
Exercise
Smoking
Drinking
Weight
Stress
```

The fitness leader engages in behavior modification by helping people to begin and continue regular exercise as part of their lifestyles. Fitness participants often look to the fitness leader to assist them in changing the behaviors they perceive to be unhealthy. Most individuals have one or more habits that prevent them from achieving the highest level of fitness and health. This chapter describes a model of behavior change with implications for five behaviors that are directly related to positive health. For many people, the healthy life includes one or more of the following: reducing smoking, alcohol intake, weight, and stress or increasing exercise. To help individuals adopt and maintain a healthier lifestyle, the fitness leader should understand the basic principles of behavior change and develop the skills to put these principles into practice.

Transtheoretical Model of Behavior Change

This model views change in one's behavior as a dynamic process through which attitudes, decisions, and actions evolve through different stages over a period of time—not an all-or-nothing one-time event.

Stages of Change

Many attempts at changing behavior assume that the individual is ready to change. This model recognizes that individuals are at different stages regarding change. These stages are as follows:

1. Precontemplation
2. Contemplation
3. Preparation
4. Action
5. Maintenance

Figure 15.1 describes the different strategies for the various stages.

Precontemplation. In this stage, an individual is not thinking seriously about changing a health behavior any time in the next 6 months and may deny the need to change. Encourage people at this stage to have their health risks and fitness levels assessed and to learn about the benefits of healthier behaviors.

Contemplation.   The second stage finds the individual seriously considering making changes within the next 6 months. Positive role models and clear guidelines on how to start the different behaviors are helpful at this stage.

Preparation.   The individual has decided to take action within the next month and is making plans. Goal setting, evaluation of benefits and barriers, a behavioral contract, and specific recommendations for the new behaviors can aid the person at this stage.

Action. This stage includes the first 6 months after modifying behavior. Social support, self-reinforcement, self-monitoring, and relapse prevention are important during this period.

Maintenance.   Maintenance of the modified behavior begins after 6 months of the action stage. Social support and self-reinforcement are still needed. In addition, review and revision of goals, with periodic assessment are helpful during this final stage.

Methods of Behavior Change

Later in the chapter, we discuss the problems of inactivity, smoking, alcoholism, excess fat, and stress and recommend some specific procedures for resolving them. The general plan outlined in table 15.1 has several components, but an individual won't necessarily use each step for every habit being changed. An individual's current stage of change will change the emphasis at different steps.

The fitness leader who is a good role model for the desired behavior and is supportive as the participant changes can help the participant throughout the behavior modification process. The first step is to analyze the problem. Analysis includes facing such questions as when the behavior started, what the conditions were, why it continues, when it last happened, and the conditions under which it usually occurs. You and the participant need to reach a mutual understanding of the problem. Collecting some baseline data concerning the extent of the behavior over a period of several days often aids the analysis. After the initial analysis, you and the participant should be able to clearly describe the current status of the problem.

Once you have analyzed the past and present, address the future by discussing goals. Goal statements concern future conditions and often include time constraints. Assist the person

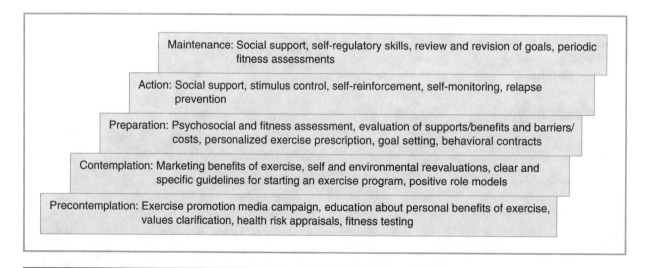

Figure 15.1 Intervention strategies for various stages of change.
Reprinted from Howley and Franks 1997.

Table 15.1 General Model for Changing Behavior

Step	Activity
1	Acknowledge desire to change.
2	Analyze history of problem.
3	Record current behavior.
4	Analyze current status.
5	Set long-term goals.
6	Set short-term goals.
7	Sign contract with friend(s).
8	List many possible strategies that could be used.
9	Select one or two strategies to use.
10	Learn new coping skills.
11	Establish regular contact with helper.
12	Once goal reached, outline potential maintenance problems.
13	Learn new coping skills.
14	Maintain periodic contact with helper.

Adapted from Howley and Franks 1986.

in making the desired goal realistic and clear. If the participant desires a great deal of behavior change, he should set subgoals. Achieving the goal of successful behavior for a single day may lead to 2 successful days, then 3, a week, and so on. To increase the chances of achieving the goal, he can earn a reward contingent on the successful accomplishment of the goal. He receives the reward only if the goal is reached.

A signed, written contract can also help a participant achieve goals. A written agreement, specifying the conditions to be met and the rewards or consequences if it is or is not met, is more successful if it is made between the individual who wants to change and a close friend. In some cases, groups contract to provide support to each other and increase everyone's level of commitment.

Once you and the participant have analyzed a problem and agreed to a goal, the next step is to determine a plan for reaching the goal. The first step in developing a plan is for you and the individual to brainstorm, listing as many different plans as possible without taking time to

evaluate each one. From this list, help the individual pick the one or two strategies that seem to have the best chance of success. Depending on the strategy selected, she may need to learn new coping behaviors, such as improving social skills, increasing professional competence, and learning how to relax or be assertive. The focus on particular coping behaviors depends upon what goals and strategies are selected.

An individual who has had difficulty in changing behavior in the past may experience feelings such as fear and helplessness about trying to change again. Help the individual express these feelings to you, thereby enabling him to go forward in spite of these feelings. After he has reached an initial goal, he enters a very difficult stage, namely, how to maintain the results in the long run. At this point the individual needs to recognize the environmental conditions under which old behaviors are likely to occur. Being able to recognize the onset of these potentially dangerous conditions increases the likelihood that he can take steps to avoid them. Long-term contact between you and the individual can maintain the change over time. This contact can become less frequent as the new behaviors become part of the individual's lifestyle.

Increasing Exercise

There is general agreement that exercise is good for people. The *Healthy People 2000* goals for the U.S. and the recent report from the Surgeon General on physical activity and health recommend regular physical activity. Exercise seems to be good both physiologically and psychologically. Earlier chapters in this book dealt with specific factors (e.g., intensity) needed for improvement in health and fitness as well as a variety of activities that you can have participants use to achieve these goals.

The current emphasis on and interest in fitness has brought many people into fitness programs. A major problem for many new fitness participants is sticking with it; indeed, up to 50% of participants quit within 6 months of starting a program. People more likely to drop out include those who smoke, have low self-motivation, lack social reinforcement, or believe that additional exercise is not needed. Reasons often given for quitting exercise are inconvenience and lack of time. Several strategies have been suggested that can help increase and maintain regular exercising:

1. Availability of program. Change is facilitated by accessible programs. Provide a program with convenient times and locations.

2. Social support. It is important to include the participant's family and (or) "significant others" (important persons such as spouse, work colleagues, or friends), so that they can encourage and support participation in the fitness program.

3. Emphasis on enjoyment. Learning new behaviors must be pleasurable if the participant is to discard old behaviors. Offer an upbeat fitness program and activities that create an enjoyable atmosphere in which fitness changes are more likely to take place. The performance approach (e.g., military or athletic) that aims only at producing results while making participants hate the exercise will not entice participants to adopt a lifelong fitness program. Emphasize the potential gains of new behavior rather than any negative aspects.

4. Program attributes. Qualified and enthusiastic personnel, regular assessment of important fitness components, relevant personal and general communication, and a variety of group and individual exercises, games, and sports that interest the participant are all qualities of a good fitness program. Physical exercise and socialization make a profitable combination, as evidenced by the success of many dance and physical fitness groups. Many people enjoy the social interaction with others, and a support group develops to help everyone continue the exercise.

5. Role models. People learn from each other and from others they admire. As a fitness leader, you should display healthy behaviors, enjoying a healthy lifestyle yourself.

In addition, an example of a contract to increase regular exercise is shown in table 15.2. As with all such forms, you can modify it to be more effective for a specific participant.

Stopping Smoking

There is little disagreement (outside cigarette-producing circles) that smoking is bad for your health. Indeed, there are ample data to show that smoking is the largest avoidable cause of death in the United States. Through warning labels on packages and in advertisements, virtually all American citizens are now aware of the dangers of smoking. Millions of people have quit smoking, but as smokers know, it is a hard habit to break.

Reasons for Smoking

Remember, our first step in changing behavior is to analyze the problem. Perhaps a brief summary of some of the reasons people smoke will help individuals understand their own reasons. Many smokers start and continue the habit because they smoke with friends or in certain situations. Others smoke while solving a problem, during a work break, watching a game, or after dinner. When does the individual smoke? Who else is around? What is he or she feeling?

The so-called "rewards" of smoking include the effects experienced when nicotine reaches the brain a few seconds after inhaling, giving the smoker a series of "highs." The decreasing aversion to the smoke itself is a positive reinforcement

Table 15.2 | Sample Contract to Begin Exercise

I, _____, do agree with _____
　　　　　　　　(your name)　　　　　　　　　　　　　　　　　　　　　　　　　(helper's name)

that I will begin the following walking program as of January 1, 2000:

1. I will walk from 7:00 to 7:30 A.M. on Monday, Wednesday, and Friday of each week.

2. I will record in writing my walking distance covered, and comments on a weekly form.

3. I will take this form to _____ each Sunday afternoon and discuss
　　　　　　　　　　　　　　　(helper's name)

    any problems I had as we walk together at 5:00 P.M.

4. In May, I will join the Plainview Fitness Center and attend a Tuesday-Thursday fitness class
   of my choice, continuing my Sunday afternoon walks with _____.
   　　　　　　　　　　　　　　　　　　　　　　　　　　　　　　　　　(helper's name)

I will reward myself with the purchase of one new cassette each week of perfect attendance in my program. At the end of each month of perfect attendance, I will buy a new compact disc of my choice. At the end of one year of perfect attendance, I will treat my helper and myself to a Broadway show in New York.

For each exercise session I miss, I will send a $25 contribution to the person who in my opinion is the most hypocritical politician.

_____　_____　_____
　　　　(Signed)　　　　　　　　　　　　　(Date)　　　　　　　　　　　(Witness)

---

of smoking. An addiction to smoking is similar to addiction to other drugs. There is a "craving" for a cigarette, and withdrawal symptoms make it a habit resistant to change. But individuals can break the habit, as millions have done.

Smoking Cessation Plan

The following plan for stopping smoking includes preparation, cessation, and maintenance.

Stage 1: Preparation. The individual needs to gain confidence that he can be successful in quitting smoking. Foster his self-confidence by setting clear goals and determining procedures to follow. During the first stage, have him monitor the current frequency of smoking. This self-observation often helps to temporarily reduce the smoking behavior.

Stage 2: Cessation. Ending the smoking behavior abruptly has been found to be more effective than gradually cutting down. An effective method for stopping smoking is to have the individual sign a contract to quit on a specific

date. The behavioral contract involves a specific agreement between you and the smoker. Be sure to specify the goal in precise behavioral terms. Clearly describe the behavior, or the lack of the behavior, and link it to a time constraint. The contract should also specify what contingency comes into effect if the contract is broken. The contract should be individually tailored to the individual's capabilities and needs. Determine the answer to the question "How long does the individual have to refrain from smoking to feel that the habit has been broken?" Help develop the contract so it contains the contingencies that are most likely to help the person abide by the conditions of the contract. Maintain frequent contact with the individual during the early part of the contract for encouragement and discussion of unanticipated problems.

Another smoking cessation strategy that has a good record of success is rapid smoking. This strategy is based on the principle of satiation whereby an individual is encouraged to smoke as rapidly and continuously as possible until becoming sick and having to quit. Because of the possibility of nicotine poisoning along with physiological abnormalities, this must only be done under medical guidance or supervision.

Stage 3: Maintenance. Once again, an old joke makes a good point. The person says, "Stopping smoking is easy—I've done it hundreds of times!" The real problem, of course, is to find ways to keep from starting to smoke again after quitting. Your continuing contact with the individual and help developing new behavioral skills are essential ingredients in maintaining the behavioral change.

How? Help the participant learn the advantages of a smokeless life (e.g., lower risk of major health problems, less stress in daily activities). The individual may have to learn new skills to deal with old stimuli that were associated with cigarette smoking. If drinking coffee at the end of a meal was an old cue to light up, then perhaps avoiding coffee and drinking tea instead may eliminate that cue. If cigarette smoke in the lobby of a basketball arena during halftime provided a cue for lighting up, then either remaining seated in the arena or chewing gum in the lobby might be a new behavior. Once again we emphasize that determining what new behaviors are needed and what will be effective often involves talking about potential problem situations with the individual.

Table 15.3 is a sample contract for stopping smoking. You can modify this form to be more effective for a particular individual or to serve as a contract for other behavior change.

Reducing Alcohol Consumption

Alcoholism is one of our nation's leading public health problems. It is estimated that there are between 5 and 15 million alcoholics in the United States. The problems of family disruption, lost time at work, bodily injury, and death that are directly and indirectly due to excessive drinking are not disputed even by the producers of alcoholic beverages. Indeed, drinking

---

Table 15.3	**Sample Contract to Stop Smoking**

I, _____ , do agree with _____ to the following:
    (your name)   (helper's name)

1. Stop smoking as of 6:00 A.M., January 1, 2000.

2. I will call my helper each night at 7:00 P.M. during January, every Thursday night from February through May, and on the first of each month starting in June. We will discuss the problems I have had since our last call and set a time to meet if I need to talk with her in person.

3. During January, I will do the following at those times when, based on my past experience, I am most tempted to smoke:

   (a) Rub my pet rock with my right hand while talking with friends at social affairs

   (b) Eat fruit following dinner each night

   (c) Play a game of solitaire prior to going to sleep each night

I will reward myself with the purchase of one new cassette each week that I go without smoking. At the end of each smokeless month, I will buy a new compact disc of my choice. At the end of one year without smoking, I will treat my helper and myself to a Broadway show in New York.

For each cigarette I smoke during the year, I will send a $25 contribution to the person who in my opinion is the most hypocritical politician.

_____   _____   _____
        (Signed)   (Date)   (Witness)

problems exact a heavy toll on the health and financial well-being of the people of our nation.

Though there is agreement on the reality of the alcoholism problem, debate on appropriate goals for treating the problem is heated. Should an alcoholic strive for controlled moderate drinking or complete abstinence? Those who feel that abstinence is the correct goal tend to conceptualize the problem as a disease. The successful treatment approach of Alcoholics Anonymous (AA) is based on the disease concept. One fundamental precept of AA is that a person who has the disease of alcoholism will always have it: there is no cure. AA believes that combating the "disease" requires total abstinence. Alcoholics Anonymous helps individuals to achieve this goal with the support of other alcoholics via person-to-person contacts and regular group meetings.

Others contend that alcoholism is not a disease and that no crucial difference distinguishes the social drinker from the problem drinker besides the amount of alcohol consumed. Four factors that determine the probability of whether an individual will indulge in excessive drinking have been proposed: (a) the degree to which the individual feels controlled, (b) the availability of an adequate coping response, (c) expectations about the results of the drinking, and (d) availability of alcohol and situational constraints. For example, (a) at a New Year's Eve party, there is strong pressure to drink; (b) there may not be an adequate coping response, for example, the individual is unable to ask for a soft drink and requests liquor instead; (c) there may be pleasant memories of previous New Year's Eve parties that included excessive drinking; and (d) there is plenty of alcohol available, and party-goers are expected to consume it.

Abstinence or Controlled Drinking

The individual must decide which choice is appropriate. In general, someone with a history of chronic alcohol abuse who has developed serious life problems associated with drinking may be more suited to the complete abstinence approach. A younger person who is open to learning new social skills may respond well to the controlled drinking approach.

Controlled Drinking

If individuals believe that they can control their drinking, the following ideas may help. Social skills training to reduce excessive drinking normally includes instruction in assertive response, refusing alcohol, relapse prevention, and ways to obtain reinforcement other than from drinking. In assertiveness training people learn how to communicate their feelings in a productive, caring manner. This type of training may help those whose excessive drinking behavior is related to an inability to communicate feelings to intimates and other associates. Learning how to refuse alcoholic drinks is also important. Some alcoholics simply do not know what to say to refuse a drink. Help individuals learn and practice ways of refusing a drink.

Many techniques can enable an individual to abstain or drink less for a given period of time. It is difficult, however, to maintain these improvements over a long period. Thus, relapse prevention is probably the most important component of the social skills training plan. One of the key elements in maintaining the desired behavior is to be able to anticipate problem situations. Planning ways to avoid problems before the problems actually arise can help participants discover behaviors other than excessive drinking that can provide positive reinforcement from peers and important others. For example, improving conversation or storytelling skills can substitute for excessive drinking in some situations. You can have participants practice new skills and responses through role-playing to help them avoid relapses. Help individuals learn to discuss their feelings and coping behaviors in potential problem situations.

Achieving Desired Weight

Obesity seems to be more difficult to overcome than either smoking or problem drinking. Fewer than 5% of obese individuals successfully maintain a lower weight, whereas 20% to 25% report success at quitting smoking or alcohol abuse. One problem seems to be emphasizing "negative change" goals rather than developing healthy substitute behaviors. For example, instead of concentrating on eating less cheese, have the individual choose a positive change, such as planning to eat fruit at snack time. Another problem is the disregard for either energy intake or energy expenditure. Both decreased caloric intake and increased exercise (caloric expenditure) are normally essential for maintaining desired weight. Either one by itself dooms most people to failure (see also chapter 5). Another problem is the direct attack on the behavior rather than on the indirect reasons for the behavior. If a particular cue results in poor eating behavior, then an individual must learn to either avoid the cue or react to it differently. To this end, keep in mind that the ready access of food and drink and media messages promoting a relationship between happiness and what is consumed contribute to the problems people have trying to change their eating behaviors.

Chapter 5 deals with methods of determining percent fat and estimating ideal weight. It is important that individuals work toward the goal gradually in ways they can accept physiologically and psychologically.

You should not recommend a single weight loss program to everyone. The following seven components, however, appear to be common ingredients in all successful programs. Much of an individual's success depends on deciding what steps to take and what is likely to work for the individual to make it happen.

1. Self-monitoring. Before any specific steps are implemented, have the person keep a daily diary for 2 weeks. The diary should describe the quantity of food eaten and the eating environments (see chapter 6, table 6.5, for a form).

2. Treatment goals. Help the person determine the ultimate goal of ideal weight, then set weekly goals (from 1/2 to 2 lb per week). Medical supervision should be provided for extremely obese persons (>40% fat if female; >30% fat if male).

3. Diet selection. Assist the individual in selecting a dietary plan that specifies food type, portions, and calorie amounts. Several sound diets are available (see chapter 6).

4. Stimulus control. Certain situations or cues often are strongly related to eating patterns (e.g., watching a movie or television). Have the person decide to eat only at certain places (e.g., the dining room table, the cafeteria at work) and at certain times (e.g., breakfast, lunch, supper, and one snack time).

5. Self-reward. Some people are helped by giving themselves small rewards for progress toward their goals (e.g., a new audiotape for each 3-lb loss) and a larger reward (e.g., tickets to a Broadway show) when they reach the final goal. The rewards should be consistent with healthy behaviors, something the individual enjoys, and things for which there are no acceptable alternatives.

6. Exercise. An earlier section of this chapter dealt with ways to begin and continue regular exercise. Although everyone who begins an exercise program does not necessarily need to begin a weight reduction program, remember, most people who need to lose fat should begin diet and exercise programs simultaneously.

7. Support. The awareness and support of a spouse or other important person can greatly assist the person in staying with the program. Involving friends or family members early in the program enhances its probability of success.

Reducing Stress

Attempts to understand human stress and to develop plans to alleviate it are relatively recent. Although some have emphasized the stress response or the condition causing the stress (stressor), we recommend that you help individuals pay attention to their interactions with potential stressors as a way to reduce excessive stress. Help people work through the following suggested steps.

Three stages of stress reduction are preparation, skill acquisition, and practice. In the preparation stage, the individual is prepared mentally for a coming stressful situation. She keeps a diary regarding the frequency of and conditions surrounding the chosen stressor.

The skill acquisition stage mainly emphasizes learning basic cognitive and behavioral coping skills. One of the skills is "private speech," for which the individual learns sentences to repeat privately prior to, during, and following the stressor. For example, prior to a major test or presentation of a report the person tells himself, "It's going to be hard, but I have prepared for it." During the event: "If I stay calm I will be less likely to block on a question," and (or) "I'm going to relax and take it easy." Following the event: "I did as well as I could because I stayed calm."

A second component of the skill acquisition stage is relaxation training. An example of tensing and relaxing specific muscle groups was presented in chapter 11. With practice, an individual can rapidly achieve a relaxed state in a potentially stressful situation.

In the final or practice stage, individuals are presented with a series of practice situations that help them learn to apply the previously taught skills. The sequence of situations progresses from relatively mild to more severe stress so that they can experience success and gain confidence in using the skills.

Summary

One of the primary responsibilities of a fitness program is to help participants modify lifestyle behaviors. Understanding the stages of behavior change can assist you in choosing a strategy to help individuals. Although the focus is on increasing exercise, you should make it clear that participants need to decrease unhealthy behaviors as well. These behaviors include smoking, excessive alcohol consumption, overeating, and stress. Each of these behaviors is discussed in terms of what causes them and the methods a person can use to change the specific behavior. As you saw, some common characteristics exist among the behavior change techniques. Following these guidelines can assist you in helping people change their behavior if they so desire.

If a participant wishes to change a behavior, analyze the history of the problem and record the current status of the behavior. Help the individual set a long-term goal and several short-term goals, then have him or her sign a contract. List as many strategies as possible to resolve the problem, helping the individual select one or two that will be most effective. In this way, the fitness leader can help the individual learn new coping skills. Once the individual reaches the goal, help him or her outline a maintenance schedule that includes periodic contacts.

PART V
Scientific Foundations

Exercise Science
Measurement and Evaluation

This fifth part of the *Fitness Leader's Handbook* provides a brief overview of the scientific bases for fitness programs.

Chapter 16 deals with aspects of physiology and biomechanics directly related to fitness. Chapter 17 deals with measurement and evaluation concepts that are related to physical fitness testing.

Chapter 16
Basic Exercise Science

Physiology of Fitness
Functional Anatomy and Biomechanics

The purpose of this chapter is to provide the scientific information on which we have based most of our fitness recommendations. The chapter is divided into two major sections: physiology of fitness and anatomy and biomechanics. In the first section, we will discuss the energy for muscle contraction, how the cardiorespiratory system responds to exercise, and how men and women differ in their responses to the same exercise. In the second section, we will present information on anatomy as it relates to physical activity. Though some people, like our friend in figure 16.1, may find this information overwhelming, we hope that we can tie some things together.

Physiology Related to Fitness

Relationship of Energy to Work

The body needs energy to do work, any kind of work. There are different kinds of energy in the body:

- *Electrical energy* is involved in the transmission of impulses in nerves and muscles.
- *Chemical energy* is stored during the synthesis of large molecules from smaller molecules, for example, proteins from amino acids.
- *Mechanical energy* is the result of a muscle causing a bone to move.

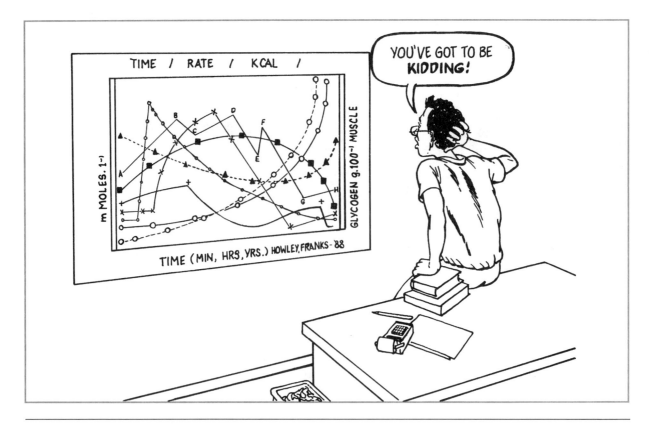

Figure 16.1 Scientific base.

- *Thermal (heat) energy* is derived from all these processes to keep the body warm.

Where do we obtain the energy for all these processes? The sun is the ultimate source of this energy; plants capture the sun's energy and use it to convert carbon, oxygen, hydrogen, and nitrogen into carbohydrates, fats, and proteins. It is this food energy that provides all the energy the body uses to breathe, think, and run.

Energy is contained in the chemical bonds of carbohydrates, fats, and protein, but for that energy to be used by the nerves, muscles, and other cells, it must first be converted into *adenosine triphosphate* (ATP), because that is the only form of energy that cells use. It is important to remember that ATP must be delivered to a cell as fast as it is used or the cell slows down or dies. ATP must be delivered to muscles at extremely high rates when a person runs a short distance and for hours on end as in a 26-mi, 385-yd marathon. To simplify our discussion of how this is done, we have divided the energy supply to the muscle into three categories based on how fast and how long it can continue to deliver ATP to the muscles.

Immediate Sources of Energy

Our muscles have a very small store of ATP that would last about 1 s during intensive exercise. In addition, we have another high energy compound called *creatine phosphate* (CP) that can replace ATP almost instantaneously. However, CP lasts only about 3 to 5 s during intensive activity. As you can see, these immediate sources provide quick energy when we need it but do not last long. Oxygen is not required for this, so we classify these as *anaerobic* (without oxygen) sources of energy.

Short-Term Sources of ATP

As our immediate sources of ATP are running out, we can obtain additional ATP at a rapid rate through the breakdown of muscle glycogen (the glucose store in muscle). This process is also anaerobic and can supply ATP for strenuous activities lasting less than 2 min. The by-product of the anaerobic breakdown of glucose is *lactic acid*, which may interfere with this energy-producing process as well as with the actual means by which a muscle contracts. Though this obviously presents problems, this anaerobic source of ATP allows us to run at a high rate of speed when we must. A goal in fitness programs is to minimize the use of this process, because it contributes to fatigue.

Long-Term Sources of Energy

Most of the ATP used by the body is derived from using fats and carbohydrates in the presence of oxygen. This is sometimes referred to as *aerobic* (with oxygen) energy production, in contrast to anaerobic energy production. On the one hand, this aerobic process does not produce ATP at as fast a rate as the anaerobic processes, taking as long as 3 min or so to meet the ATP demand of the muscle. On the other hand, the aerobic processes can supply ATP on a "pay-as-you-go" basis, allowing activity to continue for long periods of time. The oxygen needed for this process is delivered by the blood that is pumped to the muscles by the heart. This is the crucial link between the type of energy production at the muscle and the cardiovascular training effect that occurs in fitness programs. Thus, the emphasis in fitness programs should be on using submaximal activities that will require aerobic energy-producing processes in the muscle, which, in turn, stimulate the heart to deliver the necessary blood. But which of these anaerobic or aerobic energy-producing processes is most important in physical activity?

The answer depends on the type of physical activity. In maximal activities lasting less than a minute the anaerobic (immediate and short-term) sources of ATP supply most of the energy. In all-out activities lasting 2 min, the anaerobic and aerobic processes supply equal amounts of ATP, while for activities lasting 10 min, the contribution of ATP from anaerobic energy processes accounts for only 15% of the total.

Part of the reason for this variation in the use of aerobic and anaerobic energy production processes is found in the type of muscle fiber used in the activity. In very intensive, high-speed activities we use *fast twitch* muscle fibers, which produce ATP primarily through anaerobic processes, resulting in the production of lactic acid. *Slow twitch* muscle fibers produce only small amounts of tension but are extremely resistant to fatigue due to the fact that most of

their energy comes from aerobic processes. These slow twitch muscle fibers have more *capillaries* to carry oxygen to the muscle and more mitochondria to produce ATP with oxygen. With endurance training both fast and slow twitch muscle fibers improve their capacity to produce energy by aerobic means due to an increase in capillaries and mitochondria. This results in less lactic acid production and accumulation and therefore a greater resistance to fatigue.

Metabolic, Cardiovascular, and Respiratory Responses to Exercise

Fitness activities are used to provide an adequate stimulus to the cardiorespiratory system to improve or maintain function and to expend calories. This section presents basic information on how energy production and the cardiorespiratory system respond to both submaximal exercise and a graded exercise test taken to the subject's limits.

Submaximal "Steady-State" Exercise

The oxygen used for ATP production comes from the blood that is delivered to the muscles by the cardiovascular system. The respiratory system (lungs and respiratory muscles) moves the oxygen from the atmosphere to the blood. It is the coordinated activity of these two systems that results in the correct amount of oxygen reaching the muscles, allowing us to continue our workout over a period of 30 to 40 min. As oxygen delivery to the muscles cannot increase instantaneously in the first seconds of exercise, how do we meet the energy requirement during this time?

Let's consider, for example, an individual standing at rest alongside a treadmill with its belt running at 6 mph. On command, the person jumps onto the belt. Figure 16.2 shows the oxygen uptake over the course of the 5-min run that is followed by a 3-min recovery. The symbols on the graph show what the oxygen uptake is at each minute. While the person stands alongside the treadmill, the resting oxygen uptake value is .25 $L \cdot min^{-1}$, but this value increases rapidly during

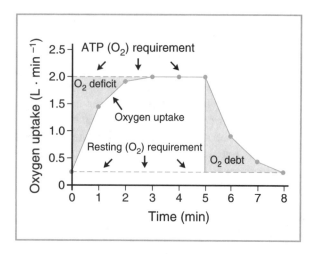

Figure 16.2 Changes in the respiratory exchange ratio during prolonged steady-state exercise. Reprinted from Howley and Franks 1997.

the first minute and more slowly over the next 2 min. By the third minute the oxygen uptake meets the steady-state oxygen requirement needed to continue the exercise, with virtually all the ATP produced by aerobic processes. As the oxygen uptake does not increase immediately during the first seconds of exercise, the body is said to incur an *oxygen deficit* during this period. During the oxygen deficit the immediate and short-term sources of ATP provide the ATP that the aerobic processes cannot. This is a good example of how the three energy sources of ATP (immediate, short-term, and long-term) work together to allow us to gradually make the transition from rest to exercise and continue the activity for 30 to 40 min. If we did not have these anaerobic sources of ATP at the start of the treadmill run, we would not be able to meet the ATP requirement and would have drifted off the back of the treadmill! When the run is completed, the person jumps off and stands alongside the treadmill. Oxygen uptake does not immediately return to the resting level; this "extra" oxygen consumed over and above the resting level is called the *oxygen debt* or excess postexercise oxygen consumption (EPOC). The body uses some of the additional oxygen to make the ATP needed to restore the creatine phosphate (immediate source of ATP) store back to normal. Meanwhile, the body uses about 20% of the "extra" oxygen to convert some of the lactic acid back to glucose in the liver. The remainder is used to support the activities of the various systems that do not immediately recover

at the cessation of exercise—like heart rate and breathing.

If a person can reach the steady-state oxygen requirement sooner after the initiation of exercise, a smaller oxygen deficit is incurred and the person depletes less CP and produces less lactic acid because the body relies less on the anaerobic sources of energy. Participation in a fitness program causes changes in the capillaries and mitochondria of muscles as well as the cardiovascular system so that oxygen uptake increases to the steady state more rapidly at the onset of exercise. People with low levels of cardiorespiratory fitness take longer to reach the steady state, producing more ATP from anaerobic processes with a higher lactic acid level the result.

This link between cardiorespiratory fitness and the ability to use oxygen should be no surprise given the purposes of these systems. Figure 16.3 shows heart rate (HR) and ventilation (liters of air breathed per minute [L·min⁻¹]) responses to the treadmill test. As you can see, neither HR nor ventilation increases immediately at the start of exercise; both follow a pattern very similar to the oxygen uptake curve. This gradual increase in both helps to explain the "lag" in oxygen uptake at the onset of work. Another part of the lag is explained by the mitochondria, which cannot instantaneously increase their ATP-generating ability. The more mitochondria you have, however, the faster the oxygen uptake can increase at the onset of work. That is the mark of an endurance-trained person.

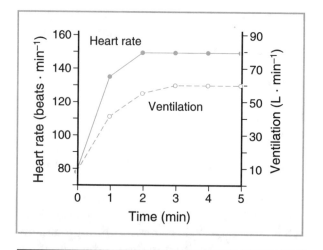

Figure 16.3 Heart rate and pulmonary-ventilation responses during a 5-min run on a treadmill. Reprinted from Howley and Franks 1997.

Graded Exercise Test. Given that our ability to do sustained exercise depends on the cardiovascular system's ability to deliver oxygen to the working muscles, it should be no surprise that we use exercise tests to determine cardiorespiratory function. In a *graded exercise test* (GXT), the subject completes a series of progressively more difficult exercise tasks until a defined end point, such as 85% of maximal HR or voluntary exhaustion, is reached. The GXT can be done on a treadmill with the walking speed constant and the grade increasing 3% each 3 min, or a cycle ergometer (a stationary cycle on which the workload can be set) on which the pedaling resistance increases at 3-min intervals. During each stage (3-min work period) of the GXT, a wide variety of physiological measures can be monitored: heart rate (HR), blood pressure (BP), electrocardiogram (ECG), oxygen uptake, ventilation, and blood lactic acid. Each of these measures provides an indication of how well a person is adjusting to the exercise, which is related to the subject's present level of fitness.

Oxygen Uptake and Maximal Aerobic Power. Oxygen uptake can be measured at each stage of the GXT. In figure 16.3, oxygen uptake is expressed in milliliters of oxygen per kilogram per minute ($ml \cdot kg^{-1} \cdot min^{-1}$) instead of $L \cdot min^{-1}$. This allows comparison of people with different body weights. As you can see in figure 16.4, oxygen uptake increases in a regular pattern with each stage of the test and levels off as the oxygen requirement is met. This pattern continues until the body reaches its cardiorespiratory system limits. At that point, oxygen uptake does not increase when the grade of the treadmill is increased. The point at which oxygen uptake levels off is called the subject's *maximal aerobic power*. This term describes the following:

1. The maximal rate at which the cardiorespiratory system can deliver oxygen to the working muscles. In this way, maximal oxygen uptake (or maximal aerobic power) is a measure of cardiorespiratory fitness.

2. The maximal rate at which ATP can be produced aerobically. This indicates how well someone can perform in long-distance runs, swims, cycle competitions, and cross-country skiing.

An untrained person participating in an endurance training program can increase maxi-

mal aerobic power about 5% to 25%; the less fit the individual, the larger the gains. The dashed line in figure 16.4 shows oxygen uptake after a training program. Steady-state oxygen uptake reached at each stage is about the same, but the person achieves the steady-state value a little sooner following training. At the end of the test, oxygen uptake increases when the treadmill grade is raised to 18%, indicating that the person's cardiovascular system can now deliver more blood to the working muscles than before training, when the leveling-off point was at the 15% grade. In spite of the increase in maximal aerobic power an individual can achieve through training, the average person is not likely to become a world-class endurance athlete. Table 16.1 presents average values for maximal aerobic power ($\dot{V}O_2max$) in a variety of groups, from the elite to those with serious disease. The link of maximal aerobic power to endurance performance is seen in the classes of athletes with the highest values—cross-country skiers and distance runners. Women's values are about 15% lower than those of men, independent of the group, and, not surprisingly, people with cardiovascular or respiratory disease have the lowest values. Maximal aerobic power decreases with age (about 1% per year) in the

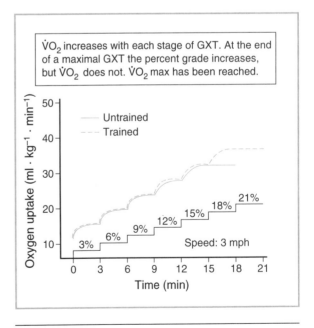

Figure 16.4 Oxygen uptake responses to a graded exercise test.

Reprinted from Howley and Franks 1997.

Table 16.1	Maximal Aerobic Power ($ml \cdot kg^{-1} \cdot min^{-1}$) Measured in Healthy and Diseased Populations	
Population	**Males VO$_2$max**	**Females VO$_2$max**
Cross-country skiers	82	66
Distance runners	79	62
College students	45	38
Middle-aged adults	35	30
Postmyocardial infarction patients	22	18
Severe pulmonary-diseased patients	13	13

Adapted from McArdle, Katch, and Katch 1986.

average population; the decrease is related to the fact that we tend to become more sedentary and heavy as we grow older. Both of these factors, independent of age, decrease maximal aerobic power. Some recent evidence suggests that in those who stay active and do not put on weight, maximal aerobic power decreases only half as fast. This certainly is another good reason to stay active, because a fit person has greater freedom to choose recreational activities later in life. Let's look, now, at what happens to some of the other measures during a GXT.

Blood Lactic Acid. Figure 16.5 shows the changes in blood lactic acid during the GXT mentioned earlier. The lactic acid level begins to increase when the intensity of the test exceeds about 60% of the person's maximal oxygen uptake. This indicates that the working muscles are now producing the lactic acid faster than other tissues (liver, heart, other muscles) can use it. This sudden increase in lactic acid concentration has been called the *anaerobic threshold* or the *lactate threshold* (LT). Figure 16.5 shows that, with training, an individual can work at higher intensities of exercise before the lactic acid level begins to increase. This is due primarily to the increase in the capillaries and mitochondria of the trained muscles, which allows the body to produce more ATP aerobically.

Heart Rate. Figure 16.6 shows the HR response to the same GXT. At very low work rates, HR

doesn't change much when the treadmill grade is increased. However, when HR reaches about 110 beats·min^{-1} it increases in a regular manner with increases in the grade of the treadmill. In this way, HR is a good indicator of how much oxygen an individual is using. This linear increase in HR is the basis for all submaximal GXTs used to predict the subject's maximal oxygen uptake. In these submaximal tests, you can measure the subject's HR at several submaximal work rates, draw a line through those points, and extend it to the subject's estimated maximal HR. You then can estimate the subject's maximal aerobic power from the grade of the treadmill that would have been achieved if the subject had been allowed to work until maximal HR was reached. Thus, you can estimate maximal aerobic power with the subject doing only submaximal work (see chapter 7 for details). Because of this linear relationship between HR and oxygen consumption, HR is the best predictor of exercise intensity and is a very sensitive indicator of the training state. Figure 16.6 shows the large change in the HR line after a training program. The subject accomplishes each submaximal stage of the GXT with a lower HR, indicating an improvement in the cardiovascular response to exercise. Two important points to remember are the following:

1. The subject's maximal HR either does not change or decreases slightly with training.

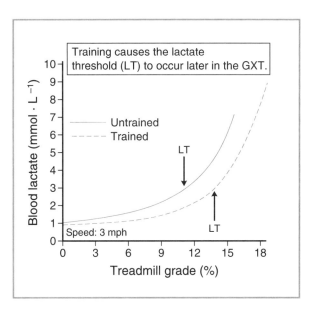

Figure 16.5 Changes in the blood lactic acid (lactate) concentration during a graded exercise test. LT indicates lactate threshold.

Reprinted from Howley and Franks 1997.

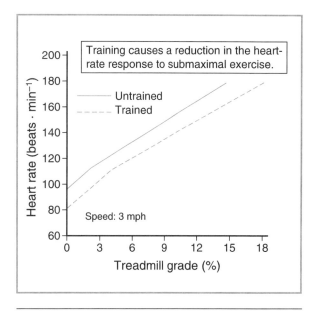

Figure 16.6 The heart rate response to a graded exercise test.

Reprinted from Ekblom, Åstrand, Saltin, Stenberg, and Wallstrom 1968.

2. If you are using the 220 – age formula for estimating maximal HR, remember that the error in estimation can be considerable. A 30-year-old could have a maximal HR of 160 to 220 beats·min⁻¹ instead of 190 beats·min⁻¹ (68% of 30-year-olds measure between about 180 and 200 beats·min⁻¹).

Stroke Volume and Cardiac Output. The volume of blood pumped from the heart per beat is called the *stroke volume.* The product of heart rate and stroke volume determines the volume of blood pumped to the tissues per minute; this is called the *cardiac output.* Figures 16.7 and 16.8 show how these measures respond to a GXT. For exercise in the upright position (e.g., cycling, walking), stroke volume increases slightly during the first few minutes of a GXT until a work rate of about 40% of maximal oxygen uptake is reached; stroke volume then levels off. This means that beyond 40% of maximal oxygen uptake, HR is the only factor causing the cardiac output to increase. It is this fact that makes HR such a good indicator of how hard the heart is working and how close it is to its maximum limits. With training, stroke volume increases, allowing the cardiac output to be higher than before in spite

of no change in maximal heart rate. In this way, the primary cardiovascular variable causing the increase in maximal aerobic power is the increase in maximal stroke volume.

Oxygen Extraction. The amount of oxygen taken up by the body depends on two factors: the volume of blood circulated to the tissues per minute (cardiac output) and the volume of oxygen extracted from the arterial blood during one pass around the circulatory system (oxygen extraction). Oxygen extraction is expressed as the number of milliliters of oxygen taken from one liter of blood (ml O_2·L⁻¹). Figure 16.9 shows the changes in oxygen extraction with increasing oxygen uptake.

As the work rate increases, the number of muscles involved also increases. This brings more and more blood into the capillaries where the oxygen can be given up to mitochondria, which use it to produce ATP. With an endurance training program, the ability to extract oxygen increases, explaining about 50% of the increase in maximal aerobic power that occurs with training.

In table 16.1, we showed the tremendous variability that exists in maximal aerobic power among different groups, some groups having

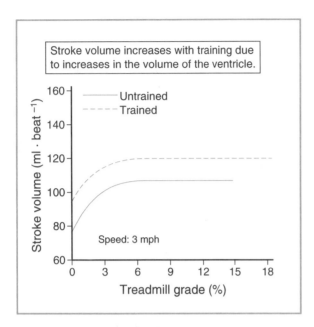

Figure 16.7 The stroke volume response to a graded exercise test.

Reprinted from Ekblom, Åstrand, Saltin, Stenberg, and Wallstrom 1968.

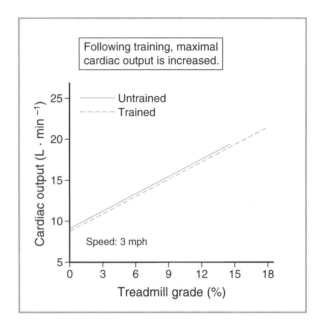

Figure 16.8 The cardiac output response to a graded exercise test.

Reprinted from Ekblom, Åstrand, Saltin, Stenberg, and Wallstrom 1968.

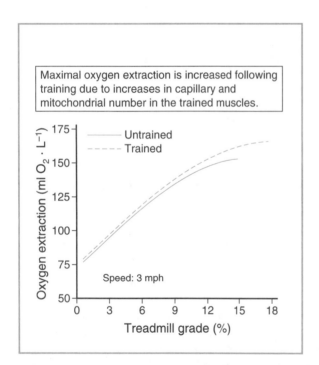

Figure 16.9 The changes in oxygen extraction (difference between the oxygen content of arterial blood and the mixed venous blood in the right heart) during a graded exercise test.

Reprinted from Ekblom, Åstrand, Saltin, Stenberg, and Wallstrom 1968.

levels twice as high as others have. What causes such variability? For the most part the variability can be explained by variations in maximal cardiac outputs among the different groups, because maximal oxygen extraction is only slightly higher in trained subjects. Highly trained subjects may have cardiac outputs more than 50% higher than those of their sedentary counterparts. But is maximal cardiac output in the trained person due to a higher maximal HR or a higher stroke volume? The following examples will answer this question:

Maximal Cardiac Output =

Maximal Heart Rate · Maximal Stroke Volume

Trained athlete: 30 L·min⁻¹ = 190 beats·min⁻¹ x .16 L·beat⁻¹

Untrained person: 20 L·min⁻¹ = 200 beats·min⁻¹ x .10 L·beat⁻¹

As you can see, the higher maximal cardiac output in the trained athlete is due exclusively to the higher stroke volume. This higher stroke volume is due to both genetic factors as well as the training effect that causes the ventricle of the heart to be larger. This is a functional enlargement of the heart, because the heart has a greater capacity to pump oxygen-rich blood to the muscles.

Blood Pressure. Figure 16.10 shows the blood pressure response to the GXT used in the previous figures. The *systolic pressure* increases in a regular manner with increasing exercise intensity, and the *diastolic pressure* remains about the same or decreases slightly. If during a GXT the systolic pressure *fails to increase* or the diastolic pressure increases when the grade is increased, this indicates that the subject is approaching the limits of the cardiovascular system. An endurance training program tends to lower the blood pressure of those who were borderline hypertensive prior to the program.

When HR and BP are elevated during exercise, the heart is working hard and is consuming oxygen at a high rate. A measure of the work of the heart is the *double product*, which is the product of the HR and the systolic BP. As we have seen, following an endurance training program, the HR response to a work task is lower, indicating that the work of the heart is decreased (HR x systolic BP). This is important, especially for those with a compromised coronary artery circulation that must supply blood to the heart. If the oxygen demand of the heart is less because of the lower HR, the arteries are more likely to be able to meet that demand.

Pulmonary Ventilation. The volume of air breathed per minute is called the pulmonary ventilation. Figure 16.11 shows that ventilation increases in a linear manner until about 60% of the person's maximal work rate is reached and then rises more quickly. This sudden increase in ventilation (a slight hyperventilation) is called the *ventilatory threshold,* and some use this as a noninvasive indicator of the lactate threshold (noninvasive means that no blood is taken). With training, the ventilatory response is less at each work rate and the ventilatory threshold is shifted to the right.

Summary of the Effects of Endurance Training and Detraining. A wide variety of physiological (HR), structural (mitochondria), and biochemical (enzyme) changes occur as a result of participation in endurance exercise:

• The number of mitochondria and capillaries increase in all active muscle fibers. This results in an increased ability to transport oxygen from the blood to the muscle and an increased capacity of the muscle to use oxygen for energy production.

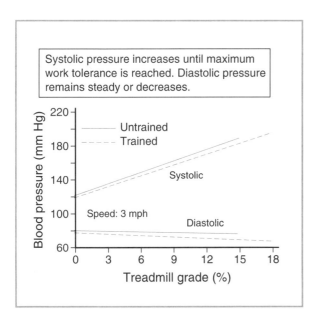

Figure 16.10 The systolic and diastolic blood pressure responses to a graded exercise test. Reprinted from Howley and Franks 1997.

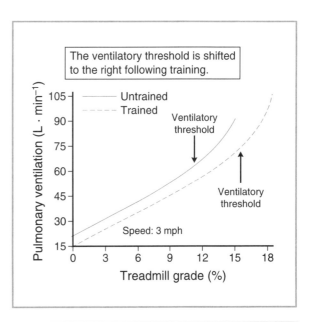

Figure 16.11 The pulmonary ventilation response to a graded exercise test. Reprinted from Howley and Franks 1997.

• The time it takes to get to the steady state in submaximal work is decreased. This reduces the oxygen deficit and the production and accumulation of lactic acid in the muscle and blood.

• The size (diameter) of the ventricle of the heart is increased, allowing more blood to be pumped with each beat of the heart (stroke volume). This results in the "classic" training effect seen when an individual can do the same work rate after training at a lower heart rate (and perception of effort).

• Cardiorespiratory fitness ($\dot{V}O_2$max) is increased as a result of the increased stroke volume (able to pump more blood to the muscles during maximal work) and the increased number of capillaries and mitochondria in the trained muscles (able to extract more oxygen from the blood).

An individual can maintain these training effects as long as she continues to participate in endurance exercise. If she stops training, the adaptations listed return toward their pretraining values. If, however, the person chooses to simply reduce the duration or frequency of training (by 1/3 or 2/3), $\dot{V}O_2$max is not affected very much. In contrast, when the intensity of the workout is reduced by 1/3 or 2/3, $\dot{V}O_2$max is decreased. The data suggest that it is easier to maintain a training effect if exercise intensity is maintained at a high level. This, however, can cause problems for the occasional exerciser (see chapter 18 on injury prevention).

Cardiovascular Responses to Exercise for Males and Females.
Earlier in this chapter we mentioned that maximal aerobic power is about 15% lower for females than for males. This is true for all ages after puberty and for all levels of physical ability. Why? The answer is found primarily in three factors: heart size relative to body size, body fat, and hemoglobin levels in the blood.

Heart Size. At adolescence, females develop a smaller heart size relative to their increase in body size. As a result, they cannot transport as much blood during maximal exercise compared to a male of the same size. This limits oxygen delivery and, consequently, oxygen uptake at the tissues.

Body Fat. At puberty, the female increases body fat percentage more than the male, which results in about 10% higher essential fat for females. Given the fact that maximal aerobic power is expressed in units relative to body weight (you must divide body weight into the measured oxygen uptake), the value for females will be lower than that of males, everything else being equal. We mentioned this effect of added fat earlier in our explanation of why maximal aerobic power decreases with age.

Hemoglobin. Oxygen is transported in the blood bound to hemoglobin, which is found in the red blood cells. The female has about 130 g of hemoglobin in a liter of blood, compared to 150 g for the male. Thus, the male can transport more oxygen per liter of blood.

Submaximal Exercise. These three factors also affect how a woman responds to submaximal exercise compared to her male counterpart. When a male and female exercise at the same work rate on a cycle ergometer, each has to transport the same amount of oxygen to tissues. As a result of the differences between males and females listed above, there will have to be higher physiological responses for the female compared to the male for the following reasons:

1. Due to the lower stroke volume (related to a smaller heart size), the female's heart rate has to be higher to compensate.

2. Due to the lower hemoglobin level, the female's cardiac output has to be slightly higher during submaximal work to deliver the same amount of oxygen to the tissues (as there is less oxygen per liter of blood). This increase in cardiac output is brought about by a higher HR.

The difference in body fatness between the sexes also causes a difference in the physiological responses to exercise when body weight is being carried along, as in walking or running. In these activities, the amount of oxygen used in the activity is proportional to body weight. If a male runs at 6 mph, approximately 35 ml of oxygen is required per kilogram of body weight per minute (35 ml·kg^{-1}·min^{-1}) to maintain that speed. If we now add 10 kg to that person's back, the oxygen requirement is still the same per kilogram of weight (35 ml), but the total amount of oxygen required to continue the activity with the higher weight is 350 ml more per minute (10 kg x 35 ml·kg^{-1}·min^{-1}). The average female carries relatively more fat than the male; this extra weight requires additional oxygen to carry it along, necessitating a higher HR to deliver that additional oxygen to the muscles.

Cardiovascular Responses to Isometric (Static) Exercise. We have primarily dealt with the physiological responses to aerobic exercise and have shown the effect of training on those responses. Before we finish this discussion, however, we must address isometric exercise, a form of exercise that can have a very different effect on the cardiovascular system. Figure 16.12 shows BP responses to dynamic exercise with the increase in systolic BP and HR and the decrease in diastolic pressure. There is very little change in the "mean," or average, pressure during this dynamic form of exercise. In contrast, a simple hand grip held at a tension equal to only about 30% of the person's maximal voluntary contraction strength (MVC) causes a systematic rise in diastolic and systolic BP with only a small increase HR. This is viewed as an inappropriate form of exercise for older people or those with heart disease because it increases the work of the heart and may compromise the ability of the coronary circulation to meet the heart's oxygen requirements.

Movement Anatomy and Functional Biomechanics Related to Physical Activity

Here we will summarize the most important information on anatomy as it relates to physical activity. We will outline the different types of bones, the joints that are the linking points between bones, and the muscles that move the bones as the joints allow.

Bones

The skeleton consists of more than 200 bones that provide protection for the internal organs and a leverage structure for muscles. The skeleton also allows for growth and houses the largest store of calcium in the body. There are four classes of bones:

- *Long bones* are found in the arms and legs, and are associated with movement.

- *Short bones* are found in the hands and feet.

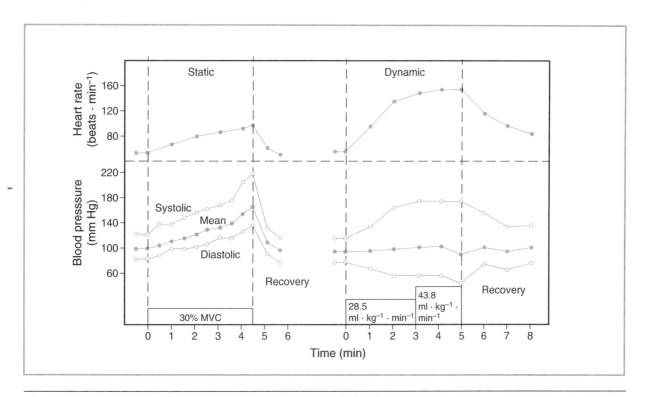

Figure 16.12 Static and dynamic exercise heart rate and blood pressure.
Adapted from *CMAJ* 1967.

Some short bones are irregular in shape like the bones in the vertebral (spinal) column.

- *Flat bones* are found in the upper part of the skull.
- *Irregular bones* are found in vertebrae and the pubic area.

Figure 16.13 shows the front (anterior) and back (posterior) views of the skeleton and identifies the major bones, groups of bones, and anatomical landmarks.

Joints

A joint is the point at which bones link or connect. Joints are also called *articulations*, and items associated with joints usually begin with the prefix arthr-, as in *arthr*oscope, a device that doctors use to look into joint spaces of a person with *arthr*itis. Joints are classified on the basis of how much movement is permitted between the bones:

- *Synarthrodial joints* are immovable joints or those with limited movement, such as the joints between the bones in the skull.
- *Amphiarthrodial joints* are joints with slight movement, as seen in the connections between vertebrae in the spinal column.
- *Diarthrotic or synovial joints* are joints possessing great potential for movement, as in the knee.

The diarthrotic or synovial joint is most important in physical activity. Movement occurs when the muscles move the bones through a range of motion within the limits of these joints. These joints are held together by connective tissue: ligaments, which cross over the joint, and tendons, which attach muscles to bones, also cross over joints to lend additional support.

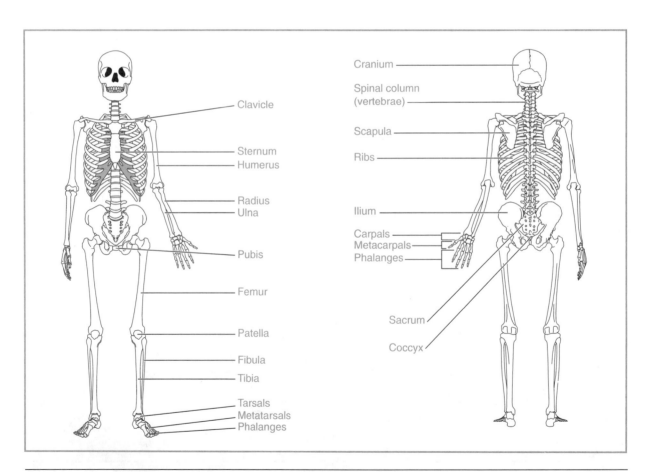

Figure 16.13 Front and back views of the human skeleton.
Adapted from Howley and Franks 1986.

Because these joints move a great deal, the structure also provides slippery surfaces and a lubricant. The slippery surface in each movable joint is the articular *hyaline cartilage* that covers the ends of the bones. This cartilage also absorbs some of the shock of impact to reduce the chance the bony surface will wear out. *Synovial fluid* is the lubricant secreted by the *synovial membrane* within the joint housing or capsule. In addition, *bursae,* or sacs containing synovial fluid outside the joint space, help to lubricate the movement of tendons, ligaments, and muscles over bony structures. Some of these joints (e.g., the knee) have additional cartilage in the joint space between the bones to take up some of the shock of impact. This is the type of cartilage that can be torn as a result of high-impact forces, while the smooth articular cartilage is the type that can be damaged by arthritis.

Diarthrodial (movable) joints are classified on the basis of the type of movement permitted:

- *Ball and socket joints* allow movement in all directions (e.g., where the head of the humerus [the bone of the upper arm] fits into the shoulder).

- *Hinge joints* allow movement in one plane of motion (e.g., the elbow).

- *Saddle joints* allow movement in all directions (e.g., metacarpal-carpal joint of the thumb).

- *Pivot joints* allow rotation around the long portion of the bone (e.g., the radio-ulnar joint: as we rotate a wrist to make the hand face up [supinated position] or down [pronated position]).

- *Gliding joints* allow only gliding or twisting (e.g., the joints between the wrist bones [carpals] or the ankle bones [tarsals]).

Movements

The type of movements possible at each joint depends on the type of joint. It is important to know the terms that describe these movements before we present a summary of the muscles involved:

• *Flexion and extension.* Flexion describes a motion that decreases the angle of a joint, and extension is a movement that increases the joint angle. If your arm is hanging straight down,

flexion is the movement of your hand toward your shoulder around the elbow joint; lowering the hand back to its starting position is extension. The term hyperextension refers to a movement beyond a joint's ordinary resting position.

• *Abduction and adduction.* Abduction describes a movement away from the center line of the body; adduction is a return to the ordinary anatomical position. Moving the leg to the side away from the body is an example of abduction.

• *Rotation.* Rotation is movement around the long axis of a bone and describes a movement either toward (*inward,* or *medial* rotation) or away from (*outward,* or *lateral* rotation) the center of the body. With your forearm at a 90° angle relative to your upper arm, and your hand in front of your body, movement of the wrist and lower arm toward the center line of the body is an example of medial rotation.

• *Pronation and supination.* If you hold your forearm at a 90° angle relative to your upper arm, hand in front of the body with thumb up, pronation describes a movement of the forearm such that the palm turns downward; and supination is the reverse. We also use these terms to describe the manner in which the foot lands when walking or running. A person who lands with the inside, or medial, aspect of the foot striking first is said to be a "pronator." Many running shoes are designed to control this problem.

• *Dorsiflex and plantarflex.* These terms describe the movement of the foot from its normal position either toward the lower leg (dorsiflex) or toward the bottom of the foot (plantar flex).

Muscles

Muscles are composed of muscle fibers, which are individual muscle cells. Each cell possesses the capacity to contract when stimulated by a motor neuron, or nerve cell. A single motor neuron may stimulate as few as 10 to more than 100 muscle fibers, and when it does, all the fibers attached to that single motor neuron fire at once. This complex of a single motor neuron and its muscle fibers is called a *motor unit.* A muscle possesses many motor units, and the tension that a muscle develops depends primarily on the number of motor units called into play. If more tension is needed, more motor units are recruited. When a muscle contracts, the ends of the muscle move toward the center, pulling the tendons (attached to the bones) toward each other. A variety of terms describe the different types of contractions:

• *Concentric contraction.* If the force of contraction is greater than the resistance offered, movement occurs as the bones to which the tendons are attached move toward each other. This type of contraction used to be called an *isotonic*, or "same-tension," contraction suggesting that tension is maintained throughout the range of motion. However, as the muscle shortens and the bones change position, the amount of tension needed to move a weight varies; more tension must be developed at some joint angles than at others to cause the same movement. This led to the development of variable resistance, or accommodating resistance, machines to provide a better match between resistance and the ability of a muscle to exert tension.

• *Eccentric contraction.* If you hold your forearm at a 90° angle relative to the upper arm and a weight (resistance) that is greater than the force your muscles can develop is placed in your hand, extension occurs at the elbow. This is an eccentric contraction in that the joint angle increases even though tension is being developed.

• *Isometric contraction.* This is also called a *static contraction* in that there is no movement even though the muscles are developing tension. Standing in a doorway and pushing against the door jamb is an example of this type of contraction.

Figure 16.14 describes the major muscle groups, and table 16.2 lists the prime movers at each joint. The term *prime mover* refers to the muscle that is primarily involved in the movement at that joint.

Muscles Involved in Selected Activities. In this section we will summarize the muscle groups involved in some of the most common physical activities. We will cover both activities of daily living and typical fitness endeavors.

Walking, Jogging, and Running. Walking, jogging, and running have a lot in common; they differ, however, in terms of the muscular force needed to move forward at different speeds. During walking, one foot is in contact with the ground at all times, but in jogging or running there is a period of "flight" when both feet are off the ground. If a period of flight is involved, a person must expend a greater amount of energy to both take off and land. The primary muscle groups involved in each phase of these activities include the following:

• Push-off phase—This phase involves concentric contraction of the *hip extensors, talocrural plantar flexors,* and *foot metatarsophalangeal flexors.*

• Bringing the push-off leg forward—Concentric contraction of the *hip flexors* initiates movement that is modified by the lateral hip rotators. The *knee flexors* first cause knee flexion, then the *knee extensors* straighten the knee. The knee flexors continue to act via an eccentric contraction, to control the rate of knee extension prior to the foot touching down. The foot is dorsiflexed prior to landing.

• Landing—The *hip extensors* that initiated the push-off now contract eccentrically to slow the swing of the forward leg. When the foot touches down the *knee extensors* also contract eccentrically to control the motion of the foot on the ground.

Cycling. Given that cycling is a restricted activity in that the pedals move in a fixed manner, it should be no surprise that the muscle groups involved in cycling are also somewhat limited. The *hip* and *knee extensors* develop the force to move the pedals downward, and, if toe clips are used by a cyclist skilled in their use, *hip* and *talocrural dorsiflexors* are involved in the return to the starting position.

Jumping. The force needed to propel the body off the ground is generated by the *knee* and *hip extensors* as well as the *plantar flexors.* To absorb the forces of impact, these same muscles contract eccentrically.

Lifting and Carrying. When a person lifts an object, the large, strong *knee and hip extensors* should be the primary muscles involved, not the muscles in the arms or along the spine. Keeping the object close to your body reduces the stress on your back.

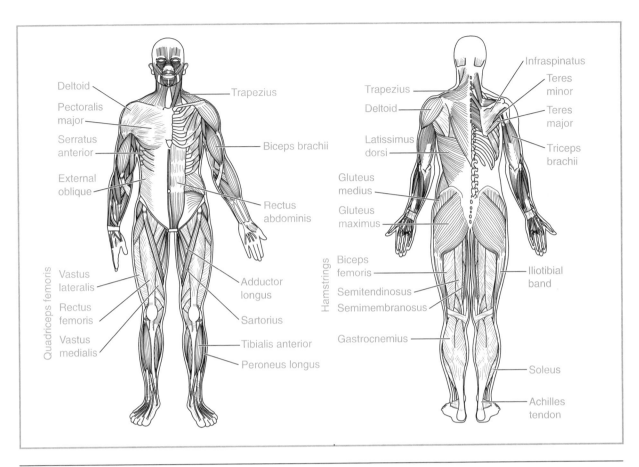

Figure 16.14 Front and back views of the surface muscles of the human body.

Adapted from Howley and Franks 1997.

Table 16.2	Muscles That Are Prime Movers
Joint	**Prime movers**
Intertarsal joint	Invertors—tibialis anterior, tibialis posterior
	Evertors—extensor digitorum longus, peroneus brevis, peroneus longus, peroneus tertius
Talocrural joint	Dorsiflexors—tibialis anterior, extensor digitorum longus, peroneus tertius
	Plantar flexors—gastrocnemius, soleus
Knee joint	Flexors—biceps femoris, semitendinosus, semimembranosus
	Extensors—rectus femoris, vastus lateralis, vastus medialis, vastus intermedius
Hip joint	Flexors—psoas, iliacus, pectineus, rectus femoris
	Extensors—gluteus maximus, biceps femoris, semitendinosus, semi-membranosus
	Abductors—gluteus medias

(continued)

Table 16.2 *(cont'd)*

Joint	Prime movers
Hip joint (cont.)	Adductors—adductor brevis, adductor longus, adductor magnus, gracilis, pectineus
	Lateral rotators—gluteus maximus, six deep lateral rotators
	Medial rotators—gluteus minimus
Spinal column (thoracic and lumbar areas)	Flexors—rectus abduminis, external oblique, internal oblique
	Extensors—erector spinae group
	Rotators—internal oblique, external oblique, erector spinae group
	Lateral flexors—internal oblique, external oblique, quadratus lumborum, multifidus, rotatores
Shoulder girdle	Abductors—pectoralis minor, serratus anterior
	Adductors—middle fibers of trapezius, rhomboids
	Upward rotators—upper and lower fibers of trapezius, serratus anterior
	Downward rotators—rhomboids, pectoralis minor
	Elevators—levator scapulae, upper fibers of trapezius, rhomboids
	Depressors—lower fibers of trapezius, pectoralis minor
Shoulder joint	Flexors—anterior deltoid, clavicular portion of pectoralis major
	Extensors—sternal portion of pectoralis major, latissimus dorsi, teres major
	Abductors—middle deltoid, supraspinatus
	Adductors—latissimus dorsi, teres major, sternal portion of pectoralis major
	Lateral rotators—infraspinatus, teres minor
	Medial rotators—latissimus dorsi, teres major, pectoralis major, subscapularis
Elbow joint	Flexors—biceps brachii, brachialis, brachioradialis
	Extensors—triceps brachii
Radio-ulnar joint	Pronators—Pronator teres, pronator quadratus, brachioradialis
	Supinators—supinator, biceps brachii, brachioradialis
Wrist joint	Flexors—flexor carpi ulnaris, flexor carpi radialis
	Extensors—extensor carpi ulnaris, extensor carpi radialis longus and brevis
	Abductors—flexor carpi radialis, extensor carpi radialis longus and brevis
	Adductors—flexor carpi ulnaris, extensor carpi ulnaris

Reprinted from Howley and Franks 1986.

General Biomechanical Concepts

Understanding a variety of basic principles and laws governing the movement of objects and people can help you determine proper and improper movements. In this section, we will discuss the concepts of stability, rotational inertia, torque, and angular momentum.

Stability. The center of gravity for an average person is near the navel. The stability of an individual is greater the closer the center of gravity is to the ground and the wider the base of support. A person standing with both feet close together is less stable than when standing with feet spread apart, and bending the knees to lift an object brings the center of gravity closer to the ground.

Rotational Inertia. The concept of rotational inertia as applied to the body describes the tendency of a body segment to remain at rest and not rotate around a joint. The larger the body segment and the farther the mass of the segment is from the joint (e.g., arm versus leg), the more rotational inertia the body segment has and the greater the energy required to move that segment through a range of motion. A person can reduce the energy requirement by bringing the mass of the body segment closer to the joint of rotation; for example, bringing the flexed rear leg forward during running is an application of this principle.

Torque. This is the effect produced when a muscle contraction (force) causes rotation. We will look at forearm flexion as an example, with the forearm at a 90° angle to the upper arm and a 10-lb weight held in the hand. The resistance is the product of the 10-lb weight and the distance from the center of the weight to the elbow joint. The muscular force needed to move that weight depends on the distance from the elbow that the tendon of that muscle is inserted into the bones of the forearm. The closer the biceps' insertion is to the hand, the smaller the muscular force needed to move the resistance. In the same way, if the person moves the 10-lb weight closer to the joint (to reduce the length of the lever arm), less muscular force is needed to move the resistance. This concept can be extended to the carrying of objects. The reason for carrying an object close to the body is to maintain stability and reduce the force of the back muscles needed to carry the load. If the person holds the object with arms outstretched, however, the back muscles must exert more force, which can cause back problems.

Angular Momentum. This term describes the amount of motion that takes place as a limb moves around a joint or a body rotates and is equal to the product of angular velocity and rotational inertia. The *conservation of angular momentum* states that once motion is initiated, angular momentum remains constant until an outside force changes it. This means that a decrease in rotational inertia during a movement results in a higher angular velocity. For example, when an ice skater spins around in place, as he brings his arms closer to his body to decrease rotational inertia, the velocity of rotation increases.

Summary

Muscles use ATP for contraction. Muscles must supply the ATP as fast as it is being used if work is to continue. Muscles can supply ATP from stored creatine phosphate, the anaerobic breakdown of glucose, and the aerobic metabolism of carbohydrates and fats. Although there is an oxygen deficit at the onset of work, at 2 to 3 min into submaximal work the oxygen uptake meets the entire ATP demand of the task. A graded exercise test (GXT) can be used to evaluate how the various physiological systems respond to gradually increasing work demands. Oxygen uptake increases with each stage of the test until the maximal capacity of the circulatory system to transport oxygen (maximal aerobic power) is reached. This increased oxygen delivery is achieved through increases in heart rate, stroke volume, oxygen extraction, and pulmonary ventilation. With endurance training maximal oxygen uptake increases, due primarily to increases in maximal stroke volume and oxygen extraction. Keep in mind, however, that females have a higher heart rate response to submaximal work than do males because of smaller heart size and the lower amount of hemoglobin in each liter of blood.

The human skeleton consists of more than 200 bones; it provides protection for internal organs and a leverage structure for muscles.

Bones are classified as short, long, flat, or irregular, with the long bones being primarily involved in movements. Joints are the linking points of bones, and the most important ones for movements are the diarthrotic or synovial joints. The ends of the bones are covered with a smooth articular (hyaline) cartilage, and synovial membranes secrete a fluid into the joint to reduce friction. Diarthrodial joints are classified as ball and socket, hinge, saddle, pivot, and gliding. Joint movements include flexion and extension, abduction and adduction, rotation, pronation and supination, and dorsiflexion and plantar flexion. Muscles are composed of many motor units, which are the basic units of muscle contraction. A motor unit is composed of a single motor neuron and the muscle fibers (from 10 to more than 100) stimulated by that neuron. Muscle contractions include concentric, eccentric, and isometric (static). Primary muscle groups involved in selected activities were presented.

Chapter 17
Measurement and Evaluation

| Validity |
| Accuracy |
| Interpretation |

Fitness programs combine knowledge from several aspects of our field. Previous chapters in this book have presented information based on exercise physiology, biomechanics, and behavior modification. This chapter summarizes aspects of measurement and evaluation related to fitness testing.

Validity

The most important question to raise about a test is validity; that is, does it measure the characteristic you're interested in evaluating? The first criterion for validity is consistency. Consistency includes the reliability of the test and the objectivity of the testers. If the test is repeated without a change in fitness of the person being tested, does it provide the same score both times (reliability)? If different people administer or score the test, do they record the same results (objectivity)?

Although a test can be reliable and objective and still not be valid, unreliable and nonobjective tests can never be valid. For a consistent test, three major criteria determine if the test measures what it is supposed to: content validity, concurrent validity, and construct validity. Content validity indicates that the test seems to be a good one based on logic, expert testimony, and widespread use. Concurrent validity indicates that the test being used is highly correlated to an "accepted" test of the same characteristic. Construct validity is provided by showing that a test responds in the same ways that one would expect based on the theoretical understanding of that characteristic.

The fitness tests recommended in this book (part III) have all been shown to be reliable and objective when carefully administered by trained professionals. They all have content validity, in that it appears that endurance runs, skinfold fat tests, curl-ups, sit-and-reach tests, and push-ups or modified pull-ups measure cardiorespiratory fitness, relative leanness, abdominal endurance, low-back flexibility, and upper arm strength and endurance, respectively. Fitness experts have recommended these tests, and they have been used for these variables in numerous fitness programs and research projects. Endurance runs and skinfold fat tests have concurrent validity, because they are closely related (correlated) to the "gold standards" of aerobic power (maximal oxygen uptake) and relative leanness (underwater weight). There is some construct validity for all of the tests—they have been shown to be related to other tests of the same fitness component, they improve with the type of physical conditioning that improves the characteristic, and they get worse with detraining.

Tips for Increased Testing Accuracy

A test score includes the individual's true score, plus or minus error. The error can result from the testing environment, the equipment, normal performance variations of the person being tested, and the tester. Fitness leaders can do a number of things to obtain more accurate results (less error) from testing, including preparing the person to be tested, organizing the testing session, and paying attention to details.

Preparing the Subject

The most accurate test results come from subjects who understand what test procedures you are going to use, have previously practiced any unusual or novel aspects of the test, have complied with pretest instructions in terms of rest, food, drink, drugs, and exercise, and are physically and mentally prepared to take the test. Table 17.1 provides a checklist to help you determine if an individual is ready to be tested.

Organizing the Testing Session

Preparing the subject is part of organization. In addition to the items listed in table 17.1, the fitness tester must ensure that everything is ready to test subjects accurately and efficiently. Table 17.2 provides a checklist for the tester.

Table 17.1	Checklist to Determine if Subject Is Ready to Be Tested
Step	**Item**
1	Has read and understands test procedures
2	Has signed informed consent
3	Has practiced the test and is comfortable with it
4	Understands starting and stopping procedures
5	Understands expectations before, during, and after test
6	Has complied with all pretest instructions: Rest Food and drink Smoking and drugs Clothes and shoes
7	Is not ill or injured
8	Is not on medication (except as planned with physician)
9	Has had proper warm-up

Table 17.2	Checklist for Fitness Tester
Step	**Item**
1	Test(s) to be administered determined for each person
2	Equipment in working order and calibrated
3	Scoresheet(s) and other supplies ready
4	Testing assistants clearly understand responsibilities
5	Testing assistants checked out on task they are to do
6	Timing and sequence of testing set
7	Starting and stopping instructions clear to tester and subjects
8	Subjects ready for test
9	Emergency equipment and procedures ready
10	Warm-up consistent for all
11	Posttest activities and responsibilities set
12	Temperature, humidity, and barometric pressure recorded and within acceptable limits
13	Fields, mats, and areas clean, marked, and ready for testing
14	Atmosphere is calm, private, and relaxed

Attention to Details

A tester can improve the accuracy of the testing situation by paying close attention to all the details (such as those listed in tables 17.1 and 17.2). Preparing the subject, organizing the testing situation, and precise data collection are possible only when the tester attends to each aspect of the testing protocol (see figure 17.1).

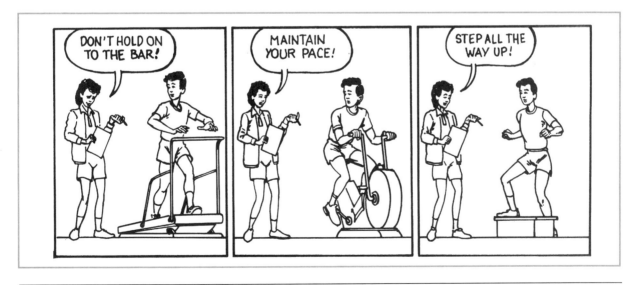

Figure 17.1 Tips for testers.

Interpreting Test Scores

The following can assist you in interpreting fitness test scores:

- Emphasize health status rather than comparison with others.
- Emphasize change rather than current status.
- Provide specific recommendations based on the test data and your understanding of the individual.

As shown in figure 17.2, it's important to avoid overwhelming the participant with too much data and too many statistics.

Health Status

One common approach is to compare the fitness participant with others of the same gender and similar age (e.g., the subject performed better than 60% of people of his or her age and sex on the 1.5-mi run). Although participants may ask for this type of feedback, it is probably the least useful in terms of fitness. This type of comparison with others is heavily influenced by a person's heredity and early experience. There are limits to how much a person can change relative to others even with a lot of effort.

It is unfortunate that many people emphasize the "performance" model of being "number one" in fitness programs. You should not emphasize who can run the fastest or who has the lowest cholesterol, but rather helping all people understand and try to obtain and maintain healthy levels of cardiorespiratory fitness, body composition, and low-back function. Therefore, in the first testing session, base your feedback on whether participants meet the health standards rather than what percent of the population they can "beat" on a test. This is the approach that we have used in this book. We have set fitness standards for people to try to obtain based on what is needed for good health. For example, we would like all women to have between 15% and 25% fat (children and men, between 10% and 20%). It doesn't matter what percent of the population currently is in that range. What does matter is that a person who has less fat than the lower portion of the range has health risks associated with having too little fat. A person with more fat than the upper part of the range risks developing (or making worse)

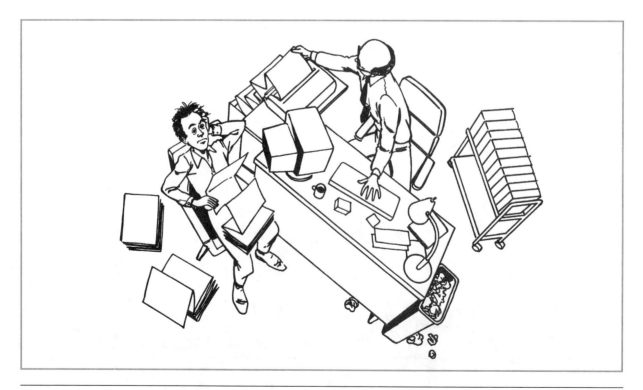

Figure 17.2 Feedback on fitness test results.

major health problems. The fitness leader should encourage all participants to try to reach and maintain the health standards for cardiorespiratory fitness, body composition, and low-back function. Table 17.3 provides health standards for different ages. Note that more research is necessary so we can refine these standards; therefore, these standards may change as we find out more about the relationship between test scores and positive health.

Improvement

The most important question for a fitness participant is not what her or his status is at this moment in life, but rather what it will be 6 months, 2 years, and 20 years from now! By encouraging participants to deal with their status compared with health standards, you help the individual set reasonable goals for the next testing period.

Table 17.3 Fitness Test Standards

Test item	6-9	10-12	13-15	16-30	35-50	55-70
	Age (years)					

Mile run (min)

Males						
Good	14	12	11	10	11	12
Borderline	16	14	13	12	13	15
Needs work	≥18	≥16	≥15	≥14	≥15	≥17
Females						
Good	14	12	13	12	13	14
Borderline	16	14	15	14	15	17
Needs work	≥18	≥16	≥17	≥16	≥17	≥19

Percent fat (%)

Males						
Good	10-20	10-20	10-20	10-20	10-20	10-20
Borderline	23	23	23	23	23	24
Needs work	<5	<5	<5	<5	<5	<5
	>26	>26	>26	>26	>26	>27
Females						
Good	10-20	10-20	15-25	15-25	15-25	15-25
Borderline	23	23	27	27	27	28
Needs work	<5	<5	<14	<14	<14	<14
	>26	>26	>30	>30	>30	>31

Curl-ups (#)

Good	≥20	≥25	≥30	≥35	≥35	≥30
Borderline	12	15	22	25	25	20
Needs work	≤5	≤10	≤13	≤15	≤15	≤10

(continued)

Test item	6-9	10-12	13-15	16-30	35-50	55-70
Table 17.3 (cont'd)						
Age (years)						
Sit-and-reach (in.)						
Good	10	10	10	10	10	9
Borderline	8	8	8	8	8	7
Needs work	≤6	≤6	≤6	≤6	≤6	≤5
Modified pull-ups (#)						
Males						
Good	8	15	22	30	30	25
Borderline	3	5	9	12	12	8
Needs work	2	3	7	10	10	5
Females						
Good	8	15	12	12	12	8
Borderline	3	5	5	5	5	3
Needs work	2	3	3	3	3	1
90° Push-ups (#)						
Males						
Good	9	18	30	35	35	30
Borderline	4	7	15	20	20	15
Needs work	2	5	10	15	15	10
Females						
Good	9	18	15	15	15	10
Borderline	4	7	7	7	7	5
Needs work	2	5	5	5	5	3

Setting Specific Fitness Goals

Another way that you can use test results is to help individuals meet specific goals. Sometimes, health standards are inappropriate or unreasonable for a particular individual. For example, the mile run standards are inappropriate for someone who is swimming for their fitness workouts or someone in a wheelchair. However, you can establish individual goals for covering a certain distance in the water or in a wheelchair. Or you may want to set subgoals for an individual who is very unfit. For example, it is discouraging to discuss mile run standards with a person who can walk only a quarter of a mile without stopping. The initial goal for that person may be to work up to being able to walk a mile without stopping. As indicated in chapter 15, it is important to set goals and subgoals to help people begin and continue healthy behaviors.

Healthy Behaviors

Fitness behaviors (exercise, diet, rest, no substance abuse, coping with stress) and fitness test scores are related. You should, however, emphasize the fitness behaviors over the fitness test scores themselves. It is more important that people begin and continue regular physical activity than that they achieve a certain time on an endurance run. It is more important that people eat properly than that they attain a certain body fat percentage. By emphasizing the healthy behaviors, you can recognize people for their efforts, and in the long run, positive reinforcement is the best way to improve fitness test scores. Indeed, overemphasizing test scores can discourage some participants.

Feedback

The health standards and emphasis on improvement and behavior should provide the basis for the specific feedback you give each participant. The other factor involved in feedback is the individual's own nature and likes. The key to effective feedback is to provide the best recommendations concerning activities (type, total work, intensity, frequency) that will be healthy, helpful, and interesting to this particular individual and thus more likely to be done. Assistance is especially important early in the fitness program.

Deciding on Program Revision

Analysis of test scores from the different fitness classes can help you decide how to revise the fitness program (see figure 17.3). How many people drop out of various classes? What kind of aerobic, fat, and low-back changes are participants making? How many injuries are related to the various classes? Answers to these questions can help you improve the fitness activities you offer in a program.

Another use of test scores is to help educate the public and get positive attention for your program (see figure 17.4). What percentage of the participants stays with the program long enough to make important fitness gains? What is the total amount of fat participants lost this past year? How many miles have the participants run during the year? Careful testing, record keeping, and analysis can provide the public with helpful information about your program.

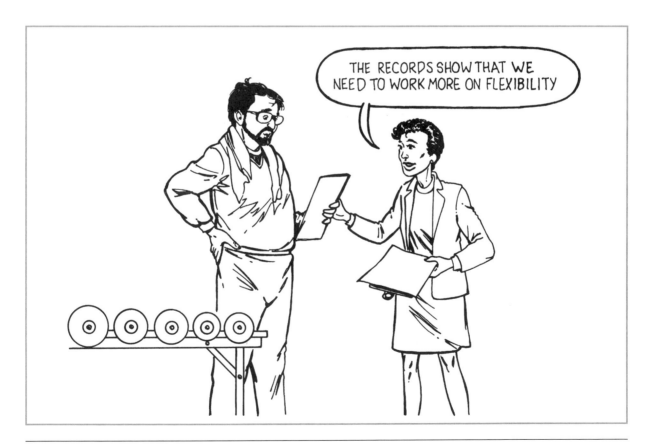

Figure 17.3 Modifying an individual's fitness program.

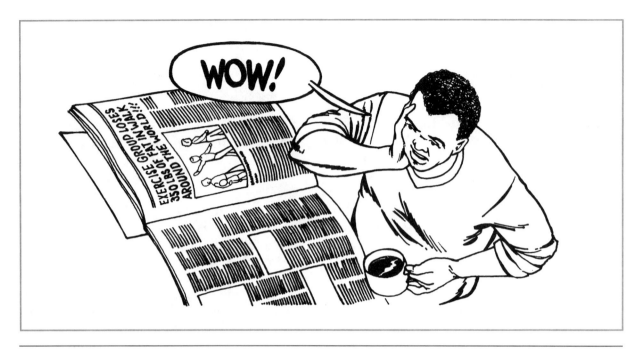

Figure 17.4 Publicity.

Summary

Validating fitness tests includes ensuring consistency in tests and testers and checking content, concurrent, and construct validity. You can enhance testing accuracy by preparing the subject, organizing the testing situation, and paying attention to details. Interpretation of test scores should emphasize health status, improvement, and specific feedback based on both the results and nature of the individual. Emphasize the fitness behaviors, not the test scores themselves, in helping individuals enhance their positive health. Fitness test evaluation can help individuals assess health status by comparing current test scores with desired health standards. Your fitness program can benefit from your analyzing test results to discover needed program revisions as well as improve public relations.

PART VI

Safe and Effective Programs

Injury Prevention
Special Conditions
Management
Human Relations

This final part of the *Fitness Leader's Handbook* describes ways that the fitness program can be safe, efficient, and effective.

Chapter 18 describes ways to prevent injury. Easy-to-use charts present the causes of and treatments for common exercise-related injuries. Chapters 19 and 20 describe ways to deal with special personal conditions and environmental factors. Chapter 21 offers suggestions for administering a fitness program. Finally, chapter 22 provides some tips concerning effective human relations.

Chapter 18
Preventing and Treating Injuries

Risk of Injury
Prevention of Injury
Treatment of Injury

There is some risk of injury in crossing the street, driving a car, operating a lawn mower, or climbing a ladder. If even these common tasks pose a risk of injury, it should come as no surprise that participation in a physical activity program, even one designed to improve health status, includes risks as well. Evidence shows that the risk of injury increases for workouts conducted at high intensities, durations longer than 40 min, and frequencies greater than four times per week (see figure 18.1).

Activities such as running and exercise to music cause more muscle and skeletal trauma than riding a stationary cycle or swimming. Games, especially competitive ones, are associated with more injuries than are controlled, low-intensity, cooperative activities. However, the potential for injury goes beyond the type, intensity, frequency, and duration of the activity. The environment and the characteristics of the par-

ticipant also contribute to the overall injury risk. Exercising in a hot, humid environment predisposes one to heat injury, while exercising in the cold can lead to frostbite and hypothermia. Not surprisingly, older, less fit individuals are more susceptible to skeletal injuries than are young, fit people. Finally, people with a medical condition such as asthma or diabetes require special attention to avoid a situation that could result in serious trouble.

The purpose of all this is not to scare you to the point of deciding not to lead an exercise program; rather, we wish to set forth issues that you must address to minimize the risks associated with exercise programs. Inform your participants of the risks and teach them how to minimize the possibility of injury. In addition, show them how to treat common injuries and how to modify their exercise programs when problems occur.

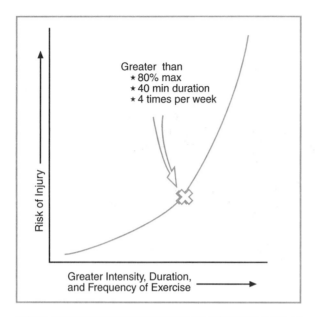

Risk of Injury

Greater than
★ 80% max
★ 40 min duration
★ 4 times per week

Greater Intensity, Duration,
and Frequency of Exercise

Figure 18.1 Increased risk of injury with too much activity.

Minimizing Injury Risk

As we have indicated throughout the preceding chapters, one of the most important things to do to minimize risk is to screen participants prior to their entry into an exercise program. On the basis of the screening you may refer persons for additional tests, recommend a medically supervised program, or indicate that exercising in a graduated program like the one described in parts I and IV of this book represents a low risk. Our recommended exercise program focuses attention on starting slowly, progressing in an orderly fashion from low to higher intensities, and avoiding more uncontrolled activities until an individual has achieved a solid fitness base. Figure 18.2 shows that it is important to teach fitness participants to listen to their bodies, paying attention to signals that indicate they may be doing too much, and slow down. In spite of this advice, however, some participants may still experience injuries during exercise. Therefore, we must move beyond these recommendations and discuss the treatment of common injuries associated with exercise.

One of the most common problems associated with starting an exercise program is muscle soreness. It is important to understand that muscle soreness is a normal sensation associated with any new physical activity. If an individual has been an avid jogger, putting in 12 mi a week, and

decides to participate in a game of soccer, which emphasizes sudden bursts of speed, changes of direction, and explosive kicks, it is not surprising that muscle soreness shows up 24 to 48 hr after the game. The soreness is related to actual tissue damage in the active muscles and the inflammation (swelling) that follows. Once the participant has experienced soreness, it usually does not recur in those muscles as a result of the same activity unless a long period of time (6 to 9 weeks) elapses between exposures. The following signs and symptoms associated with injury are listed here to call your attention to circumstances that may require some special attention. We encourage you to discuss these with your fitness participants. Though these signs and symptoms can also appear in an extreme case of muscle soreness, in general, this is not the case.

Signs of Injury

1. Extreme tenderness when body part is touched
2. Pain while at rest; pain that will not disappear after warming up; joint pain; increased pain when moving or exercising that body part
3. Swelling or discoloration
4. Changes in normal body function

Treatment of Common Injuries

The most common injuries associated with exercise programs are sprains and strains. Sprains are caused by the stretching of the connective tissue (ligaments) surrounding a joint, while strains occur when muscles or tendons are stretched. Figure 18.3 shows that the immediate treatment of both conditions is summed up by the acronym PRICE, which stands for *protecting* and *resting* the injured body part and using *ice* with *compression* on the body part, which should be *elevated* to reduce fluid accumulation.

The steps described next will tend to reduce the swelling associated with an injury and reduce the time needed for normal function to return. Ice helps to reduce the blood flow to the injured site as well as the sensation of pain. Follow this same set of steps when a muscle is

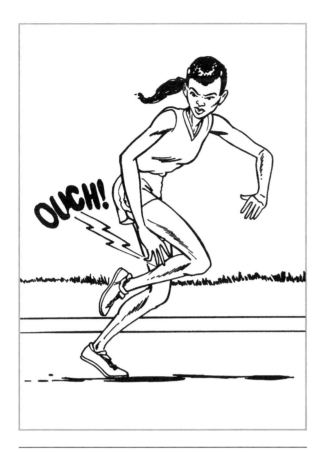

Figure 18.2 Listen to your body.

damaged by a direct blow (contusion), or when the heel of the foot strikes a hard surface, causing a "stone bruise." For a contusion, the individual should usually stretch the muscle before applying ice. Put a soft pad under the heel to reduce the force of impact for a heel bruise.

Immediate Treatment of Common Injuries

1. *Protect* the body part from further damage.

2. *Rest* the body part; do not try to "walk it off."

3. *Ice* (crushed or cubes in a plastic bag) is applied for 20 to 30 min; repeated on a regular basis: hourly or when pain occurs. Ice treatment should continue for 24 to 72 hr, depending on the degree of injury.

4. *Compression* bandages should be used to hold the ice bag in place and when the ice is removed. Wrap the bandage firmly, but not too tightly, to help minimize swelling.

5. *Elevate* the injured body part whenever possible.

Moderate injuries (exhibiting swelling, discoloration, and joint tenderness) to severe injuries

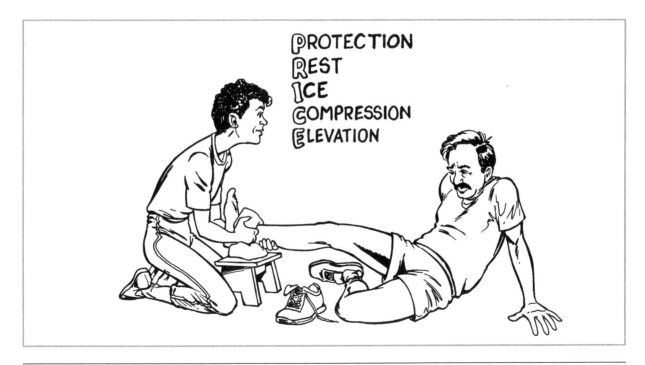

Figure 18.3 The PRICE method for treating sprains and strains.
Reprinted from Howley and Franks 1997.

(exhibiting extreme tenderness and swelling, discoloration, and deformity of body part) should be examined by a physician. Always remember to follow the PRICE steps for any acute (recent) injury. Heat may be applied later in the recovery process when the swelling and the chance of more bleeding (which causes more swelling) are reduced. In addition, for those with chronic problems like tendinitis or bursitis, heat may be applied prior to activity. If you are ever in doubt, use ice.

Heat Illness

Though sprains and strains may be common, they are seldom life-threatening. This is not the case for heat injury. Normally, body temperature increases with exercise due to the heat the muscles produce, but it stabilizes at a safe level as heat loss mechanisms (particularly the evaporation of sweat) catch up and equal the rate of heat production. This balance can be upset if the body gains too much heat from the environment or can't evaporate enough sweat to get rid of the heat. In chapter 20, we discuss the problems involved in exercising in heat and humidity as well as in the cold, and we suggest modifications for exercise under these conditions. When the body cannot adequately handle the heat load, a variety of problems, classified as heat injuries, can occur. These are listed as follows from least to most dangerous:

Classification	Signs and symptoms
Heat syncope	Headaches, nausea, light-headedness
Muscle cramps	Spasms in single muscles; more dangerous when more than one muscle is affected
Heat exhaustion	Lots of sweating, cold and clammy skin, pale skin, dizziness, nausea, headache, loss of consciousness
Heat stroke	No sweating, hot and dry skin, extremely high body temperature, rapid and strong pulse

You must attend to the following signs and symptoms that may indicate that a participant is getting into trouble:

1. Hair standing on end on arms, back, and chest
2. Chills
3. Throbbing in the head or headache
4. Vomiting or nausea
5. Dry lips or "cotton mouth"
6. Muscle cramping
7. Light-headedness
8. No sweating

You need to be aware of these signs and symptoms, and if they occur, to act on them immediately. If an individual feels light-headed and is experiencing nausea, stop, get the person to a cool place, have her or him sit or lie down with feet elevated, and give fluids to drink. Treat a muscle cramp by putting direct pressure on the muscle, massaging it, and stretching it gently. With multiple cramps or the symptoms of heat exhaustion, have the person go to a cool place, lie down with feet up, drink lots of fluids, and, when feeling better, see a physician. Heat stroke is a medical emergency—get the affected person to a hospital as soon as possible, remove the person's clothing, and cool him or her down starting at the head with ice, cold wet towels, fans, and so on.

Common Orthopedic Problems

A number of orthopedic problems have a common denominator: overuse. Skeletal muscles, connective tissue (both tendons and ligaments), and tissues in or around joints can be affected. We do not mean that overuse is the only cause of orthopedic problems; infection and direct physical trauma can also cause them. Some common conditions include the following:

- Bursitis—inflammation of the bursa (a fluid-filled sac between muscle and bone that aids in movement)
- Tendinitis—inflammation of a tendon (the tissue tying a muscle to a bone)
- Myositis—inflammation of a muscle
- Synovitis—inflammation of the synovial membrane (forms the inner lining of joint cavities and secretes synovial fluid to aid in the movement of the bones in the joint space)
- Plantar fasciitis—inflammation of the connective tissue on the bottom of the foot

The common factor in all of these definitions is the process of inflammation, which is the body's normal reaction to infection or trauma. Tennis elbow and shin splints (more on these later) are examples of inflammation involving muscles and connective tissue. Inflammation involves special white blood cells as well as chemicals that expand the pores in capillaries to let large proteins enter the injured area. This influx of protein brings along water, causing the swelling.

Treatment

The immediate treatment for these problems is the same as for sprains: ice and rest. If the problem is a chronic (long-term) one, warming the area before physical activity and using ice afterward can help reduce pain and discomfort. An obvious recommendation is to stop doing the activity that causes the problem and shift to another activity. For joggers who develop problems with their knees, swimming or deep-water running is a good substitute. For swimmers who develop shoulder problems, cycling is a good substitute. A physician should examine any chronic inflammatory condition that limits normal daily function.

Stress fractures to the lower leg and the foot are also caused by overuse. This problem occurs when the bone's ability to adapt to a chronic load is exceeded. The area over the fracture is very tender to the touch. Pain is present most of the time but is increased when standing. Stress fractures need a physician's care and take a long time to heal (6 to 10 weeks). Any supplemental exercises used during the recovery process should be approved by a physician.

Shin Splints

Shin splints refer to an inflammation of the muscle-tendon unit on the front side of the lower leg. This injury has a wide variety of causes, including overuse. It is more common in runners and dancers (including participants in exercise-to-music programs) because of the high loads these participants place on the lower leg during exercise. However, weak arches, hard surfaces, inadequate shoes, structural abnormalities, and improper exercise techniques can all cause shin splints. The recommended ways to deal with this injury are as varied as the list of causes:

- Overuse—cut back on the total amount of running or dancing, or simply substitute something else.
- Surface—running or dancing on softer surfaces will help absorb the shock of impact.
- Shoes—well-cushioned and properly designed exercise shoes will help to dissipate the shock of impact.

Don't be fooled into believing that the simple purchase of an excellent (and expensive!) pair of exercise shoes will make shin splints disappear. Shoes can help reduce the problem, but good judgment must be exercised about overuse. Some people use good shoes and a soft floor as a justification for even more exercise, aggravating the problem. Instead, adding variety to a participant's workout will reduce the chance of overstressing any single area of the body.

Exercise Modification

Table 18.1 summarizes the classifications of injury with the terms mild, moderate, and severe, and offers some suggestions on how to deal with them. Please recognize that this list is not a prescription to follow. If there is a "pop" or a deformity or when conservative recommendations do not result in a relief of the problem after 2 to 4 weeks, have the participant contact a physician.

CPR and Emergency Procedures

You must maintain current cardiopulmonary resuscitation (CPR) certification. In addition, you must learn and follow the emergency procedures that are used in your program.

Summary

The risk of injury associated with physical activity increases for workouts conducted at high intensity, for durations longer than 40 min, and for frequencies greater than four times per week. Risks are greater in competitive games compared to stationary cycling, and for older, less fit persons compared to younger, more fit individuals. The risk of injury is minimized by

Table 18.1	Injury Classification Criteria and Exercise Modifications
Criteria	**Modifications**
Mild injury	
Performance is not affected. Pain is experienced only after athletic activity. Generally, no tenderness is felt on palpation. No or minimal swelling is present. No discoloration is apparent.	Reduce activity level, modify activity to take stress off of the injured part, treat symptomatically, and gradually return to full activity.
Moderate injury	
Performance is mildly affected or not affected at all. Pain is experienced before and after athletic activity. Mild tenderness is felt on palpation. Mild swelling may be present. Some discoloration may be present.	Rest the injured part, modify activity to take stress off of the injured part, treat symptomatically, and gradually return to full activity.
Severe injury	
Pain is experienced before, during, and after activity. Performance is definitely affected because of pain. Normal daily function is affected because of pain. Movement is limited because of pain. Moderate-to-severe point tenderness is felt on palpation. Swelling is most likely present. Discoloration may be present.	Rest completely and see a physician.

Reprinted from Howley and Franks 1997.

participation in a screening prior to an exercise program, starting at low levels, progressing in small steps, and developing a fitness base before engaging in less controlled activities.

It is important to distinguish simple muscle soreness from serious injury. Acute injuries, including sprains, strains, contusions, and bone bruises should be treated with the PRICE approach: protect and rest the injured part, use ice with compression, and elevate the injured part. Heat injury's signs and symptoms can vary from headaches and nausea to extremely high body temperatures that are life threatening. Prevention is the key, and you must focus on providing exercise in an environment that facilitates the evaporation of sweat and does not impose a large heat load.

Besides strains and sprains, most common orthopedic problems are inflammation reactions caused by overuse. The treatment of an acute inflammation includes ice and rest, similar to the treatment for a sprain. For chronic problems, however, the inflamed area may be warmed before a workout to help relieve discomfort during the activity. Use the ice treatment after the workout. A better choice is to change activities to rest the injured area. If daily function is limited by such inflammation injuries, the individual should consult a physician. Shin splints is a condition affecting the front part of the lower leg and is found primarily in runners and dance-exercisers. The condition is relieved by changing activities, decreasing the intensity or duration of the current activity, and using well-cushioned surfaces and shoes.

Chapter 19
Special Personal Conditions

How to Modify Exercise for Specific Health Problems
Exercise for Special Populations

You need to modify an exercise program or use special caution in its planning for those who are injured or have a special medical problem. This chapter addresses a variety of conditions that dictate a modification of an individual's exercise program.

Orthopedic Problems

If a participant complains of pain in the ankle, knee, or hip when walking, jogging, or running, recommend a change in exercise intensity or duration, the surface on which it is done, or the activity itself. If a participant is working at the top part of the THR zone, suggest that the intensity be reduced by focusing on the lower part of the THR zone. If a person is jogging for 40 continuous min, recommend a change to 20 min of walking and 20 min of jogging, done in 10-min intervals. If an individual is walking, jogging, or

running on an uneven surface or one that has little cushioning, recommend a change to a smooth, even surface that absorbs shocks better. If these recommendations do not bring relief, encourage the participant to try another activity that will relieve the load on the involved joint. For example, substituting swimming, deep-water running, or riding the cycle ergometer (in which body weight is supported by the seat) may relieve the problem. However, if the condition persists for several weeks, suggest that the participant see a physician or other healthcare professional.

Diabetes

Blood glucose is the primary fuel for the brain, and the concentration of blood glucose must be maintained within narrow limits if the brain and other organs are to function properly. After a person eats a meal, the level of glucose increases in the blood (due to the glucose in the small intestine entering the bloodstream), and the pancreas releases insulin, which is needed for the blood glucose to enter the cells; the blood glucose then returns toward the normal value. Between meals, when blood glucose falls as tissues use it for fuel, the liver releases glucose to keep the blood glucose concentration constant.

The pancreas of the *insulin-dependent* or *Type I diabetic* does not produce insulin, so insulin must be injected to keep the blood glucose concentration under control. The Type I diabetic must balance food intake and insulin injections in order to achieve this "control," and for many, that in itself is a difficult task. Exercise has the potential to both complement and complicate this balancing act.

If the Type I diabetic exercises when blood glucose is in control, exercise causes glucose to leave the blood at a faster rate, as muscles can use it as a fuel. But if the person exercises at a time when the blood glucose is either too high (*hyperglycemia*) or too low (*hypoglycemia*), problems can develop. On the one hand, if the glucose concentration is too high before exercise due to inadequate insulin, exercise causes a release of glucose from the liver faster than the muscles can take it up. This worsens the situation in that the diabetic goes further out of control, and it can lead to *diabetic coma*. On the other hand, if the diabetic takes too much insulin before exercise, blood glucose is taken up by tissues during exercise faster than the liver can supply it, and the blood glucose concentration falls to extremely low values, leading to *insulin shock*. So, though exercise can be helpful in that the diabetic may need less insulin to maintain control of glucose, exercise complicates things in that the diabetic must now balance three things: diet, insulin, and exercise. In spite of these potential problems, participation in sports and exercise by Type I diabetics is a normal part of life. What steps, then, should the Type I diabetic follow in developing an exercise program?

The Type I diabetic should have a comprehensive medical exam, including a graded exercise test (GXT), to evaluate nerve, kidney, eye (retina), and cardiovascular function. Because the Type I diabetic may suffer from a wide variety of problems (depending on the length of time the diabetes has been present and the degree to which blood glucose has been con-

trolled), this is crucial. Following this, the Type I diabetic usually works with a physician or nurse-educator to develop an injection and meal-consumption pattern to maintain control of blood glucose and avoid hypoglycemia. This is achieved by careful monitoring of the blood glucose concentration before, during, and after exercise, and varying insulin and carbohydrate intake depending on the intensity and duration of exercise, and the fitness of the individual:

- Before exercise, if blood glucose is below 80 to 100 mg/dl, the person should consume carbohydrates. If it is above 250 mg/dl, the person should delay exercise until it is below 250 mg/dl.

- The person should not exercise at the time of peak insulin action, and she should inject the insulin into a nonexercising muscle or skinfold. The quantity of insulin injected is usually decreased, depending on the activity.

- The person should consume additional carbohydrate in recovery from exercise to replace the glycogen stores and provide enough to maintain the blood glucose concentration.

You will have to carefully individualize exercise sessions for Type I diabetics, depending on the state of the disease, which can vary greatly. For example, Type I diabetics are marathon runners and professional athletes. Yet some must do weight-supported activities because of peripheral nerve and blood vessel damage. Clearly, it is crucial to follow a physician's directions.

Type I diabetics represent only 10% of all diabetics. The remainder are *Type II* or *noninsulin-dependent diabetics*. This type of diabetes is associated with obesity, and because it usually occurs later in life, it is also called *adult onset diabetes*. Some Type II diabetics may take an oral medication that stimulates the pancreas to produce more insulin, but many of these diabetics are treated simply with a combination of exercise and diet to achieve weight loss and normalize blood glucose. The exercise is helpful because it helps to remove glucose from the blood without additional insulin and in addition makes the tissues more responsive to the insulin that is available. As with the Type I diabetic, a medical exam is recommended for a Type II diabetic prior to undertaking a new exercise program. Part of the reason for this is that many Type II diabetics have multiple risk factors: high blood pressure, high serum cholesterol, and obesity. Encourage Type II diabetics to do moderate exercise (about 50% $\dot{V}O_2$max) 5 to 7 days per week to promote the improved sensitivity to insulin and to facilitate weight loss. Remind Type II diabetics that achieving the goals of normal body weight and blood glucose control requires more than exercise. A diet low in fat and high in carbohydrates (see chapter 6) is also recommended. The combination of the diet and exercise not only improves the chance that Type II diabetics will achieve blood glucose control, they are likely to improve blood lipids, blood pressure, and $\dot{V}O_2$max, all of which reduce the risk of cardiovascular disease.

The previous information is important to help you understand what diabetes is and how exercise fits into the plan to deal with the problem. The following are reasonable recommendations that an exercise leader should consider with regard to diabetes:

- Determine if there are any diabetics in your exercise class, through initial screening as in chapter 4.
- Ask if the diabetics received instructions from a physician or nurse-educator on how to alter carbohydrate and insulin (or other medications) prior to exercise to maintain blood glucose control during exercise. If not, refer them back to their physicians before allowing participation in the fitness program.

- Ask if the diabetics have a readily available form of glucose with them in case of hypoglycemia.
- Have each diabetic participant work with a "buddy" to help out in case of a problem.

Asthma

Asthma is a condition in which the airways suddenly decrease in diameter, making breathing more difficult. A variety of factors can cause this problem in susceptible individuals: pollen, aspirin, pollutants, and, for some, exercise itself. A condition called *exercise-induced asthma* occurs when a person breathes large volumes of dry air that cools and dries the respiratory tract. This results in a series of reactions by special cells in the respiratory tract, leading to the secretion of fluid and a constriction of the airway. The net effect is that the person has a difficult time breathing, and in some cases it can lead to death. Though this is a problem, there is no question that asthma can be controlled. The best evidence for this is found in the large number of asthmatics who have won Olympic medals. The condition is controlled by medications taken *prior to exercise* that prevent the problem from occurring. In addition, many asthmatics carry with them an aerosol drug that causes an immediate bronchodilation if an asthma attack occurs during exercise. It is certainly a good idea for the exercise leader to follow our figure 19.1 friend's lead.

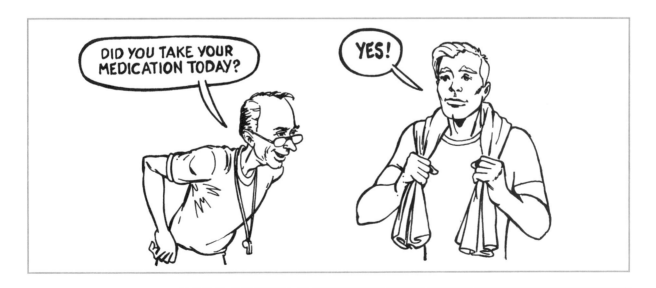

Figure 19.1 Take medication as prescribed.

It is generally recommended that an asthmatic use a long warm-up period (more than ten minutes) prior to exercise and exercise in an intermittent fashion, with exercise bouts lasting 5 min or less. Because breathing warm, moist air reduces the chance of an attack, swimming is a preferred activity for asthmatics. Wearing a scarf or mask over the mouth and nose while running or cycling outdoors tends to trap moisture and reduce the chance that the respiratory tract becomes dry and cool. The following are reasonable recommendations that an exercise leader should consider in regard to asthma:

- Determine if there are any individuals with asthma in your exercise class as part of the initial screening (see chapter 4).
- Ask if they have taken their medication prior to class.
- Ask if they have their aerosol bronchodilators with them.
- Inform them about doing a long warm-up and interval-type exercise. Have each participant with asthma exercise with a "buddy" who can help in an emergency.

Obesity

A combination of diet and exercise is recommended for achieving weight loss in overweight and obese individuals. Chapters 5 and 6 provided the details on this recommendation, and this section simply highlights and emphasizes the need to begin slowly and progress gradually toward a weight loss goal. The obese individual probably has a low level of cardiorespiratory fitness due to both the body fatness and a sedentary lifestyle. The emphasis in an exercise program must be on starting slowly with a walking program to build up the habit of exercise and to gradually condition the muscles involved. If the person has orthopedic problems, cycling and aquatic activities are excellent choices, as both relieve the load on the ankles, knees, and hips. The number of kilocalories expended for a given amount of exercise decreases as the obese individual loses weight; the quantity of exercise the individual does per session has to increase if the rate of energy expenditure is to remain constant across a weight loss program.

Hypertension

A large number of people have borderline hypertension (high blood pressure) or take medication to keep it under control. Given that a blood pressure measurement is one of the recommended tests for a fitness participant to complete prior to an exercise program, the exercise leader should be aware of the problem. We recommend that blood pressure be evaluated on a regular basis, and if it is elevated, the individual should contact a physician. The physician may prescribe a special diet low in sodium (salt), weight loss, exercise, or medication. The primary goal is to get the blood pressure within normal limits. An exercise program involving large muscle groups in dynamic activities is recommended for borderline hypertensives. The fitness leader should avoid activities that involve small muscle groups or require people to hold their breath. As in the case of the diabetic or the asthmatic, encourage the hypertensive participant to take the prescribed medication on a regular basis, at the same time each day. If it is possible, we recommend that the blood pressure of these individuals be monitored on a frequent basis, as the combination of weight loss, diet, and exercise may cause the blood pressure to decrease independent of the medication. In this way, the blood pressure value provides a guide for the individual to return to the physician for a change or elimination of medication.

Blood pressure medications work in different ways to achieve the same effect. Diuretics work by causing a loss of sodium and water from the body. Given that exercise can bring about the same effect by causing a large sweat loss, it is important for the fitness leader to educate fitness participants who take diuretics to be especially aware of the need to replace fluids during and after exercise. Hypertensive individuals who are treated with a beta adrenergic blocking drug (e.g., Inderal) cannot use the 220 – age formula to estimate maximal heart rate. The drug lowers maximal heart rate, making the usual THR zone calculation incorrect. The following are reasonable recommendations that a fitness leader should consider regarding participants with controlled hypertension:

- Identify all individuals with controlled hypertension in the class, through initial screening, and find out what kind of medication they are using.
- Monitor resting blood pressure on a regular basis.
- Encourage those taking medication to do so on a regular basis.
- Emphasize large muscle dynamic activities done at moderate intensities (40% to 60% of maximal oxygen uptake or RPE = 10 to 12) for long durations, most days of the week.

Seizure Disorders

Those with seizure disorders (like epilepsy) are encouraged to participate in a regular activity program and lead a normal life. The exercise leader needs to be aware of those in class who may have such a problem and should inquire about the types of circumstances or events that can trigger a seizure.

Generally, no special restrictions are necessary, but the exercise leader should try to assign a "buddy" to work alongside each seizure-prone individual. The following are reasonable recommendations that an exercise leader should consider regarding seizure disorders:

- Identify those in the class who have seizure disorders through the initial screening (see chapter 4).
- Encourage those individuals to take medication on a regular basis.
- Use the "buddy" system to ensure additional safety.

Exercise Prescription Across the Ages

Physical activity is needed for optimal growth and development in early childhood. In addition, physical activity is crucial in the prevention of and rehabilitation from a wide variety of problems encountered by older individuals. Consequently, the fitness leader needs to be aware of the unique needs of individuals across the age span, when exercise is prescribed.

Exercise Prescription for Children

Childhood is a special time for the development of the major gross motor skills (e.g., throwing, jumping, running, swimming). Children are inherently active and given the opportunity to play, they will. This need for children to develop motor skills must be kept in mind when discussing fitness programming for children. Compared to adults, children are similar in terms of cardiorespiratory fitness (per unit body weight) and can perform endurance tasks well; they are also similar in terms of muscle stores of creatine phosphate and ATP, allowing them to do well in brief, explosive activities. They are lower than adults in the ability to generate energy through the anaerobic pathways, dissipate heat via evaporation, and in the economy of walking or running. This all means that they have a lower capacity to do all-out activities lasting 10 to 90 s, have an increased potential for heat-related problems, and use more energy per unit body weight to walk and run. They are well suited to intermittent activities in that they get to a steady state faster and recover faster.

Cardiovascular Fitness. You can use the same exercise prescription for cardiovascular fitness for children as you do for adults; however, there is some debate about whether or not they will experience the same increases in $\dot{V}O_2max$ with training. Many believe that the focus of the exercise prescription should be on establishing the behavior of "regular exercise" in children, in that such a behavior is most important in gaining the health-related benefits of physical activity. Therefore, encourage children to become involved in individual continuous activities (e.g., running, swimming, in-line skating), team sports (e.g., basketball, soccer), individual and dual sports (e.g., tennis, racquetball), and recreational activities (e.g., hiking). You may be able to facilitate this in your role as a fitness leader by working with parents, schools, and community organizations to promote an active lifestyle for children.

Muscular Strength and Endurance. Children can participate safely in formal weight training programs, but you must take precautions:

- Trained personnel should supervise each session.

- Teach children proper lifting techniques, with no breath-holding.

- Emphasize controlled lifting techniques, avoiding ballistic movements.

- Children should do one or two sets of 8 to 10 different exercises (with 8 to 12 reps per set) and include most major muscle groups.

- Limit training sessions to two times per week to encourage the development of other skills.

- Teach children that if they cannot lift a weight 8 times, they should use a lower weight.

- Have children avoid performing exercises to the point of momentary fatigue due to risks of harming developing bone and joint structures.

Elderly

One of the fastest-growing segments of the population is the elderly. Exercise is good for this population not only because of its potential to improve or maintain cardiorespiratory fitness but also for the stimulus it provides to promote bone growth. Osteoporosis, a thinning of the bones, is a major problem in this population; exercise works with diet and hormones to improve or maintain the integrity of the bones. Bone structure is maintained by the downward force of gravity (upright posture) and the lateral forces generated by muscle contraction. Although a specific exercise recommendation about how to deal with osteoporosis is not available, it is known that weight-bearing activities (walking or jogging) are better than bicycling or swimming. You must exercise caution, however, because the elderly who are not fit (see later) and those with previous fractures may need to bicycle or swim.

A wide variety of studies have shown that compared to sedentary individuals, endurance-trained older athletes have half the decrease in cardiorespiratory fitness over time, higher HDL (good) cholesterol, enhanced sensitivity to insulin (the opposite of Type II diabetes),

greater strength, and faster reaction time. Studies of elderly who have undertaken a formal exercise program have confirmed these findings and show that with training the elderly can improve strength and cardiovascular fitness similar to younger individuals (but generally at a slower rate) and can improve blood pressure and insulin sensitivity. These studies show that the elderly can participate safely in exercise programs and make improvement similar to what is expected in younger populations.

The elderly population is very diverse and was classified by Smith and Gilligan (1987) in the following manner:

- Athletic-old > 55 years with good fitness (10 METs)

- Young-old > 55 years with moderate fitness (6 to 7 METs)

- Old-old > 75 years with very low fitness (2 to 3 METs)

Exercise recommendations vary with the type of elderly individual. Those in the athletic-old group can do much of what is recommended for the average young adult, with few modifications. Those in the young-old group have a lower fitness level and are limited to activities similar to those seen in cardiac rehabilitation programs. These programs emphasize large muscle dynamic activities at low exercise intensities. Walking, cycling, and swimming are well within their capabilities; thus, encourage these. The old-old group has extremely limited cardiorespiratory fitness and must do most fitness activities while sitting or standing with support. The idea is for this group to maintain as high a fitness level as they can to make self-care activities possible. Because of the risk of skeletal injury due to osteoporosis, it is important to emphasize controlled activities such as walking, cycling, and swimming. However, the exercise leader should develop a variety of warm-up and cool-down activities that can accomplish flexibility and muscular strengthening goals while the participant has fun. An appropriate solution is to adapt children's low organized games that call for the participant to sit and stand during activity. For example, have them stand, reach for the stars, turn to look left and right, sit, and touch their toes.

Pregnancy

Pregnancy is a special case to consider because it puts additional stress on the woman, over and above that of exercise alone. As in the case of the person with diabetes or asthma, the pregnant woman should discuss her exercise plans with her physician prior to beginning a program and again at different stages during the pregnancy. Exercise does not deprive the fetus of oxygen and, judging by the fetus's heart rate response, there are no signs of distress during exercise. Exercise guidelines for pregnant women are gradually developing as new research results become available. Currently, the American College of Obstetricians and Gynecologists recommends that the pregnant participant should do the following:

- Talk with her physician to plan an exercise program.
- Follow the 3 days per week pattern, with warm-ups and cool-downs.
- Avoid performing any activity while lying on the back after the first trimester.
- Avoid exercising to exhaustion.
- Avoid activities with potential for trauma or in which loss of balance is likely.
- Augment heat dissipation by ensuring adequate hydration, appropriate clothing, and optimal environment.

- Consider weight-supported activities as a way to continue exercising throughout pregnancy.

American College of Ostetricians and Gynecologists (1994).

Summary

Many health problems or personal characteristics influence the kinds of activity individuals can do in a fitness program. This chapter provided some suggestions to assist you, as you work with appropriate medical personnel, to select appropriate exercise for participants with orthopedic problems, diabetes, asthma, obesity, high blood pressure, or seizure disorders, as well as those who are children, elderly, or pregnant. General recommendations for anyone who has questions about exercise are to check with a personal physician; use longer warm-ups; slow the progression to the main part of the workout; lower the intensity of the activity; use longer cool-down activities; pay attention to environmental conditions; recognize signs of overexertion; exercise with others; be regular with food, water, and prescribed medication; and use common sense in deciding to modify or stop an activity.

Chapter 20
Environmental Problems

Exercising in
Heat
Cold
High Altitude
Pollution

The target heart rate (THR) zone identifies the safe and proper intensity of exercise that both creates a cardiovascular training effect and allows an individual to continue long enough for the exercise to be an effective part of a weight reduction program. The exercise leader must be aware, however, that environmental factors such as heat, humidity, high altitude, and pollution can elevate the HR, thus requiring a reduction in exercise intensity. In addition, the exercise leader has to recognize the health risks of exercising in the cold. The purposes of this chapter are to provide information about how each of these factors interact with an exercise program and recommend ways to deal with these factors.

Exercising in Heat and Humidity

Ordinarily, the workload associated with exercise provides the primary stimulus for HR to increase; the environment, however, can play an important role in determining the overall HR response to exercise. For example, if the environmental temperature is higher than skin temperature (>90° F), the body gains heat from the environment rather than loses heat to it. High relative humidity reduces an individual's ability to evaporate sweat, making it still more difficult to lose heat from the body. Both of these conditions cause body temperature to rise, and along with it, HR. Table 20.1 estimates heat stress using a combination of environmental temperature and relative humidity. The proper way to deal with a high environmental heat load is to decrease the intensity (MET load) of the activity, shift the activity to a cooler part of the day, or exercise in an air-conditioned facility.

In addition to environmental heat and humidity, the type of clothing worn and the degree of hydration influence the HR response. Clothing that does not allow sweat to reach the surface of the skin causes body temperature and heart rate to increase. Sweat that merely runs down into your socks does you no good in cooling your body. Recommend that participants wear as little as possible and choose cotton or mesh materials. Another problem aggravated by choosing the wrong kind of clothing is the degree of hydration, or water balance. The normal sweating response is important to the process of losing heat during exercise; high heat, humidity, and improper clothing cause a higher sweat loss and increase the chance that an individual will become dehydrated. Fitness participants must drink water in *anticipation of, during, and after exercise.* One of the best ways to reinforce this point is to have the participant weigh in each

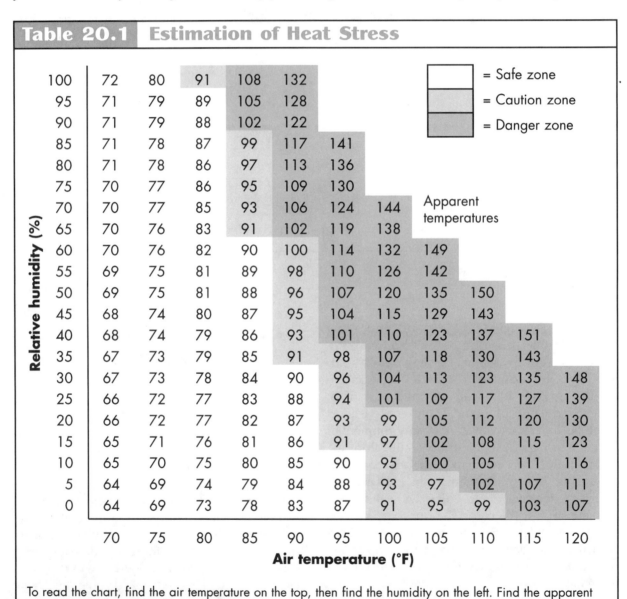

Table 20.1 Estimation of Heat Stress

Relative humidity (%)	70	75	80	85	90	95	100	105	110	115	120
100	72	80	91	108	132						
95	71	79	89	105	128						
90	71	79	88	102	122						
85	71	78	87	99	117	141					
80	71	78	86	97	113	136					
75	70	77	86	95	109	130					
70	70	77	85	93	106	124	144				
65	70	76	83	91	102	119	138				
60	70	76	82	90	100	114	132	149			
55	69	75	81	89	98	110	126	142			
50	69	75	81	88	96	107	120	135	150		
45	68	74	80	87	95	104	115	129	143		
40	68	74	79	86	93	101	110	123	137	151	
35	67	73	79	85	91	98	107	118	130	143	
30	67	73	78	84	90	96	104	113	123	135	148
25	66	72	77	83	88	94	101	109	117	127	139
20	66	72	77	82	87	93	99	105	112	120	130
15	65	71	76	81	86	91	97	102	108	115	123
10	65	70	75	80	85	90	95	100	105	111	116
5	64	69	74	79	84	88	93	97	102	107	111
0	64	69	73	78	83	87	91	95	99	103	107

Air temperature (°F)

= Safe zone
= Caution zone
= Danger zone

Apparent temperatures

To read the chart, find the air temperature on the top, then find the humidity on the left. Find the apparent temperature where the columns meet.

Reprinted from Corbin and Lindsey 1991.

day. Any rapid weight loss has to be due to dehydration and should be corrected before the participant continues exercise. You must emphasize water replacement in times of high sweat losses. Even though salt is lost in sweat along with water, the quantity is small, and most people already eat more salt than they need. So for those participants who ask about taking salt tablets, suggest that they simply shake a little more salt on their food at mealtime instead.

Given this concern about high heat and humidity, should anyone even consider exercising under such conditions? We believe so, but you as the exercise leader should provide appropriate information to reduce the risk of heat injury. Because many people do exercise or engage in recreational activities on their own in high heat and humidity, helping participants learn how to adapt to such conditions is a reasonable goal. Emphasize using the THR as the best indicator of the combined heat and exercise load. Heart rate is influenced by the workload, humidity, temperature, clothing, and state of hydration. Participation in a supervised exercise program can help those who wish to exercise on their own in high heat and humidity achieve some degree of acclimatization. As you acclimatize, your body "learns" to sweat more without losing more salt. The result is that you are better able to deal with the heat with a lower body temperature, heart rate, and risk of heat injury. A fitness leader should consider these recommendations for exercising in the heat and humidity:

- Use THR as the best guide to reduce the chance of heat injury.
- Suggest that participants exercise during the cooler part of the day to reduce heat gain from the sun.
- Gradually introduce fitness participants to heat and humidity; acclimatization takes 7 to 10 days.
- Educate participants to wear appropriate clothing and use sunblock.
- Educate participants to drink water in anticipation of, during, and after exercise.
- Educate participants to avoid taking salt tablets.
- Educate participants about signs of heat illness (such as cramps or light-headedness) and how to deal with the problem: Stop exercising, get out of the heat, drink water, and cool down with wet towels, fans, and so forth (see chapter 18)

Exercising in the Cold

Cold air causes the blood vessels in the skin to constrict to prevent warm blood from reaching the surface and reduces heat loss from the body. This response, if prolonged, can lead to frostbite, and for some susceptible individuals, cold air can cause angina (chest pain) or bring on an asthma attack. Air temperatures of –20° F or less create a risk of frostbite, and the dryness of the cold air can irritate the respiratory tract. You must educate participants about dressing properly for the cold and how to deal with frostbite. Treat superficial frostbite by immersing the affected body part in warm water (100-105 degrees fahrenheit) without massaging it. Individuals with deep frost bite should be referred to a physician.

Although frostbite is certainly a problem associated with exercising in the cold, hypothermia is potentially more dangerous. Hypothermia is a condition in which the body loses heat faster than it is produced; body temperature falls as a result. Strangely, most cases of hypothermia occur at temperatures above 30 °F, due to the effect of wind, dampness, and cold water immersion. When a person is immersed in water, heat is lost from the body about 25 times faster than when a person is in air at the same temperature.

Windchill is a major factor in the rate of heat loss in cold temperatures. Table 20.2 shows the effect of wind velocity on the temperature experienced by the body. Wind increases the number of cold, dry air molecules that come in contact with the skin, and, as a result, the body loses heat at a faster rate. The fall in body temperature triggers violent shivering and can impair basic neuromuscular function and a person's ability to make good decisions. For example, one poor decision made under these conditions would be to lie down and rest. This usually results in death, as the body's heat production slows down as a person rests and the rate of heat loss increases. This is where fitness comes in: The fit person is able to keep going for a longer period of time (if necessary), thereby reducing the chance of hypothermia.

A fitness leader should recommend the following to prevent hypothermia:

- Do not exercise in extreme cold or high winds; exercise indoors or skip a workout.
- Wear appropriate clothing in layers that provide insulation.

Table 20.2	Windchill Index										

Wind speed in MPH	Actual thermometer reading (°F)											
	50	40	30	20	10	0	−10	−20	−30	−40	−50	−60
	Equivalent temperature (°F)											
Calm	50	40	30	20	10	0	−10	−20	−30	−40	−50	−60
5	48	37	27	16	6	−5	−15	−26	−36	−47	−57	−68
10	40	28	16	4	−9	−21	−33	−46	−58	−70	−83	−95
15	36	22	9	−5	−18	−36	−45	−58	−72	−85	−99	−112
20	32	18	4	−10	−25	−39	−53	−67	−82	−96	−110	−124
25	30	16	0	−15	−29	−44	−59	−74	−88	−104	−118	−133
30	28	13	−2	−18	−33	−48	−63	−79	−94	−109	−125	−140
35	27	11	−4	−20	−35	−49	−67	−82	−98	−113	−129	−145
40	26	10	−6	−21	−37	−53	−69	−85	−100	−116	−132	−148

(Wind speeds greater than 40 mph have little additional effect)

Little danger (for properly clothed person)

Increasing danger

Great danger

Danger from freezing of exposed flesh

Adapted from Sharkey 1984.

- Remove layers of clothing as you warm up to minimize sweating and maintain the insulating quality of the clothing.
- Stay as dry as possible, as evaporation of water from the skin can cause body temperature to fall at a rapid rate.
- If hypothermia occurs, get the person out of the cold, wet, and wind; remove wet clothing; and provide warm drinks and a warm sleeping bag.

Exercising at High Altitude

The partial pressure of oxygen decreases with increasing altitude. This means that there is less oxygen bound to the hemoglobin in the blood, which reduces the heart's ability to transport oxygen to the working muscles. Figure 20.1 shows that maximal aerobic power (cardiorespiratory fitness) decreases with increasing altitude. This means that a person cannot run at the same rate of speed at high altitude as at sea level in long-distance races. More than maximal aerobic power is affected, however. Because there is less oxygen in the blood at high altitude, the heart must beat more often to deliver the same quantity of oxygen to the muscles. This is shown in figure 20.2, demonstrating that HR is higher at any level of oxygen consumption at high altitude.

This means that when exercising at high altitude, the fitness participant must slow down in order to stay in the THR zone. Again, the fitness leader should focus the participant's attention on the importance of the THR, which provides a means of adjusting exercise intensity to a wide range of environmental circumstances.

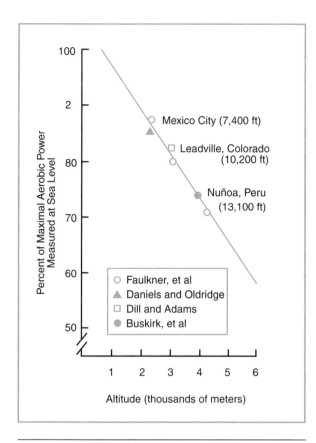

Figure 20.1 Effect of altitude on maximal aerobic power.

Reprinted from "Effect of Altitude on Physical Performance" by E.T. Howley. In *Encyclopedia of Physical Education, Fitness, and Sports: Vol. 2. Training, Environment, Nutrition, and Fitness (p. 182)* by G.A. Stull and T.K. Cureton, Jr. (Eds.), 1980, Salt Lake City, UT: Brighton. © 1980 by Brighton.

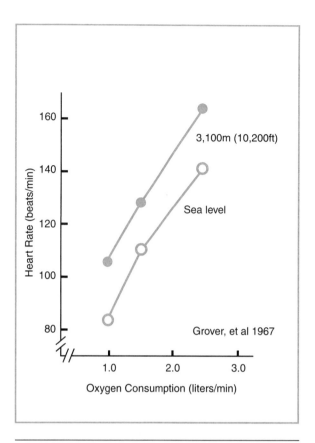

Figure 20.2 Effect of altitude on the heart rate response to submaximal work rates.

Reprinted from "Effect of Altitude on Physical Performance" by E.T. Howley. In *Encyclopedia of Physical Education, Fitness, and Sports: Vol. 2. Training, Environment, Nutrition, and Fitness (p. 182)* by G.A. Stull and T.K. Cureton, Jr. (Eds.), 1980, Salt Lake City, UT: Brighton. © 1980 by Brighton.

Pollution

A variety of pollutants can decrease performance, including carbon monoxide, ozone, and sulfur dioxide. Carbon monoxide has an immediate effect on oxygen transport because it binds about 200 times more readily to the hemoglobin molecule in the blood than does oxygen, reducing the blood's oxygen-transporting capacity. The normal carbon monoxide level in blood is 1% for nonsmokers and 10% for smokers; however, a nonsmoker who lives in a polluted urban area may have a level of 5%. Performance is affected at 3%, and maximal aerobic power decreases when carbon monoxide levels in the blood reach 4.3%.

Ozone and sulfur dioxide can affect performance by causing bronchoconstriction, an increase in airway resistance, that can lead to a wheezing sound associated with asthma. Long-term exposure to ozone can decrease lung function, and high heat and humidity compound the problem.

The fitness leader must monitor the "pollution index" available in communities with major pollution problems. Those exercising in an area with air pollution should do the following:

- Reduce exposure to the pollutant prior to exercise.

- Stay away from areas where one might receive a large dose of carbon monoxide, such as smoking areas and high vehicle traffic areas.

- Avoid scheduling activities during the times when pollutants are at their highest levels (usually rush hour—7 to 10 A.M. and 4 to 7 P.M.).

Summary

This chapter described safety tips you should remember when leading exercise in hot, humid, cold, or polluted environments or at high altitude. It's important to prevent heat injury; instruct participants to exercise in an environment that facilitates the evaporation of sweat and does not impose a large heat load. Encourage participants to wear cotton (or mesh) fabrics to allow sweat to evaporate. Gradually increase their exposure to a hot environment so their bodies adapt by sweating more. Have participants drink water before, during, and after a workout. Most exercisers do not need to increase salt intake with fluid loss because they take in more than they need in their normal diet.

Hypothermia results when heat is lost from the body faster than it is produced. Instruct participants to wear clothing in layers during cold weather and to shed layers as they begin to sweat. Wind increases the loss of body heat during cold temperatures, and participants may wish to exercise indoors on cold and windy days. Increasing altitude reduces the oxygen content of blood, and increases the rate at which the heart must pump blood to deliver the required oxygen to tissues during exercise. Instruct participants to monitor THR and to reduce exercise intensity at altitude. Pollution can influence a participant's response to exercise, and fitness leaders should provide exercise guidelines relevant to local conditions.

Chapter 21
Program Organization

Screening
Testing
Activities
Communication

The fitness leader is not normally the same person as the fitness program administrator. However, understanding the organization assists everyone working in the program to put their own responsibilities into the broader perspective of the program's goals. This chapter provides an overview of program organization.

The key concept in administration is planning. Many different programs can be successful if they are carefully planned. In contrast, almost nothing works well over the long-term without prior thought. Components of the long-range plan include policies and procedures for screening, testing, activity, and communication (see figure 21.1).

Screening

All fitness programs should screen participants so that they engage in appropriate fitness programs. Chapter 4 discussed criteria for admis-

sion to various programs. For example, people with known or suspected health problems are not placed in fitness programs aimed at increasing the positive health of apparently healthy people. You, as the fitness leader, need to understand the criteria for exclusion or referral so you can take appropriate action based on test results, signs, and symptoms that indicate problems.

Any fitness program should follow informed consent procedures established to protect participants. Informed consent has several components. The first component is a clear description of the fitness program and all the procedures to be used. This description should be in writing; the individual reads it and receives a copy to keep. In addition, each person gets a chance to have any questions answered. The second component, which should be included in the written description of the program, is a list of the possible benefits and risks of such a program. The

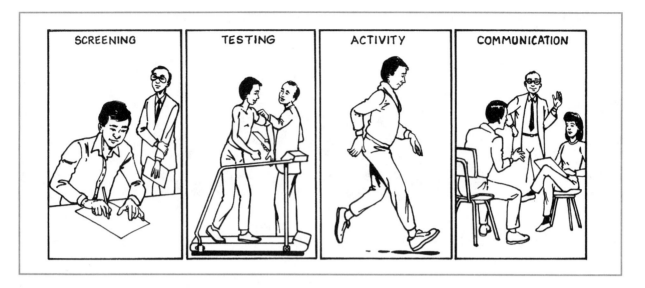

Figure 21.1 Administrative responsibilities.

fitness benefits are extensive; however, there is also increased risk of certain kinds of injuries, and heart attacks do occasionally happen during or after exercise. After reading the program description outlining the potential benefits and risks, the individual signs the form. This signature indicates he is participating voluntarily and can stop a test or any activity at any time without penalty or coercion to continue. The last component is confidentiality. Each participant's data will be confidential, unless he gives permission to release it. People will normally agree to have their test scores used in fitness reports and research, but these reports should use a format that preserves confidentiality of an individual's test score. An exception to this guideline is using test scores to recognize participants in newsletters or news releases—in these cases, you should request permission (which is usually granted) from the participant before publication. Table 21.1 illustrates a sample form that you can use in a fitness program. You should modify specific procedures to fit the particular fitness program.

Testing

Testing is an important aspect of fitness programs (see figure 21.2). You will use test results to decide whether persons should be excluded from a fitness program, can enter the program only with medical clearance, or can begin immediately. For participants in the program, periodic testing is important to determine progress toward their individual objectives. Test results can motivate people to continue and support a progressive modification of activities. Part III included our recommended fitness testing procedures. Table 21.2 shows a sample score sheet that facilitates comparison between testing periods.

Activities

After the screening and the initial testing, you will provide fitness participants with a variety of activities appropriate for their fitness levels. Part of the feedback from the screening and testing is to encourage participants to choose activities suitable for them at their own fitness levels. The fitness leader can help reinforce appropriate activities and suggest alternatives for those who seem out of place in a particular activity.

The main objective for the fitness program is that it be conducted safely for all persons permitted to participate in it. Fortunately, the same factors that make the program safe also help protect it legally. Chapter 18 included detailed procedures to prevent and deal with injuries and emergencies; this is essential information for all staff members who will be in contact with fitness participants.

Table 21.1	Sample Consent Form: Generic Fitness Program*

Informed Consent for Physical Fitness Test

In order to more safely carry on an exercise program, I hereby consent, voluntarily, to exercise tests. I shall perform a graded exercise test by riding a cycle ergometer or walking or running on a treadmill. Exercise will begin at a low level and be advanced in stages. The test may be stopped at any time because of signs of fatigue. I understand that I may stop the test at any time because of my feelings of fatigue or discomfort or for any other personal reason.

I understand that the risks of this testing procedure may include disorders of heartbeats, abnormal blood pressure response, and, very rarely, a heart attack. I further understand that selection and supervision of my test is a matter of professional judgment.

I also understand that skinfold measurements will be taken at (number) sites to determine percentage of body fat and that I will complete a sit-and-reach test and an abdominal curl-up test to evaluate factors related to low-back function.

I desire such testing so that better advice regarding my proposed exercise program may be given to me, but I understand that the testing does not entirely eliminate risk in the proposed exercise program.

I understand that information from my tests may be used for reports and research publications. I understand that my identity will not be revealed.

I understand that I can withdraw my consent or discontinue participation in any aspect of the fitness testing or program at any time without penalty or prejudice toward me.

I have read the statement above and have had all of my questions answered to my satisfaction.

_____
Signed

_____
Witness

_____
Date
(Copy for participant and for program records.)

*Replace title with name of your program

Note. From *Fitness Leader's Handbook* (2nd ed.) by B.D. Franks and E.T. Howley, 1998, Champaign, IL: Human Kinetics. This form may be copied by the fitness leader for distribution to participants.

A fitness program needs a written emergency procedure and must train staff members to carry it out. While establishing the emergency procedure, contact local emergency services to help establish the procedure and to make sure they know and agree with the procedure. Table 21.3 includes a sample form you can modify for your specific situation.

The program and its staff have a responsibility to watch for any danger signs that may indicate a problem, take appropriate actions to stop the activity before problems occur, and perform emergency procedures in a professional manner. If problems should occur, the fitness leader must take appropriate action to deal with minor problems and get immediate help for major

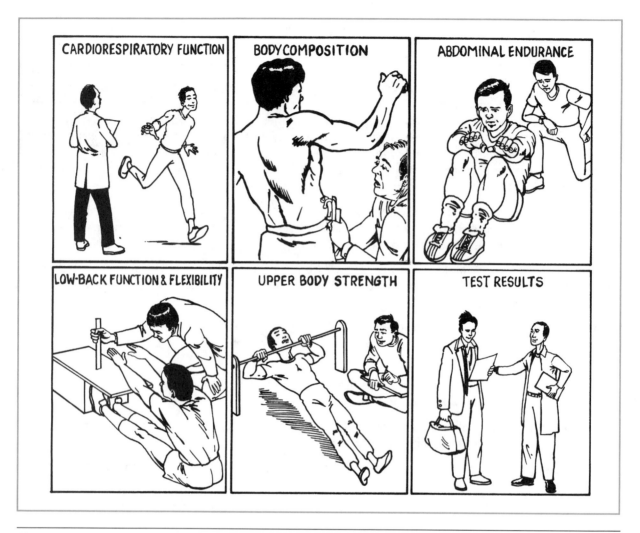

Figure 21.2 Types of testing.

problems. Professional organizations (such as the American Alliance for Health, Physical Education, Recreation and Dance and the American College of Sports Medicine) have liability insurance available for individuals, and staff members should have this type of insurance. In addition, the organization should include liability insurance for the fitness leader and facilities in its insurance coverage.

Although getting participants' consent does not prevent legal actions or protect the facility against negligence, it does indicate that the program is concerned with the participant and has acted in good faith. However, no amount of informed consent procedures can justify negligence. People and areas need supervision. Staff members need training in appropriate emergency procedures. Supervision and emergency

procedures must be followed. Failure to do so, or failure to act in a manner befitting a fitness professional, is negligence. If injury or death occur as a result of the negligence, then the fitness professional and the program are legally liable.

Safety procedures include regular checks of equipment and facilities, as well as periodic reviews of the staff's procedures in both testing and fitness sessions. The program must keep adequate records detailing when the review, training, and practice occurred.

Personnel

The most important aspect of any program is the quality of its staff. Recruiting, hiring, supporting, and evaluating personnel to help achieve the organization's goals are extremely

Table 21.2	Youth Fitness Sample Scoresheet*			

Name (or code number): _____ Birthdate: _____

Test item	Date of test			
	Test 1 / /	Test 2 / /	Test 3 / /	Test 4 / /
1-mi run (min:sec)				
Triceps skinfold (mm)				
Calf skinfold (mm)				
Sum of skinfolds (mm)				
Percent fat (%)				
Modified curl-ups (#)				
Sit-and-reach (in.)				
Modified pull-ups (#)				
*Replace title with name of your program				

important, time-consuming, and often sensitive. What types of persons does a program need to carry out the program that has been planned? In fitness programs, staff must be able to present and supervise the fitness activities. A typical fitness center needs the following personnel:

Full-time	Part-time
Program director	Medical advisor
Health and fitness instructor	Nutritionist
Fitness leaders (or part-time)	Psychologist
Educational coordinator	Physical therapist
Secretary	Equipment technician
	Fitness leaders (or full-time)

It is important to provide a good working environment and to accurately describe the working conditions to prospective staff members. The physical environment should be safe, clean, and cheerful, with equipment that works, supplies available, and quick repairs when needed. The professional environment is one in which the expectations for each staff member are clearly described, with enough supervision to assist professional growth and ensure quality performance. The psychological environment ensures that employees are valued, are communicated with openly and honestly, have support for any problems that might arise, and solicits and welcomes their input.

A clear, mutually understood job description provides the basis for periodic evaluations. The main purpose of the evaluation should be to assist the staff member in self-improvement. However, the evaluation may also be used to determine whether to promote or retain professionals in their positions and whether to offer merit raises. Evaluation of a fitness leader includes the content of the fitness program; the manner in which the program is conducted; the leader's rapport with fitness participants, other

Table 21.3	Sample Emergency Procedures: Generic Fitness Center*

Cardiac emergency

1. Do NOT move the victim, except to try to get him or her into a lying position.
2. Check for breathing and pulse; if absent, begin CPR immediately.
3. Call, or have someone call, the Emergency Room at _____(name)_____ Hospital, _____(phone number)_____, ext. ____(number)____.
4. Read the statement above the phone to the person:

   (Statement to be posted by all phones:)

   This is _____(name)_____ at the _____(name)_____ Fitness Center. We have a cardiac emergency, please send an ambulance to the _____(name)_____ Street entrance of the _____(name)_____ building, at _____(address)_____.
5. Send someone to get Dr. _____(name)_____, whose schedule is posted by the phone (this is for the centers that have medical personnel on the site).
6. Continue CPR until medical personnel arrive, then follow their instructions.

Other serious accidents or injuries

For any of the following:

   Airway problems other than choking
   Unconsciousness
   Head injury
   Bleeding from ear, nose, or mouth
   Neck or back injuries
   Limb injury with obvious deformity
   Severe chest pains

   1. Do NOT move the person, except to try to get him or her into a lying position, with feet elevated (unless you suspect back injuries).
   2. Contact ambulance and medical personnel—same as cardiac emergencies.
   3. Treat for shock.
   4. Control bleeding.

Other injuries or accidents

1. Do not allow a sick or injured person to sit, stand, or walk until you are sure that his or her condition warrants it.
2. Do not encourage a person who is "feeling bad" to begin or continue working out.
3. Check on people who have questionable symptoms in the locker room.
4. For less serious injuries, a first aid kit is available at _____(place)_____.

As soon as the situation is under control, inform _____(person)_____ about the accident, complete accident report, and turn in to _____(name or place)_____ within 24 hr.

Your suggestions for improving these instructions and the emergency procedures are welcome—talk to _____(name)_____.

*Replace title with name of your program

Note. From *Fitness Leader's Handbook* (2nd ed.) by B.D. Franks and E.T. Howley, 1998, Champaign, IL: Human Kinetics.

staff, and the fitness director; response to emergency and unusual situations; accurate collection and recording of test data; and prompt and professional manner of carrying out other assigned responsibilities. Table 21.4 outlines the types of questions the fitness leader might be asked in an annual evaluation conference.

Communication

The most important components of a fitness program are planning and communication (see figure 21.3). Any organization—whether private, public, or nonprofit—needs to clearly indicate what it wants to accomplish. The long-range plan includes

Table 21.4	Sample Evaluation Checklist: Generic Fitness Program

Evaluation of a Fitness Leader

Attainment of current goals

Did the fitness leader
- adhere to Center procedures?
- make proper screening decisions?
- administer tests efficiently with accurate results and good records?
- provide appropriate content for the exercise sessions?
- conduct the sessions with enthusiasm?
- provide a variety of fitness activities?
- relate well with the clients?
- relate well with the staff?
- provide comprehensive training and supervision of new staff members?
- understand and carry out emergency procedures?
- make suggestions for improvement in all aspects of the Center's activities and procedures?
- make efforts to improve in identified areas of weakness?
- accomplish things not listed as specific goals for this year?

Evaluation of past activities

What responsibilities were carried out (be specific)
- very well?
- adequately, but could be improved?
- below expectations that must be corrected?

Future goals

What responsibilities should be
- continued?
- added?
- deleted or handled by someone else?

What additional knowledge, skills, and so forth are needed? How will they be obtained?

How can the evaluation process be improved?

Reprinted from Howley and Franks 1997.

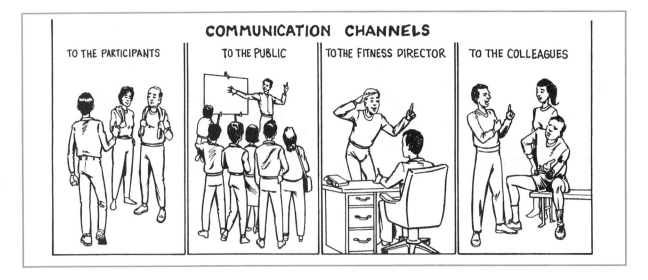

Figure 21.3 Communicating information clearly.

what should be accomplished, what is needed to accomplish these goals, how the organization will move from where it is to where it wants to be, and the processes for implementing the program.

There must be open and honest communication between program administrators and the staff so that staff members know what is expected and how they are evaluated. The staff needs to feel appreciated and encouraged to try to find better ways to accomplish the goals. Many advances in organizations come from staff members who help find better ways to improve the content and procedures of the program.

Participants need basic information concerning what the fitness program can (and cannot) do for them, with periodic progress reports and educational information that enhances their positive health knowledge and status. Fitness programs have used minilectures during warm-ups, information posted on bulletin boards, and newsletters to help educate participants. Keep in mind that the information needs to be accurate, brief, and to the point.

Fitness programs have a responsibility to help educate the public concerning positive health, including its definition, components, and recommendations for its achievement. To this end, fitness programs should share the effects of fitness programs on health, with corresponding benefits for the family, the community, and work performance, in the mass media and with interested groups, such as local industry.

Records

Careful collection of personal and testing information, systematically collected, recorded, and filed, provides the basis for much of the communication with the board, staff, and participants. In addition, the fitness program uses this information to evaluate the effectiveness of various programs and achievement of long-range goals. As already mentioned, the program will also keep staff training records, including a demonstration of competence in emergency and safety procedures.

Accident and Injury Reports

Table 21.5 is a sample form that you can use to record all accidents and injuries. Such a form must be carefully completed as soon as possible after the accident (and after the participant has been taken care of). It is essential to keep this kind of a record so that you can follow up to ensure that the individual is recovering.

Evaluation

This chapter has repeatedly mentioned evaluation. Successful fitness programs will make value judgments, based on the best data available, concerning its achievement of pro-

Table 21.5	Sample Accident or Injury Form

1. Name of victim _____ Date _____

2. Describe, in detail, the nature of the injury or health problem:

3. Describe, in detail, how the accident occurred:

4. List, in order, the things you or other staff members did in response to the incident:

5. Describe any problems encountered in dealing with the situation:

6. List the names of people who witnessed the accident or emergency procedures being performed:

Turn in this form, within 24 hr of accident, to _____(name or place)_____.

Your suggestions concerning safety, emergency procedures, and/or this form are welcome; please talk to _____(name)_____.

Reprinted from Howley and Franks 1997.

gram objectives. Evaluation should answer many questions. How many people are included in the fitness program? What kind of body composition, CRF, and low-back function changes have participants made? Do the participants enjoy the activities? How many dropouts were there? Why? How many injuries? Why? What can the program do to help more people make better fitness gains with fewer dropouts and injuries? Are some staff members better than others in some of these areas? What can the program do to help the staff maintain strengths and improve weaknesses?

Summary

This chapter helped you understand the organization of the fitness program in which you are working. The program includes screening of individuals to ensure that people can participate safely and that special help and activities are available to those who need them. A comprehensive fitness testing plan not only assists with the screening but also allows participants and program leaders to determine what fitness changes are being made as a result of the program. A team of qualified personnel who communicate openly with each other and are evaluated fairly in a positive atmosphere are essential ingredients in an effective program.

Chapter 22
Human Relations

Importance
Suggestions

This chapter attempts to help the fitness leader look beyond the skinfold calipers and the warm-up activities to focus on fellow human beings, including bosses, support staff, fitness participants, and those in the public who have not yet chosen to become fitness participants.

Beyond Exercise

Just as it is impossible to achieve the optimal quality of life without paying attention to health status, failing to look beyond oneself can also prevent its realization. This element of fitness, which many view as the spiritual component, may have religion, humanism, or enlightened self-interest as its basis. The world's major religions have a common element: An individual derives meaning from life by going beyond him- or herself. Other people come to the same conclusion from their concern for basic human values. Some recognize that their own freedom and well-being depend on the existence of a society in which all people have both their basic needs fulfilled and the opportunity to achieve their potential.

The interest in one's fellow human beings leads to a concern for societal problems and, more importantly, to involvement in solutions to these problems. Indeed, it is not enough to define the many things that interfere with quality of life; we must help find ways to improve the environment in which we all live. This problem solving will extend from our behavior in interpersonal relations to working with others on local, state, national, and international levels to address the interrelated problems of equal access to the full life.

As we go beyond ourselves and attempt to solve problems that prevent some of our sisters and brothers from attaining fitness, we recognize that no one is free until we all are. This means more than just keeping an "open door." We must look at creating conditions that will truly allow opportunities for full participation in all aspects of life.

Suggestions

The most important way a program can serve the community, as well as its participants, is to set up procedures that ensure high quality in all information, personal contact, and activities conducted in the name of the fitness program. Ensuring inclusiveness of the program is one aspect of establishing high standards (figure 22.1). All individuals should feel welcome in the program regardless of their gender, ethnic background, or social class.

The administrator can do several things to achieve this atmosphere, including the following:

- Maintaining a staff with varied backgrounds
- Training the staff to be sensitive to individuals from different backgrounds
- Scheduling programs at convenient times and places
- Contacting various community groups
- Providing ways for low-income people to participate
- Making it clear that inappropriate (e.g., sexist or racist) comments or actions by staff members or participants will not be tolerated

Summary

Fitness programs can assist relations among people by promoting concern that each of us has an opportunity to live a high-quality life. You can express this concern by offering an inclusive program of the highest quality.

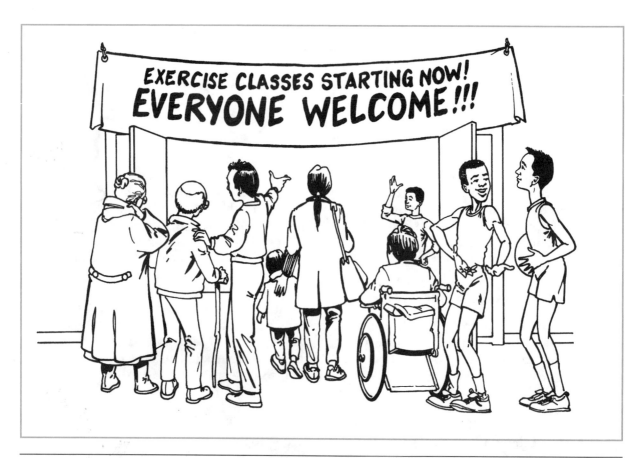

Figure 22.1 An inclusive exercise program.

Appendix

Recommended Dietary Allowances and Intakes

Table A.1	Estimated Safe and Adequate Daily Dietary Intakes of Selected Vitamins and Minerals[a]							
		Vitamins		Trace elements[b]				
Category	Age (years)	Biotin (µg)	Pantothenic acid (mg)	Copper (mg)	Manganese (mg)	Fluoride (mg)	Chromium (µg)	Molybdenum (µg)
Infants	0-0.5	10	2	0.4-0.6	0.3-0.6	0.1-0.5	10-40	15-30
	0.5-1	15	3	0.6-0.7	0.6-1.0	0.2-1.0	20-60	20-40
Children	1-3	20	3	0.7-1.0	1.0-1.5	0.5-1.5	20-80	25-50
and	4-6	25	3-4	1.0-1.5	1.5-2.0	1.0-2.5	30-120	30-75
adolescents	7-10	30	4-5	1.0-2.0	2.0-3.0	1.5-2.5	50-200	50-150
	11+	30-100	4-7	1.5-2.5	2.0-5.0	1.5-2.5	50-200	75-250
Adults		30-100	4-7	1.5-3.0	2.0-5.0	1.5-4.0	50-200	75-250

[a]Because there is less information on which to base allowances, these figures are not given in the main table of RDA and are provided here in the form of ranges of recommended intakes.

[b]Because the toxic levels for many trace elements may be only several times usual intakes, the upper levels for the trace elements given in this table should not be habitually exceeded.

Reprinted from *Recommended Dietary Allowances* 1989.

							Fat-soluble vitamins				Water-soluble vitamins						
	Age (years) or condition	Weight[b] (kg)	Weight[b] (lb)	Height[b] (cm)	Height[b] (in)	Protein (g)	Vitamin A (μg R.E.)[c]	Vitamin D (μg)[d]	Vitamin E (mg α-T.E.)[e]	Vitamin K (μg)	Vitamin C (mg)	Thiamin (mg)	Riboflavin (mg)	Niacin (mg N.E.)[f]	Vitamin B$_2$ (mg)	Folate (μg)	Vitamin B$_{12}$ (μg)
Infants	0.0–0.5	6	13	60	24	13	375	7.5	3	5	30	0.3	0.4	5	0.3	25	0.3
	0.5–1.0	9	20	71	28	14	375	10	4	10	35	0.4	0.5	6	0.6	35	0.5
Children	1–3	13	29	90	35	16	400	10	6	15	40	0.7	0.8	9	1.0	50	0.7
	4–6	20	44	112	44	24	500	10	7	20	45	0.9	1.1	12	1.1	75	1.0
	7–10	28	62	132	52	28	700	10	7	30	45	1.0	1.2	13	1.4	100	1.4
Males	11–14	45	90	157	62	45	1000	10	10	45	50	1.3	1.5	17	1.7	150	2.0
	15–18	66	145	176	69	59	1000	10	10	65	60	1.5	1.8	20	2.0	200	2.0
	19–24	72	160	177	70	58	1000	10	10	70	60	1.5	1.7	19	2.0	200	2.0
	25–50	79	174	176	70	63	1000	5	10	80	60	1.5	1.7	19	2.0	200	2.0
	51+	77	170	173	68	63	1000	5	10	80	60	1.2	1.4	15	2.0	200	2.0
Females	11–14	46	101	157	62	46	800	10	8	45	50	1.1	1.3	15	1.4	150	2.0
	15–18	55	120	163	64	44	800	10	8	55	60	1.1	1.3	15	1.5	180	2.0
	19–24	58	128	164	65	46	800	10	8	60	60	1.1	1.3	15	1.6	180	2.0
	25–50	63	138	163	64	50	800	5	8	65	60	1.1	1.3	15	1.6	180	2.0
	51+	65	143	160	63	50	800	5	8	65	60	1.0	1.2	13	1.6	180	2.0
Pregnant						60	800	10	10	65	70	1.5	1.6	17	2.2	400	2.2
Lactating	1st 6 months					65	1300	10	12	65	95	1.6	1.8	20	2.1	280	2.6
	2nd 6 months					62	1200	10	11	65	90	1.6	1.7	20	2.1	260	2.6

[a]The allowances, expressed as average daily intakes over time, are intended to provide for individual variations among most normal people as they live in the United States under usual environmental stresses. Diets should be based on a variety of common foods in order to provide other nutrients for which human requirements have been less well defined.

[b]Weights and heights of reference adults are actual medians for the U.S. population of the designated age, as reported by NHANES II. The median weights and heights of those under 19 years of age were taken from Hamill et al. (1979). The use of these figures does not imply that the height to weight ratios are ideal.

	Age (years) or condition	Weight[b] (kg)	Weight[b] (lb)	Height[b] (cm)	Height[b] (in.)	Protein (g)	Minerals Calcium (mg)	Phosphorus (mg)	Magnesium (mg)	Iron (mg)	Zinc (mg)	Iodine (µg)	Selenium (µg)
Infants	0.0-0.5	6	13	60	24	13	400	300	40	6	5	40	10
	0.5-1.0	9	20	71	28	14	600	500	60	10	5	50	15
Children	1-3	13	29	90	35	16	800	800	80	10	10	70	20
	4-6	20	44	112	44	24	800	800	120	10	10	90	20
	7-10	28	62	132	52	28	800	800	170	10	10	120	30
Males	11-14	45	90	157	62	45	1200	1200	270	12	15	150	40
	15-18	66	145	176	69	59	1200	1200	400	12	15	150	50
	19-24	72	160	177	70	58	1200	1200	350	10	15	150	70
	25-50	79	174	176	70	63	800	800	350	10	15	150	70
	51+	77	170	173	68	63	800	800	350	10	15	150	70
Females	11-14	46	101	157	62	46	1200	1200	280	15	12	150	45
	15-18	55	120	163	64	44	1200	1200	300	15	12	150	50
	19-24	58	128	164	65	46	1200	1200	280	15	12	150	55
	25-50	63	138	163	64	50	800	800	280	15	12	150	55
	51+	65	143	160	63	50	800	800	280	10	12	150	55
Pregnant						60	1200	1200	320	30	15	175	65
Lactating	1st 6 months					65	1200	1200	355	15	19	200	75
	2nd 6 months					62	1200	1200	340	15	16	200	75

[c]Retinol equivalents. 1 retinol equivalent = 1 µg retinol or 6 µg ß-carotene.

[d]As cholecalciferol, 10 µg cholecalciferol = 400 I.U. of vitamin D.

[e]α-Tocopherol equivalents. 1 mg d-α tocopherol = 1 α-T.E.

[f]1 N.E. (niacin equivalent) is equal to 1 mg of niacin or 60 mg of dietary tryptophan.

Reprinted from *Recommended Dietary Allowances* 1989.

Table A.3	Estimated Sodium, Chloride, and Potassium Minimum Requirements of Healthy People[a]			
Age	Weight (kg)[a]	Sodium (mg)[ab]	Chloride (mg)[ab]	Potassium (mg)[c]
Months				
0-5	4.5	120	180	500
6-11	8.9	200	300	700
Years				
1	11.0	225	350	1000
2-5	16.0	300	500	1400
6-9	25.0	400	600	1600
10-18	50.0	500	750	2000
>18[d]	70.0	500	750	2000

[a]No allowance has been included for large, prolonged losses from the skin through sweat.

[b]There is no evidence that higher intakes confer any health benefit.

[c]Desirable intakes of potassium may considerably exceed these values (~3500 mg for adults).

[d]No allowance included for growth. Values for those below 18 years assume a growth rate at the 50th percentile reported by the National Center for Health Statistics (Hamill et al., 1979) and averaged for males and females.

Reprinted from *Recommended Dietary Allowances* 1989.

Definitions

The following list of words are terms related to physical fitness with which the fitness leader will come into contact. Many of these words have more general alternative meanings. The health and fitness implications of appropriate terms are noted. Refer to *Health Fitness Instructor's Handbook* (3rd ed.) for more information on these terms.

Abdominal crunch—Slow curl-up to sticking point. Recommended for testing and strengthening abdominal muscles.

Abduction—Movement of a bone laterally from the anatomical position.

Acclimatization—A physiological adaptation to a new environment. For example, a person can do the same work with less effort and more total work after becoming acclimatized to a higher altitude (or temperature).

Accommodating (variable) resistance—Providing resistance so that maximal force can be applied throughout the complete range of motion.

Acidosis—A disturbance in the acid-base balance of the body tissues in which the tissues become more acidic (i.e., pH is lowered).

Acute injury—An injury that has just occurred, needing immediate attention.

Acute muscle soreness—Muscle soreness present during exercise or in recovery immediately following exercise.

Acute stressor—A situation or condition that causes an immediate and temporary physiological reaction in excess of what is needed to carry out the task.

Adaptation—The ability to adjust mentally and physically to circumstances or a changing situation. Acclimatization is one example of adaptation.

Adenosine diphosphate (ADP)—One of the chemical products resulting from the breakdown of ATP (e.g., during muscle contraction).

Adenosine triphosphate (ATP)—A high-energy compound from which the body derives energy.

Adherence—State of continuing. Often used to describe people who continue to participate in a physical fitness program.

Adipose tissue— Tissue composed of fat cells.

Adrenal glands—Endocrine glands directly above each kidney, composed of the medulla (which secretes the hormones epinephrine and norepinephrine) and the cortex (which secretes cortisol, aldosterone, androgens, and estrogens).

Adrenalin—See epinephrine.

Aerobic activities—Activities of sub-maximal intensity that use large muscle groups with energy (ATP) supplied aerobically.

Aerobic metabolism—Processes in which energy (ATP) is supplied when oxygen is utilized while a person is working.

Aerobic power—The maximal oxygen uptake, or the greatest rate at which oxygen can be utilized during maximal physical work.

Aggression—High levels of animosity or hostility, often unprovoked, which sometimes result from frustration or a feeling of inferiority.

Agility—Ability to start, stop, and move the body quickly in different directions.

Aging—The process of becoming older. Changes associated with aging are caused by various factors, including the lapse of time. These factors include decreased physical activity and an increased number and severity of health problems.

Agonist—A muscle that is the prime mover in a contraction.

Air displacement plethysmography—Method of body composition assessment that estimates body density from body volume.

Airway obstruction—Blockage of airway; can be caused by foreign object, swelling secondary to direct trauma, or allergic reaction.

Alkalosis—An increase of pH of the body, caused by excessive alkaline substances such as bicarbonate or by a removal of acids or chlorides from the blood.

Altitude—The height above sea level for a given point. A person has a lower maximal aerobic power with increasing altitudes because of the decreased partial pressure of oxygen in the air.

Alveolus (plural, alveoli)—A tiny air sac of the lungs where carbon dioxide and oxygen are exchanged with the surrounding pulmonary capillaries.

Amenorrhea—A cessation of menses.

American Alliance of Health, Physical Education, Recreation and Dance (AAHPERD)—An organization of professionals interested in these fields.

American College of Sports Medicine (ACSM)—An organization of professionals interested in the relationship of sport (and other physical activity) to medicine (and health and performance).

Amino acids—Nitrogen containing building blocks for proteins; can be used for energy.

Amphiarthrodial joint—A type of joint that allows slight movement.

Anaerobic activities—High-intensity activities during which energy demands exceed the ability to work aerobically.

Anaerobic metabolism—Energy supplied without oxygen, causing an oxygen deficit; creatine phosphate and glycolysis supply ATP without O_2.

Anaerobic (lactate) threshold—The sudden increase in lactic acid in the blood during a graded exercise test.

Anatomy—The science that deals with the structure of the human body.

Android-type obesity—Obesity in which there is a disproportionate amount of fat in the trunk and abdomen.

Anemia—A condition characterized by a decreased ability to transport oxygen in the blood.

Aneurysm—A spindle-shaped or sac-like bulging of the wall of a blood-filled vein, artery, or ventricle.

Anger—A strong emotion of displeasure or antagonism, which is often excited by a sense of injury or insult and frequently paired with a desire to retaliate.

Angina, angina pectoris—Severe cardiac pain that may radiate to the jaw or arms. Angina is caused by myocardial ischemia, which can be induced by exercise in susceptible individuals. Exercise should be stopped, and the person should be referred for medical attention.

Angular momentum—The quantity of rotation. Angular momentum is the product of the rotational inertia and angular velocity.

Anorexia nervosa—An eating disorder in which a preoccupation with body weight leads to self-starvation.

Antagonist—A muscle that causes movement at a joint in a direction opposite to that of its agonist (prime mover).

Anthropometry—The measurement of the body and its parts.

Anticoagulant—A drug that delays blood clotting.

Antioxidants—Substances which attach to harmful metabolic products (free radicals). There is some evidence that antioxidants are effective in decreasing the risk for developing cardiovascular disease and cancer.

Anxiety—Feeling of fear, apprehension, and dread, often without apparent cause.

Aorta—The main artery coming out of the left ventricle.

Aortic valve—Heart valve located between the aorta and the left ventricle.

Apnea—Temporary cessation of breathing; often caused by an excess amount of oxygen or too little carbon dioxide in the brain.

Aponeurosis—Broad, flat, tendinous sheath that attaches muscles to each other.

Apoplexy—The loss of consciousness and paralysis caused by an inadequate blood supply to a portion of the brain. Also called a "stroke."

Apparently healthy—A term used to describe people without a known disease or illness. These people may vary widely in terms of levels of physical fitness and numbers of risk factors.

Aquatics—Physical activities performed on or in water.

Arousal—The act of becoming excited, causing a stress response (i.e., a greater physiological response than is needed to perform the task). Arousal often occurs in competitive situations.

Arteriosclerosis—An arterial disease characterized by the hardening and thickening of vessel walls.

Arteriovenous oxygen difference—the difference between the oxygen contents of arterial blood and mixed venous blood; oxygen extraction. Also called "(a-v)O$_2$

Arthritis—Inflammation of a joint.

Articular capsule—A ligamentous structure that encloses a diarthrodial joint.

Articular cartilage—Cartilage covering bone surfaces that articulate with other bone surfaces.

Assertiveness—Pursuing objectives firmly. One of the distinctions between assertiveness and aggression or hostility is that the assertive person is sensitive to others, whereas the aggressive or hostile person tends to be less concerned with others' feelings.

Asthma—A respiratory problem characterized by labored breathing (dyspnea), coughing, mucous discharge from mouth, and a shortness of breath accompanied by a wheezing sound. May be initiated by exercise, allergies, or other irritants.

Atherosclerosis—A form of arteriosclerosis in which fatty substances are deposited in the inner walls of the arteries.

Athlete's foot—A foot fungus, often accompanied by a bacterial infection, that causes itching, redness, and a rash on the soles, toes, or between toes.

ATP-CP system—Immediate source of energy for cellular function provided through the anaerobic system.

Atrioventricular—Pertaining to the atria and the ventricles of the heart, such as a node, tract, and valve.

Atrioventricular node—The origin of the bundle of His in the right atrium of the heart. Normal electrical activity of the heart passes through the AV node prior to depolarization.

Atrium—One of the two (i.e., left or right) upper cavities of the heart. Also called "auricle" (plural is "atria," adjective is "atrial").

Atrophy—A decrease in the size of skeletal muscle or other body part because of disuse associated with muscle injury or a sedentary lifestyle.

Autonomic nervous system—The nerves that innervate the heart, viscera, and glands, controlling their involuntary functions. The autonomic nervous system consists of sympathetic and parasympathetic types of nerves.

AV block—Obstruction of the nerve impulse at the AV node.

Back extension strength and endurance—Slow and controlled extension movements to strengthen the erector spinae can be used if the upper limit of normal lumbar lordosis as seen in standing is not exceeded.

Background information—Health problems, characteristics, lifestyle, habits, signs, and symptoms of a person (and family) that are related to positive health and risks of health problems.

Balance—Ability to maintain a certain posture; or, to move without falling.

Ballistic movement—A rapid movement with three phases: an initial concentric muscle contraction by agonists to begin movement, a coasting phase, and a deceleration by the eccentric contraction of the antagonist muscles.

Baroreceptors—Receptor that monitors arterial blood pressure.

Basal metabolic rate (BMR)—The minimum energy expenditure required for life in the resting, postabsorptive state.

Behavior—The manner of conducting oneself, often in relation to others or in a particular environment; usually refers to a person's activities (rather than his or her thoughts or intentions).

Behavioral contracts—Written, signed, public agreements to engage in specific goal-directed activities, including a designated time frame and clear consequences of meeting and not meeting the agreed upon objectives.

Bench—A step used to test cardiorespiratory function. The height of the bench and the number of steps per minute determine the intensity of the effort.

Beta-adrenergic—Receptors in the heart and lungs that respond to catecholamines (epinephrine and norepinephrine).

Beta-carotene—A precursor of vitamin A thought to be an important antioxidant vitamin.

Bigeminy—On ECG, alternating normal and premature ventricular contractions.

Binge eating disorder—An eating disorder characterized by consuming large amounts of food in a short period of time.

Bioelectrical impedance analysis—Method of body composition assessment based upon the electrical conductivity of various tissues in the body.

Blood chemistry—The analysis of the content of the blood, used to determine the levels of substances related to health (e.g., cholesterol) or performance (e.g., lactic acid).

Blood pressure—The pressure exerted by the blood on the vessel walls, measured in millimeters of mercury by the sphygmomanometer. The systolic pressure (SBP, when the left ventricle is in maximal contraction) is the first sound, followed by the diastolic pressure (DBP, when the left ventricle is at rest), which is recorded when there is a change of tone of the sound (fourth phase), or disappearance of sound (fifth phase).

Blood pressure cuff—The device that is wrapped around the arm and pumped up to block off the artery. The pressure in the cuff is then slowly released to determine SBP and DBP. It is important to have the right size cuff for the arm, because improperly sized cuffs may result in inaccurate readings (e.g., too small a cuff will provide an artificially elevated blood pressure reading).

Blood profile—Assessment of health-related variables found in the blood, such as cholesterol.

Blood vessel—Any vessel (i.e., artery, vein, or capillary) through which blood circulates.

Body composition—Relative percentages of various components of the body, usually divided into fat mass (% body fat) and fat free mass (% fat free mass).

Body density—The relative weight of the body compared to an equal volume of water, or weight of the body per unit volume. Body density can be used to estimate percent fat.

Body fat distribution—Pattern of fat accumulation; often inherited.

Body mass index (BMI)—Measure of the relationship between height and weight. Calculated by dividing the weight in kilograms by height in meters squared.

Bradycardia—Slow heart rate, below 60 beats·min⁻¹ at rest; healthy if it is the result of physical conditioning.

Breathlessness—The inability to breathe without difficulty. Breathlessness may indicate a pulmonary disorder or a risk of CHD if it occurs with mild exertion; a person with this condition should be referred to medical personnel.

Bronchial asthma—A condition characterized by increased airway reactivity to various agents, leading to bronchial smooth muscle contraction, mucous secretion, and narrowing of the airway.

Bronchiole—A small branch of the airway. A bronchiole sometimes undergoes a spasm, making breathing difficult, such as in exercise-induced asthma.

Bronchitis—The inflammation of the bronchi. Symptoms are a productive cough, wheezy breathing, and varying degrees of breathlessness.

Buffer—A substance in blood that binds with hydrogen ions to minimize changes in the acid-base balance.

Bulimia nervosa—An eating disorder characterized by a pattern of consuming large amounts of food followed by periods of purging (vomiting, taking excessive laxatives).

Bundle branch block—A heart block caused by a lesion in one of the branches of the bundle of His.

Bursa—A fibrous sac lined with synovial membrane that contains a small quantity of synovial fluid; found between tendon and bone, skin and bone, and between muscle and muscle. Facilitates movement without friction between these surfaces.

Bursitis—An inflammation of a bursa.

Cable tensiometry—An instrument that measures muscular strength during a static or isometric contraction.

Calcium channel blockers—A class of medications that act by blocking the entry of calcium into the cell; used to treat angina, arrhythmias, and hypertension.

Calibration—To determine the accuracy of a measuring device by comparing it with a known standard and adjusting it to provide an accurate reading.

Calisthenics—Exercise without equipment, performed for flexibility or muscular development.

Caloric cost—The number of calories used for a specific task, normally reported in calories per minute (kcal·min⁻¹).

Calorie—1 calorie equals the amount of heat required to raise the temperature of 1 g of water 1° C; 1000 calories = 1 kilocalorie (kcal).

Calorimetry—The method used to measure the number of calories in something.

Capillary—The smallest blood vessel; the link between the end of the arteries and the beginning of the veins.

Capsular ligament—The ligament lined with synovial membrane surrounding the diarthrodial or synovial joints.

Capsulitis—Inflammation of a joint capsule.

Carbohydrate—An essential nutrient composed of carbon, hydrogen, and oxygen that is an essential energy source for the body.

Carbohydrate loading—Practice of increasing carbohydrate intake and decreasing activity in the days preceding competition.

Carbon dioxide—A gas; a waste product of many forms of combustion and metabolism, excreted via the lungs.

Carbon monoxide (CO)—A pollutant derived from the incomplete combustion of fossil fuels; binds hemoglobin to reduce oxygen transport and reduces maximal aerobic power.

Cardiac cycle—One total heartbeat with one complete contraction (systole) and relaxation (diastole) of the heart.

Cardiac output—The amount of blood circulated by the heart each minute; cardiac output equals the heart rate multiplied by the stroke volume.

Cardiac rehabilitation—A program designed to help cardiac patients return to normal lives with reduced risk of additional health problems.

Cardiopulmonary resuscitation (CPR)—A combination of chest compressions and rescue breathing to promote circulation and oxygenation of blood in an unconscious victim. People working in fitness programs should be certified in CPR.

Cardiorespiratory function—Ability of the circulatory and respiratory systems to supply oxygen to muscles during sustained physical activity.

Cardiovascular—Pertaining to the heart and blood vessels.

Carotid artery—The principle artery in each side of the neck leading to the brain.

Catecholamines—Epinephrine and norepinephrine.

Catharsis—A cleansing agent for the mind and emotions. Fitness activities can be used to erase the cluttered state of mind, allowing a person to start fresh following the exercise.

Cellulite—A label given to lumpy deposits of fat commonly appearing on the back and front of the legs and buttocks in overweight individuals.

Center of gravity—The theoretical point about which the entire weight of the body (or body part) can be considered to be acting.

Cerebral vascular disease—A disease of the blood vessels of the brain.

Certification—A document that serves as evidence of a certain status or qualification. For example, several groups certify that people are qualified to conduct specific aspects of a fitness program.

Chest pain—A tightness, compression, or sharp sensation in the chest, which may be caused by myocardial ischemia. People with chest (arm, shoulder, or jaw) pain should be referred for medical attention.

Cholesterol—A fatty substance in which carbon, hydrogen, and oxygen atoms are arranged in rings; high levels are a risk factor for heart disease.

Chondromalacia—Softening of cartilage.

Chronic bronchitis—Persistent production of sputum due to a thickened bronchial wall with excess secretions.

Chronic injury—An ongoing injury that lasts for an extended period of time.

Chronic obstructive pulmonary disease (COPD)—A term used to describe a number of specific diseases that cause a chronic unremitting obstruction to flow of air in the airways of the lungs. These diseases include chronic bronchitis, emphysema, and bronchial asthma, alone or in combination. Each disease obstructs airflow, but the underlying reason is different for each. COPD can dramatically affect one's ability to perform daily activities.

Chronic stressor—A continuing condition or situation that causes physiological responses in excess of those needed to complete a task. For example, excess fat causes chronic stress responses at rest and during exertion.

Circuit training—A sequence of different exercises done one after the other in the same workout.

Circulation—The continuous movement of blood through the heart, lungs, and tissue via blood vessels.

Cirrhosis—The hardening of an organ. The term is applied almost exclusively to degenerative changes in the liver with resulting fibrosis. Damage to liver cells can be by virus, microbes, toxic substances, or dietary deficiencies interfering with the nutrition of the cells often as a result of alcoholism.

Claudication—Interference with the blood supply to the legs, often resulting in limping.

Closed-circuit spirometry—The subject breathes 100% oxygen from a "bell" while a chemical absorbs the carbon dioxide; loss of volume of oxygen from the bell is proportional to oxygen consumption.

Coagulation, blood clotting—The formation of fibrin, a threadlike clot or clump of solid material in the blood.

Collateral circulation—Additional, supplementary, or substitute vessels that increase circulation to a part of the tissue, such as in the heart.

Compartment syndrome—Increased pressure within a muscular compartment that compromises blood flow and nerve supply.

Compound fracture—Bone fracture with external exposure.

Concentric contraction—A shortening of the muscle; causes movement.

Concussion—A condition resulting from a violent jar or shock to the head, associated with the brain; may result in loss of consciousness, pallor, coldness, and an increase in heart rate.

Conditioning—Exercise conducted on a regular basis over a period of time. Also called "training."

Conduction—The transmission of energy, heat, electricity, or sound. For example, conduction is the passage of electrical currents and nerve impulses through body tissues.

Confidentiality—Act of keeping information about an individual private. One of the elements of "informed consent" of fitness participants is that the information and data will be kept in a secure place and not shared with anyone without the individual's written permission.

Congestive heart failure—Failure of the heart, caused by its inability to pump a sufficient proportion of the blood it contains, with subsequent congestion.

Constant resistance—A load that remains the same throughout a complete range of motion during a muscle contraction (e.g., free-weight workout).

Construct validity—Evidence that a test responds in the ways one would expect based on theoretical understanding of that characteristic.

Content validity—Indicates that the test seems to be good, based on logic, expert testimony, and widespread use.

Contraindication—A sign or symptom suggesting that an individual should avoid a certain activity.

Control—The power to influence the outcome. The perception of control of a situation is one of the key elements in coping with potentially stressful conditions.

Contusion—A bruise; slight bleeding into tissues while the skin remains unbroken.

Cool-down—A period of light activity following moderate to heavy exercise. The cool-down period is important because it allows the leg muscles to continue to pump blood back to the heart, whereas stopping immediately after exercise causes pooling of the blood in the legs and a lack of venous return. Also called "taper-down."

Coordination—Ability to do a task integrating movements of the body and different parts of the body.

Cope—To struggle or strive to deal with a difficult situation with some degree of success.

Core temperature—The temperature of the central portion of the body, usually estimated by a rectal probe.

Coronary arteries—Blood vessels that supply the heart muscle.

Coronary artery bypass graft surgery (CABGS)—Surgery to bypass one or more blocked coronary arteries in which a blood vessel is sewn into existing coronary arteries above and below the blockage.

Coronary artery thrombosis—An occlusion of a coronary vessel by a blood clot.

Coronary heart disease (CHD)—Atherosclerosis of the coronary arteries. Also called coronary artery disease (CAD).

Coronary occlusion—The blockage of a coronary artery.

Coronary thrombosis—Blockage of a coronary artery by a blood clot.

Coronary-prone personality—A person with Type A behavior (e.g., hard-driving, impatient, time-conscious). Someone with a coronary-prone personality may have a higher risk of CHD.

Cortisol—A hormone released from the adrenal cortex in response to stress; involved in glucose metabolism and inflammation reactions.

Cost effectiveness—Assessment of the cost versus the benefits of a program.

Creatine phosphate—A high-energy phosphate compound that represents the primary immediate anaerobic source of ATP at the onset of exercise; important in all-out activities lasting seconds.

Criteria for entry into program—Standards for deciding which people should be referred for medical attention and which should be allowed to participate in fitness testing and activities.

Criterion validity—Evidence that a test has a high relationship to a valid criterion test. For example, underwater weighing serves as the criterion measure for validating skinfold assessment of body fatness.

Cross-adaptation—The transfer of increased adaptation from one stimulus (or stressor) to another stimulus. For example, some have claimed that increased adaptation to physical work from physical conditioning carries over to better adaptation to mental or emotional stressors; however, the evidence is inconclusive.

Curl-up (crunch)—Abdminal muscle exercise in which trunk is elevated only about 30°, used as part of exercise program for improving low-back function.

Cyanosis—A bluish tinge frequently observed under the nails, lips, and skin, caused by lack of oxygen. If noted, the exercise test or activity should be stopped.

Cycle ergometer—A one-wheeled stationary cycle with adjustable resistance used as a work task for exercise testing or conditioning.

Daily caloric need—Number of calories needed to maintain current body weight. It is composed of RMR, calories for activity, and the thermic effect of food.

Defibrillator—Any agent or measure, such as an electric shock, that stops an uncoordinated contraction of the heart muscle and restores a normal heartbeat.

Degenerative disease—A disease involving gradual deterioration and impairment of a tissue or organ.

Dehydration—The excessive loss of body fluids.

Delayed-onset muscle soreness (DOMS)—Muscle soreness that occurs a day or two after the exercise bout.

Depolarization—The change of polarity, specifically the electrical stimulus changing the atrium or ventricle from the resting to the working state.

Depression—Emotional dejection greater than that warranted by any objective reasons, often with symptoms such as insomnia, headaches, exhaustion, anorexia, irritability, loss of interest, impaired concentration, feelings that life is not worth living, and suicidal thoughts.

Detrained—The result of becoming sedentary after a physical conditioning program. The effects (e.g., increased fat, decreased CRF) are opposite those of conditioning.

Diabetes—A metabolic disorder characterized by an inability to oxidize carbohydrates because of inadequate insulin (Type I) or a resistance to insulin (Type II).

Diabetic coma—A lack of consciousness caused by lack of insulin, associated with extreme hyperglycemia.

Diaphysis—The shaft of a long bone.

Diarthrodial joint, or synovial joint—A freely moving joint characterized by its synovial membrane and capsular ligament.

Diastolic blood pressure (DBP)—The pressure exerted by the blood on the vessel walls during the resting portion of the cardiac cycle, measured in millimeters of mercury by a sphygmomanometer.

Diet—Food eaten by an individual. Diet sometimes refers to a special selection of food or a food plan.

Dietary exchange lists—Lists of foods containing similar quantities of nutrients and calories that are effective in planning diets for weight control and the management of diabetes.

Dietary fiber—Substances found in plants that cannot be broken down by the human digestive system.

Digitalis—A drug that augments the contraction of the heart muscle and slows the rate of conduction of cardiac impulses through the AV node.

Direct calorimetry—A method of measuring the metabolic rate, using a closed chamber in which a subject's heat loss is picked up by water flowing through the wall of a chamber; the gain in temperature of the water, plus that lost in evaporation are used to calculate the metabolic rate.

Disk—Located between vertebrae; acts as a shock absorber and can be involved in low-back pain.

Disordered eating—Unhealthy eating pattern that can in some cases be a precursor to eating disorders.

Diurnal variation—A daily variation or change.

Dizziness—Unsteadiness, with a tendency to stagger or fall.

Double product—The product of the heart rate and systolic blood pressure; indicative of the heart's oxygen requirement during exercise. Also called the rate-pressure product.

Drug—A substance (other than food) that, when taken into the body, produces a change in it. If the change helps the body, the drug is a medicine. If the change is harmful, the drug is a poison. Drugs are often addictive.

Dry-bulb temperature—The temperature of the air measured by an ordinary thermometer.

Duration—The length of time for a fitness workout. Guidelines often include 15 to 30 min of aerobic work at a target heart rate; however, more importantly, the total work accomplished (e.g., distance covered) should be emphasized.

Dynamometer—A device used to measure static strength of the grip-squeezing muscles and leg and back muscles.

Dyspnea—Difficult or labored breathing beyond what is expected for the intensity of the work. The exercise test or activity should be stopped.

Eating disorders—Clinical eating patterns that result in severely negative health consequences.

Eccentric contraction—A lengthening of the muscle during its contraction; resists movement caused by another force.

Ectopic focus—An irritated portion of the myocardium or electrical conducting system; gives rise to "extra beats" that do not originate from the sinoatrial node.

Ectopic ventricular complex—A ventricular contraction originating at some point other than the sinoatrial node.

Edema—The excessive retention of fluid in the tissue spaces, which causes swelling.

Efficiency—The ratio of energy expenditure to work output.

Ego orientation—Trying to win at all costs.

Ejection fraction—The fraction of the end diastolic volume ejected per beat (stroke volume divided by end diastolic volume).

Elasticity—Ability of ligaments and tendons to lengthen passively and return to their resting length.

Electrocardiogram (ECG)—The graphical recording of the electrical activity of the heart, obtained with the electrocardiograph, including the depolarization of the atrium (P-wave) and the depolarization (QRS) and repolarization (T-wave) of the ventricle.

Electrode—A conductor of electrical activity, specifically, a plate attached to various parts of the body to receive and transmit the heart's electrical activity to a recorder.

Electrolyte—Particles that in solution convey an electrical charge.

Electrophysiology—The study of electrical activity in the body as it relates to functional aspects of health.

Embolism—Sudden obstruction of a blood vessel by a solid body such as a clot carried in the bloodstream.

Emergency medical system (EMS)—A system designed to handle medical emergencies; 911 or other community emergency number.

Emotion—A strong feeling, often accompanied by stress reactions and behaviors.

Empathy—Identification with thoughts or feelings of another person.

Emphysema—Loss of elastic recoil of alveoli and bronchioles and enlargement of those pulmonary structures.

End diastolic volume—The volume of blood in the heart immediately prior to ventricular contraction; a measure of the stretch of the ventricle.

Endocardium—The membrane lining that covers the chambers of the heart, including the valves.

Endorphins—A group of hormones that are similar in composition to morphine and are normally produced and released by the pituitary gland to help reduce great pain, anxiety, and stress.

Endurance run—A race of a set distance (for time) or set time (for distance). Normally used to determine a person's cardiorespiratory endurance. Runs of at least 1 mi or 6 min should be used.

Energy—The capacity for performing work, often measured in terms of oxygen consumption.

Enlarged heart—A heart bigger than average size. If an enlarged heart is the result of pathological conditions, then it is weak and unhealthy. If it results from physical conditioning, then it is strong and healthy.

Environmental factors—Aspects of the surroundings (e.g., heat, altitude, pollution) that influence the body's response to exercise.

Enzyme—An organic catalyst that aids many body processes, such as digestion and oxidation.

Epicardium—The layer of the pericardium attached to the heart.

Epicondylitis—Inflammation of muscles or tendons attaching to the epicondyles of the humerus.

Epidemiological studies—Long-term studies of the distribution of diseases in whole populations. Those characteristics, signs, and symptoms that are related to major health problems based on epidemiological studies are called "risk factors."

Epilepsy—A nervous system disorder resulting from disordered electrical activity of the brain, often resulting in a seizure.

Epimysium—The connective-tissue sheath surrounding a muscle.

Epinephrine, adrenaline—A chemical liberated from the adrenal medulla and from sympathetic nerve endings. Effects include cardiac stimulation and constriction of blood vessels, and mobilization of glucose and free fatty acids.

Epiphyseal plates—The sites of ossification in long bones.

Epiphyses—The ends of long bones.

Ergogenic aids—Substances taken in hopes of improving athletic performance.

Error—An inaccurate score that can result from the testing environment, the equipment, normal variation of the person, and the tester. Some of the error may be constant (which can be corrected with a set number) or random (which cannot be predicted or corrected).

Erythrocytes—The red blood cells.

Essential amino acids—The 9 amino acids the body cannot synthesize and therefore must be ingested.

Etiology—The study of the causes of disease.

Euphoria—An exaggerated sense of well-being.

Evaluation—The determination or judgment of the value or worth of something or someone. In a fitness setting, an evaluation determines the health or fitness status of an individual based on his or her characteristics, signs, symptoms, behaviors, and test results.

Evaporation—Conversion from the liquid to the gaseous state by means of heat, as in evaporation of sweat; results in the loss of 580 kcal per liter of sweat evaporated.

Excess postexercise oxygen consumption (EPOC)—See oxygen debt.

Exercise—Structured physical activity whose purpose is to improve some component or components of physical fitness.

Exercise components—Warm-up, main body of exercise, and cool-down (taper-down).

Exercise Leader^SM—Qualified to lead exercise "on the floor."

Exercise modification—Adjustment of a person's exercise program in terms of type of activity, intensity, frequency, and (or) total work accomplished to more nearly achieve the fitness goals.

Exercise prescription—A recommendation for a fitness program in terms of types of activities, intensity, frequency, and total amount of work aimed at producing or maintaining desirable fitness objectives.

Exercise progression—The increase in total work and (or) intensity as a person gradually goes from a sedentary lifestyle to the recommended levels of physical activity.

Exercise Specialist^SM—A person certified by the American College of Sports Medicine to work in exercise rehabilitation settings with high-risk or diseased populations.

Exercise Technologist^SM—A person certified by the American College of Sports Medicine to conduct graded exercise stress tests on a variety of populations.

Exercise-induced asthma (EIA)—A form of asthma induced by exercise; can occur 5 to 15 min (early phase) or 4 to 6 hr (late phase) following exercise.

Expiration—Exhalation of air from the lungs.

Expired gas—The air that is exhaled from the lungs, often analyzed to determine oxygen and carbon dioxide concentrations.

Extension—Increasing the angle at a joint, such as straightening the elbow.

Extrinsic—External, as in extrinsic motivation (e.g., reward) to begin or continue exercise.

Extrovert—A person who regulates self-behavior in response to others.

Facility—Something designed, built, or installed to serve a specific function, such as the facilities for a fitness program.

Fainting—A momentary loss of consciousness.

Family history—The major health problems that have been found in a person's grandparents, parents, uncles, aunts, and siblings. Heart disease in a person's family is a risk factor for CHD.

Fartlek—A form of physical conditioning, also known as speed play, which alternates fast and slow running over varied terrain for 3 to 4 mi.

Fasciculus—A bundle of muscle fibers surrounded by perimyseum.

Fast twitch fiber—A muscle fiber characterized by its fast speed of contraction.

Fat—A compound containing glycerol and fatty acids that is used as a source of energy and can be stored in the body.

Fat mass—Weight of the fat tissues of the body.

Fat weight—The absolute amount of total body weight that is body fat, calculated by total body weight times percent fat.

Fat-free mass—Weight of the nonfat tissues of the body.

Fat-free weight—Amount of total body weight that is free of fat, calculated by total body weight minus fat weight. Also called "lean body weight."

Fat-patterning—See body fat distribution.

Fat-soluble vitamin—Vitamins that are stored in fat tissue (vitamins A, D, E, and K).

Fatty acid—Molecules 16 to 18 carbons in length, such as stearic, palmitic, or oleic acid. Circulating fatty acids can be used for energy.

Fear—A distressing emotion aroused by impending pain, danger, and so forth.

Field tests—Tests that can be used in mass-testing situations.

First-degree AV block—The delayed transmission of impulses from atria to ventricles (in excess of 0.21 s).

Fitness—A state of health characteristics, symptoms, and behaviors enabling a person to have the highest quality of life. Increases in fitness components are related to positive health, whereas decreases in fitness components increase the risk of major health problems.

Fitness activities—Actions that lead to increased fitness.

Fitness Instructor—A person who assists people in evaluating and improving fitness. Certification is offered by the American College of Sports Medicine for fitness instructors who work with apparently healthy populations.

Fitness program—An organized series of activities aimed at promoting increased fitness.

Fitness testing—The measurement and evaluation of the status of all fitness components.

Fitness workout—A specific fitness session.

Flexibility—The ability to move a joint through the full range of motion without discomfort or pain.

Flexibility exercise—Exercises to maintain or improve the range of motion of a joint.

Flexion—Anterior or posterior movement that brings two bones together.

Flow meter—An instrument that measures the rate of air movement (e.g., liters of air moved per minute) in a graded exercise test.

Food Guide Pyramid—A system (designed by the United States Department of Agriculture) for making healthy food choices. It divides foods into 6 different categories and recommends daily servings from each.

Force—Any push or pull that tends to cause movement.

Force arm—Perpendicular distance from the axis of rotation to the direction of the application of that force causing movement.

Forced expiratory volume in 1 s (FEV$_1$)—The ratio of the volume of air expelled in 1 s compared to the total VC. A person who can expel less than 75% of his or her vital capacity (VC) in 1 s should be referred to a physician.

Fracture—A break in a bone.

Frequency—How often a person performs a fitness workout (usually days per week).

Friction massage—A form of massage in which the stroking motion of the hands builds up heat on the surface of the skin overlying a tight or sore muscle.

Frostbite—Freezing of the skin and superficial tissues, resulting from exposure to extreme cold.

Fun run—A race with an emphasis on participation (as opposed to winning).

Functional capacity—Maximal oxygen uptake, expressed in milliliters of oxygen per kilogram of body weight per minute, or in METs.

Functional (spinal) curves—Ability to remove a spinal curve (e.g., olordotic curve) during normal movement, allowing forward flexion.

Game—A form of playing for amusement. Games may be cooperative or competitive, involving a few or many people. Games can also be used to improve fitness.

Gas analyzer—An instrument that measures components of air. In the case of maximal oxygen uptake, a gas analyzer is used to measure oxygen and carbon dioxide in expired air.

Genetic potential—The possibilities and limits imposed by a person's inherited genes.

Globe (black globe) temperature—Measurement of radiant heat load taken in direct sunlight.

Glucagon—Hormone opposing insulin; promotes glucose entry from liver to blood.

Glucose—A simple sugar that is a vital energy source in the human body.

Glycogen—The storage form of carbohydrates in the human body.

Glycolysis—The metabolic pathway producing ATP from the anaerobic breakdown of glucose; the short-term source of ATP that is important in all-out activities lasting less than 2 min.

Goal orientation—The tendency of a person to behave on the basis of her or his goals, with an emphasis on doing the activity well.

Goal-setting—Goals are desired tasks sought to be accomplished in a specific amount of time. Effective goal-setting includes establishing objectives that can be measured, concretely defining the objectives, and ensuring goals are practical and reachable.

Good nutrition—A diet in which foods are eaten in the proper quantities and with the necessary distribution of nutrients to maintain good health in the present and in the future.

Graded exercise test (GXT)—A multistage test that determines a person's physiological responses to different intensities of exercise and (or) the person's peak aerobic capacity.

Gram (g)—A basic unit of mass in the metric system. 1000 g = 1 kg.

Gynoid-type obesity—Obesity in which there is a disproportionate amount of fat in the hips and thighs.

Hamstrings—Large muscle groups at the back of the thigh that cross both the knee and hip joints.

Health—Being alive with no major health problem, also called apparently healthy.

Health Fitness Director—A person who is certified by the American College of Sports Medicine as qualified for management of preventive programs.

Health Fitness Instructorˢᴹ **(HFI)**—A person who is certified by the American College of Sports Medicine as qualified in exercise testing, prescription, and leadership in preventive programs.

Health history—Information about a person's past health record.

Health status—Current level of disease and fitness.

Health-related attitudes—A manner of thinking associated with healthy behaviors.

Health-related behavior—A person's actions that are associated with positive or negative health. These behaviors include exercise, healthy diet, not smoking, no or slight use of alcohol, no use of nonessential drugs, adequate sleep, ability to relax and cope with stressors, and safety habits.

Health-related sign—Evidence of something with a potential health consequence.

Health-related symptom—A sensation that arises from or accompanies a particular disease or disorder and serves as an indicator of it.

Heart—The hollow muscular organ that pumps the blood through the body. The heart lies obliquely between the two lungs, behind the sternum. Composed of four chambers, left and right atria, and ventricles.

Heart attack—A general term used to describe an acute episode of heart disease; common name for myocardial infarction.

Heart disease—A general term used to describe any of several abnormalities of the heart that make the heart unable to function properly.

Heart rate—The number of beats of the heart per minute.

Heart rhythm—The regularity of the heartbeat; or components of the cardiac cycle.

Heart rate reserve (HRR)—The difference between maximal and resting heart rates.

Heat cramps—A spasmodic contraction of a muscle or group of muscles that is caused by working in extreme heat.

Heat exhaustion—Collapse, with or without loss of consciousness, suffered in conditions of heat and high humidity, largely resulting from the loss of fluid and salt by sweating.

Heat illness—A general term denoting problems caused by activity in high temperatures.

Heat stroke—The final stage in heat exhaustion, when the body is unable to lose heat, hyperpyrexia occurs, and death may ensue.

Heat syncope—Fainting or sudden loss of strength because of excessive heat gain.

Hematocrit—The volume of red blood cells per unit volume of blood, usually about 40% to 45%.

Hemoglobin—The iron-containing protein in the red blood cells. It has the reversible function of combining with and releasing oxygen.

Hemorrhage—The escape of blood from a vessel.

Hepatitis B (HBV)—A type of hepatitis (viral infection of the liver) that is transmitted via sexual contact or blood.

Heredity—The transmission of genetic characteristics from parents to offspring.

High blood pressure, hypertension—Blood pressure in excess of normal values for a specific age and gender.

High-calorie diet—Food consumption in which the caloric value exceeds the total daily energy requirement, resulting in increased adipose tissue.

High-density lipoprotein cholesterol (HDL-C)—A plasma lipid-protein complex containing relatively more protein and less cholesterol and triglycerides. Low levels of HDL-C are associated with CHD.

Homeostasis—The tendency of the body to maintain internal equilibrium of temperature, fluid content, and so forth by the regulation of its bodily processes.

Hormone—A chemical product produced by an endocrine gland and secreted into the blood; exerts a distinct and usually powerful effect on some specific body functions or organs.

Hostile—Antagonistic, unfriendly.

Human immunodeficiency virus (HIV)—A virus that destroys the body's ability to fight infection; referred to as AIDS.

Humidity—The amount of moisture in the atmosphere.

Hydrostatic weighing—Method of body composition assessment based upon Archimedes' principle that is often used as the criterion method; also called "underwater weighing."

Hypercholesterolemia—An excess of cholesterol in the blood.

Hyperextension—A continuation of extension past the normal anatomical position.

Hyperglycemia—An elevation of blood glucose that can occur in the diabetic who does not achieve a proper balance between carbohydrate intake and injected insulin.

Hyperlipidemia—Excess fat in the blood.

Hyperplasia—Increase in the size of the muscle due to an increase in the number of muscle fibers.

Hypertension—High blood pressure. Normally systolic blood pressure exceeds 140 mmHg or diastolic pressure exceeds 90 mmHg.

Hyperthermia—An elevation of the core temperature; if unchecked, can lead to heat exhaustion or heat stroke and death.

Hypertrophy—An increase in the size of a muscle, organ, or other body part caused by an enlargement of its constituent cells.

Hyperventilation—A level of ventilation beyond that needed to maintain the arterial carbon dioxide level; can be initiated by a sudden increase in the hydrogen ion concentration due to lactic acid production during a progressive exercise test.

Hypervitaminosis—A condition in which the level of a vitamin in the blood or tissues is high enough to cause undesirable effects.

Hypoglycemia—Low blood sugar, attended by anxiety, excitement, perspiration, delirium, or coma.

Hypokinetic disease—A disease that relates to or is caused by the lack of regular physical activity.

Hypotension—Low blood pressure.

Hypothermia—Below-normal body temperature.

Iliac crest—The large bony prominence at the top of each side of the hips.

Increment—A degree of increase. In a graded exercise test, a work increment exists between stages.

Inderal—A drug blocking beta-receptor in the heart, aimed at reducing cardiac arrhythmias and dysrhythmias. Its generic name is "propranolol."

Indirect calorimetry—The estimation of energy production on the basis of oxygen consumption.

Infarction—Death of a section of tissue due to lack of blood flow, as in myocardial infarction.

Inferior vena cava—The large vein that discharges blood from the lower half of the body into the right atrium of the heart.

Inflammation—A reaction to injury; signs include heat, redness, pain, and swelling.

Informed consent—A procedure used to obtain a person's voluntary permission to participate in a program. Informed consent requires a description of the procedures to be used, the potential benefits and risks, and written consent.

Inspiration—The drawing of air into the lungs.

Insulin—A pancreatic hormone secreted into the blood that influences carbohydrate metabolism by stimulating the transport of glucose into cells.

Insulin shock—A shock-like state resulting from an overdose of insulin.

Intensity—The magnitude of energy required for a particular activity, often referred to in absolute amount of energy expended (e.g., multiples of resting metabolism—METs) or relative to a percentage of one's own maximum (e.g., $\dot{V}O_2$max or HRmax).

Intermittent work—Exercises performed with alternate periods of harder and lighter physical work, or work and rest, rather than continuous work.

Internal bleeding—Bleeding within the deep structures of the body (chest, abdominal, or pelvic cavity and bleeding of any of the organs contained within these cavities).

Interval training—A fitness workout that alternates harder and lighter work or rest.

Intrinsic—Belonging to a thing by its very nature (e.g., people continue to be active based on intrinsic motivation).

Introvert—A person concerned primarily with his or her own thoughts and feelings.

Ion—An electrified or charged (positive or negative) particle.

Iron-deficiency anemia—Anemia brought on by a chronic deficiency in iron intake; the most common mineral deficiency in women.

Ischemia—Inadequate blood supply to the heart.

Isocaloric balance—The state achieved when the calories consumed equal the energy expended.

Isoelectric—Baseline, as in an ECG.

Isokinetic contraction—A muscle contraction with controlled speed, allowing maximal force to be applied throughout the range of motion.

Isometric contraction—A muscle contraction in which the muscle length is unchanged.

Isotonic contraction—A muscle contraction in which the force of the muscle is greater than the resistance, resulting in joint movement with shortening of the muscle.

J-point—On an ECG, the point at which the S-wave ends and the S-T segment begins.

Jogging—Slow running.

Joint—The articulation of two or more bones.

Ketosis—A condition brought about by restricted carbohydrate intake, resulting in excessive acetones or other ketones being secreted by the liver; stored fat becomes more available for energy.

Kidneys—Two glands situated in the upper, posterior abdominal cavity, one on either side of the vertebral column. Their function is to maintain water and electrolyte balance and to secrete urine.

Kilocalorie (kcal) or calorie (cal)—The amount of heat required to raise the temperature of 1 kg of water 1° C. This is the ordinary calorie discussed in food or exercise energy-expenditure tables.

Kilogram (kg)—A metric unit of mass; 1 kg = 1000 g.

Kilopond meters per minute (kpm·min⁻¹), kilogram meters per minute (kgm·min⁻¹)—In a normal gravitational field, these are identical. This is a measure of power used to describe the external work rate, often on a cycle ergometer.

Krebs cycle—A series of chemical reactions occurring in mitochondria in which carbon dioxide is produced and hydrogen ions and electrons are removed from carbon atoms (oxidation). The Krebs cycle is also referred to as the "tricarboxyclic acid cycle" or "citric acid cycle."

Kyphosis—An excessive posterior curvature of the upper (thoracic) spine.

Lactate—An end product of the anaerobic metabolism of glucose; the dissociated form of lactic acid.

Lactate threshold (anaerobic threshold)—The point during a graded exercise test at which the blood lactate concentration suddenly increases; a good indicator of the highest sustainable work rate.

Lactic acid—See lactate.

Leadership—The ability to influence and motivate people in a group to make decisions and to act on the basis of those decisions.

Lean body weight—Often used to refer to all nonfat weight. Fat-free weight is the correct term.

Leukocytes—White blood cells.

Liability—Legal responsibility.

Lifestyle—A person's general pattern of living, including healthy and unhealthy behaviors.

Ligament—The connective tissue that attaches bone to bone.

Limiting factor—A physiological characteristic that establishes the upper limit of performance (e.g., muscle fiber type, maximal cardiac output, maximal oxygen uptake).

Lipid—A fatty substance.

Lipoproteins—Large molecules responsible for transporting fats in the blood.

Liter—A unit of volume in the metric system, 1 L = 1000 ml.

Lordosis—The forward curvature of the lumbar spine; can be excessive, contributing to low-back pain.

Longitudinal arch—The long arch along the medial aspect of the foot.

Low blood sugar—See hypoglycemia.

Low-back function—The ability to carry on normal activities without back pain.

Low-back pain—Strong discomfort in the low-back area, often caused by lack of muscular endurance and flexibility in the midtrunk region or tissue damage associated with improper posture or lifting.

Low-calorie diet—Food intake of which the caloric value is below the total energy requirement, resulting in a loss of weight.

Low-density lipoprotein cholesterol (LDL-C)—A plasma protein containing relatively more cholesterol and triglycerides and less protein. High levels are associated with an increased risk of CHD.

Low-intensity exercise—Exercise less than three METs.

Low-organized games—Games with simple rules not requiring high levels of skill.

Lumbar—Pertaining to the low back; five lumbar vertebrae are located just below the thoracic vertebrae, immediately above the sacrum.

Lumbar lordosis—Excessive forward curvature of the lumbar spine in which the pelvis is tilted forward.

Macrominerals—The major dietary minerals, including calcium, phosphorus, potassium, sulfur, sodium, chloride, and magnesium.

Maintenance load—The amount of exercise that enables an individual to maintain her or his present level of fitness.

Malnutrition—A diet in which there is an underconsumption, overconsumption, or unbalanced consumption of nutrients that leads to disease or an increased susceptibility to disease.

Mast cell—A cell in the bronchial tube that releases histamine and other chemicals in response to certain stimuli; involved in an asthmatic attack.

Max VO₂ (VO₂max)—See maximal oxygen uptake.

Maximal—The highest level possible, such as maximal heart rate or oxygen uptake.

Maximal aerobic power—The maximal rate at which oxygen can be used by the body during maximal work; related directly to the maximal capacity of the heart to deliver blood to the muscles.

Maximal heart rate (HRmax)—The highest heart rate attainable. A person's maximal heart rate can be estimated by subtracting his or her age from 220. The normal variation in this estimate (standard deviation) = ±11 beats·min⁻¹

Maximal oxygen uptake (VO₂max)—The greatest rate of oxygen utilization attainable during heavy work, expressed in L·min⁻¹ or ml·kg⁻¹·min⁻¹.

Maximal tests—Tests that continue until a person has reached a maximal level (e.g., VO₂max) or voluntary exhaustion.

Maximum voluntary ventilation—The maximal amount of air that can be moved in and out of the lungs. A person is normally tested for 10 to 15 s, then the result is reported in liters per minute.

Mean—The average score.

Mechanical low-back pain—Low-back pain that results from poor body mechanics, inflexibility of certain muscle groups, or muscular weakness.

Medical clearance—An indication by medical personnel that an individual can safely engage in specified activities.

Medical history—A person's previous health problems, signs, and characteristics.

Medical physical exam—The systematic examination of the different parts of the body, used to determine a person's health status.

Medical referral—A recommendation that a person get medical attention, tests, or an opinion about a characteristic, symptom, or test result to determine if medical treatment is needed, and (or) to determine whether it is safe to participate in specified activities.

Medical supervision—The presence of qualified medical personnel during a fitness test or workout.

Medication—A therapeutic substance. Also called "medicine."

Menisci—Partial disks between the femur and tibia and the knee.

Metabolic load—The energy required to complete a task.

Metabolism—The process of chemical changes by which energy is provided for the maintenance of life.

Metatarsal arch—The arch of the foot located between the "balls" of the foot.

METs—Multiples of resting metabolism (1 MET is about 3.5 ml·kg^{-1}·min^{-1}).

Micromineral—Trace dietary minerals, including iron, zinc, copper, iodine, manganese, selenium, chromium, molybdenum, cobalt, arsenic, nickel fluoride, and vanadium.

Millisecond—one one-thousandth (0.001) of a second.

Minerals—Inorganic molecules that serve a variety of functions in the human body.

Mitochondria—Cellular organelles responsible for the generation of energy (ATP) through the aerobic system.

Mitral valve—Heart valve located between the left atrium and left ventricle.

Mobitz Type I AV block—On an ECG, P-R interval progressively increasing until the P-wave is not followed by a QRS complex. The site of the block is the AV node.

Mobitz Type II AV block—On an ECG, a constant P-R interval, with some but not all P-waves followed by QRS. The site of the block is the bundle of His.

Moderate-intensity exercise—Exercise at 3 to 6 METs.

Monosaccharide—A simple sugar, such as glucose.

Morbidity rate—The ratio of the number of cases of a disease to the number of well people in a given population.

Motivation—An incentive that prompts a person to act with a sense of purpose.

Motor unit—The functional unit of muscular contraction that includes a motor nerve and the muscle fibers that its branches innervate.

Movement forms—Types of physical activity, such as aquatics, dance, exercise, games, gymnastics, and sports.

Muscle fiber—Muscle cell; contains myofibrils that are composed of sarcomeres; uses chemical energy of ATP to generate tension, which, when greater than the resistance, results in movement.

Muscle group—A group of specific muscles that are responsible for the same action at the same joint.

Muscular endurance—Ability of the muscle to perform repetitive contractions over a prolonged period of time.

Muscular strength—The ability of the muscle to generate the maximum amount of force.

Myocardial infarction (MI)—Death to a section of heart tissue in which the blood supply has been cut off.

Myocardial ischemia—A lack of oxygen for heart function due to a decrese in blood flow.

Myocardium—The middle layer of the heart wall; involuntary, striated muscle innervated by autonomic nerves.

Myofibril—Found inside muscle fibers; composed of a long string of sarcomeres, the basic unit of muscle contraction.

Myoglobin—A compound in muscle that aids in shuttling oxygen to the mitochondria.

Myosin—A contractile protein in the sarcomere that can bind actin and split ATP to generate cross-bridge movement and the development of tension.

Myositis—Inflammation of a muscle.

Negative energy balance—A condition in which less energy is consumed than is expended, resulting in a decrease in body weight.

Negative health—The presence of characteristics and behaviors that prevent optimal functional capacity and increase risks of serious health problems.

Negligence—The failure to provide reasonable care, or the care required by the circumstances. The person and (or) program is legally liable for injury that results from such failure.

Neoplasm—New or abnormal growth.

Newton (N)—A unit of measure of force.

Nitrates—A class of medications used to treat angina pectoris, or chest pain.

Nitroglycerin—A vasodilator drug used to treat angina pectoris.

Noradrenalin—See Norepinephrine.

Norepinephrine—One of the adrenal medullary hormones similar in action to epinephrine. Norepinephrine is also secreted by sympathetic nervous system nerve endings.

Nutrient—A dietary substance that the body requires for the maintenance of health, growth, and repair of tissues.

Nutrient density—The amount of essential nutrients in a food in comparison to the calories it contains.

Nutrition—The study of foods and their use in the body.

Obesity—Condition of being overfat.

Objectivity—Attained if different persons administer or score the test and obtain the same results.

Obsession—An idea or emotion that persists in an individual in spite of any conscious attempts to remove it.

Oligomenorrhea—Irregular menses.

One-repetition maximum (1-RM)—The greatest amount of weight a person can lift one time in good form.

Open-circuit spirometry—The method of measuring oxygen consumption by breathing in room air, while collecting and analyzing the expired air.

Oral antiglycemic agents—A class of medications used to treat noninsulin-dependent diabetes mellitus; they stimulate the pancreas to secrete more insulin.

Orthopedic—Skeletal problem, disease, or deformity.

Orthopedically disabled—A disorder of some aspect of the locomotor system.

Ossification—The replacement of cartilage by bone.

Osteoarthritis—Most common form of arthritis (90% to 95% of all cases); affects joints whose articular cartilage is damaged or injured.

Osteoporosis—A disease characterized by a decrease in the total amount of bone mineral and a decrease in the strength of the remaining bone.

Overfat—Condition in which one has excessive adipose tissue.

Overload—To place greater than usual demands upon some part of the body (e.g., picking up more weight than normal, overloading the muscles involved). Chronic overloading leads to increased strength and function.

Overtraining—A condition in which the training (intensity, duration, frequency) is so great that it causes a decrease in physical performance.

Overweight—Condition in which one weighs more than recommended by height-weight charts.

Oxygen—A colorless, odorless, gas; necessary for life and combustion.

Oxygen consumption—See oxygen uptake.

Oxygen cost—The amount of oxygen used by body tissues during an activity.

Oxygen debt—The amount of oxygen used during recovery from work that exceeds the amount needed for rest.

Oxygen deficit—The difference between the theoretical oxygen requirement of a physical activity and the measured oxygen uptake.

Oxygen uptake—The rate at which oxygen is utilized during a specific level of an activity.

Ozone—An active form of oxygen formed in reaction to UV light and as an emission from internal combustion engines; exposure can decrease lung function.

P-wave—On an ECG, a small positive deflection preceding a QRS complex, indicating atrial depolarization, normally less than 0.12 s with an amplitude of 0.25 mV or less.

P-R interval—The time interval between the beginning of the P-wave and the QRS complex. The upper limit is 0.2 s. This segment is normally used as the isoelectric baseline.

Pallor—Unnatural paleness. Exercise should be stopped.

Palpation—Examination by touch, as in determining HR by feeling the pulse at the wrist or neck.

Palpitation—A rapid, forceful beating of the heart of which the person is aware.

Papillary muscles—Cardiac muscles that originate at the walls of the heart ventricles and attach to AV valves.

Parasympathetic nervous system—A portion of the autonomic nervous system, derived from some of the cranial and sacral nerves belonging to the central nervous system; the system produces such involuntary responses as blood vessel dilation; increased gland, digestive, and reproductive organ activity; eye pupil contraction; decreased heart rate; and others. Effects are opposite those of the sympathetic nervous system.

Partial pressure of gas—Pressure exerted by oxygen, carbon dioxide, nitrogen, or water. The sum of these partial pressures equals the barometric pressure.

Peak heart rate—The highest heart rate occurring during a specific activity.

Peak torque—The maximal force generated during an isokinetic contraction.

Perceived exertion—A subjective rating of intensity of a particular task, normally rated on one of the Borg scales for rating perceived exertion.

Percent fat—Percentage of the total weight composed of fat tissue. Calculated by dividing fat mass by total weight.

Percent maximal heart rate (%HRmax)—Submaximal heart rate divided by maximal heart rate (e.g., 70% maximal heart rate in a person with a maximal heart rate of 200 beats·min^{-1} = 140 beats·min^{-1} [200 x 0.7]).

Percent VO$_2$max (%VO$_2$max)—Submaximal oxygen uptake divided by maximal oxygen uptake; e.g., 60% maximal oxygen uptake in a person with a maximal oxygen uptake of 3 L·min^{-1} = 1.8 L·min^{-1} (30 x 0.6).

Perception—A conscious impression of objects or situations. The stressfulness of a situation depends largely on the way it is perceived by the individual.

Percussion test—A tapping test used in the evaluation of a broken bone.

Percutaneous transluminal coronary angioplasty—A procedure in which a catheter is inserted in a blocked artery and a balloon is inflated to push the plaque back toward the wall to open the artery.

Performance—Ability to perform a task or sport at a desired level. Also called motor fitness, or physical fitness.

Perimyseum—The connective tissue surrounding fasciculi within a muscle.

Periosteum—The connective tissue surrounding all bone surfaces except the articulating surfaces.

Peripheral resistance—The resistance offered by the arterioles and capillaries to the flow of blood from the arteries to the veins. An increase in peripheral resistance causes a rise in blood pressure.

pH—The symbol for hydrogen ion concentration, or degree of acidity; 7.0 is neutral, below 7.0 is acidic, and above 7.0 is alkaline.

Phases of activities—The sequence of exercise recommended to progress from a sedentary to an active lifestyle, including a gradual progression to walking 4 mi, jogging 3 mi, and including a variety of sports and games.

Phlebitis—The inflammation of a vein.

Phospholipids—Fatty compounds that are essential constituents of cell membranes.

Physical activity—Bodily movement produced by skeletal muscles requiring energy expenditure at a level to produce healthy benefits.

Physical conditioning—Chronic regular exercise aimed at obtaining or maintaining high levels of components of fitness.

Physical fitness—A set of attributes that people have or achieve relating to their ability to perform physical activity.

Physical fitness tests—Ways to measure and evaluate the components of physical fitness.

Physical inactivity—A sedentary lifestyle.

Physical stimulus—A situation or task, such as exercise, heat, or high altitude, that requires a physiological response greater than rest.

Physical work capacity (PWC)—The capacity to perform physical work, usually measured in oxygen uptake or kilopond meters per minute, while at a set heart rate (e.g., PWC_{150}).

Physiological response—The reaction of the physiological systems to a task, condition, or stressor.

Plantar fasciitis—The inflammation of connective tissue that spans the bottom of the foot.

Plaque—Strands of fibrous tissue that attach to the inside of arteries to form soft and mushy (if fat) or hard (if scar tissue) atheromatous buildup.

Plasma—The liquid portion of the blood.

Play—Physical activity for amusement or recreation.

Playfulness—An attitude of fun.

Plyometrics—A method of resistance training that emphasizes the stretching of the muscle prior to contraction.

Polarization—A changing of electrical state. An ECG reflects depolarization and repolarization of atria and ventricles.

Pollution—Potentially toxic waste products found in water and air.

Polysaccharide—A complex sugar that yields three or more monosaccharides when hydrolyzed.

Polyunsaturated fats—Fats derived from vegetables, lean poultry, fish, and cereal.

Positive energy balance—A condition in which more energy is consumed than is expended, resulting in an increase in body weight.

Positive health—A move toward optimal functional capacity; more than a mere absence of disease.

Postabsorptive—A condition in which all food in the gastrointestinal tract has been absorbed into the blood.

Postexercise energy expenditure—The amount of energy expended, above resting levels, following exercise.

Postprandial—Occurring after a meal.

Posture—The position or carriage of the body as a whole. Improper posture is related to low-back pain.

Potential benefits and risks—A description of the relative gains and dangers of a procedure or program; one aspect of informed consent for fitness participants.

Power—Ability to exert muscular strength quickly.

Predicted maximum heart rate—An estimate of HRmax; 220 minus a person's age.

Premature atrial contraction (PAC)—On an ECG, the rhythm is irregular, and the R-R interval is short; the origin of the beat is somewhere other than the SA node.

Premature junctional contraction—On an ECG, the ectopic pacemaker in the AV junctional area that causes a QRS complex, frequently seen with inverted P-waves.

Premature ventricular contraction (PVC)—On an ECG, the QRS interval is longer than 0.12 s, and the T-wave is usually in the opposite direction; the origin is in the His-Purkinje system.

Preparticipation physical—A medical physical examination prior to an increase in physical activity.

Prescribed exercise—A recommendation of type, intensity, frequency, duration, and total work needed to accomplish fitness objectives.

Pressure points—The point of application of pressure over major arteries to control bleeding.

PRICE—The acronym for the suggested treatment for minor sprains and strains: protection, rest, ice, compression, and elevation.

Primary risk factor—A characteristic or behavior that is associated with a major health problem regardless of other factors. For example, smoking is a primary risk factor of CHD.

Prime mover—A muscle that is effective in causing a joint movement.

Private speech—Talking to oneself in order to prepare for or cope with a stressor.

Program Director^{SM}—The administrator of a program. Program Directors are certified by the American College of Sports Medicine in postcardiac rehabilitation and health fitness programs.

Progression—A gradual increase from a current level to a desired level. For example, a sedentary person may gradually increase walking and jogging until she or he is able to jog 3 mi continuously without discomfort over an 8-month period of time.

Progressive resistance exercise—A systematic increase in the overload applied to the muscle to stimulate increase in muscle function.

Proprioceptive neuromuscular facilitation—A stretching procedure in which a muscle-tendon unit is stretched; the subject does an isometric contraction with that muscle against a resistance applied by a helper; the subject relaxes, and the stretch is moved farther into the range of motion by the helper.

Proteins—Nutrients composed of amino acids that facilitate a variety of functions in the human body.

Psychological stressor—A mental condition that causes physiological arousal beyond what is needed to accomplish a task.

Pulmonary artery—The artery that carries venous blood directly from the right ventricle of the heart to the lungs.

Pulmonary function—The capacity of the respiratory system to move air.

Pulmonary valve—A set of three crescent-shaped flaps at the opening of the pulmonary artery; the semilunar valves.

Pulmonary veins—Carry oxygenated blood directly from the lungs to the left atrium of the heart.

Pulmonary—Pertaining to the lungs.

Purkinje fibers—The muscle-cell fibers found beneath the endocardium of the heart; the impulse-conducting network of the heart.

Pyramid—A mode of resistance training in which the load is either increased or decreased following each set of repetitions.

Q-wave—The initial negative deflection of the QRS complex on an ECG.

Q-T interval—The time interval from the beginning of the QRS complex to the end of the T-wave. The Q-T interval reflects the electrical systole of the cardiac cycle.

QRS complex—The largest complex on an ECG, indicating a depolarization of the left ventricle, normally less than 0.1 s.

QRS interval—The time interval from the beginning to the end of the QRS complex.

Quadriceps—The large muscle group at the front of the thigh, responsible for extending the knee joint.

Quality of life—Those aspects of living that are important to meaning and enjoyment.

R-wave—The positive deflection of the QRS complex in the ECG.

R-R interval—The time interval from the peak of the QRS of one cardiac cycle to the peak of the QRS of the next cycle; 60/R-R interval = HR, beats·min^{-1}.

Radial pulse—A pulse taken at the wrist.

Radiation—The process of losing heat from the surface of one object to the surface of another object; the heat loss depends on a temperature gradient between the surfaces of the objects.

Range of motion (ROM)—A measure of flexibility; ability to take a joint through a range of movement limited by anatomic factors associated with that joint.

Rate-pressure product—The product of heart rate and systolic blood pressure; indicative of the oxygen requirement of the heart during exercise; also called the double product.

Rating of perceived exertion (RPE)—A scale, by Borg, used to quantify the subjective feeling of physical effort. The original scale was 6 to 20; the revised scale is 0 to 10.

Rationalization—The process of inventing plausible explanations for acts or opinions that actually have other causes.

Recommended Dietary Allowances (RDA)—The recommended daily intake of nutrients. These values published by the National Research Council are thought to be adequate for good nutrition in the majority of healthy people.

Recruitment—Stimulation of additional motor units to increase the strength of a muscle contraction.

Referral—A recommendation that a person consult with a professional about a particular characteristic, sign, symptom, or test result.

Regional fat distribution—Evaluation of the tendency of an individual to deposit fat above or below the waist; the waist-to-hip ratio is used to measure this, with a high ratio being associated with greater risk of coronary heart disease and diabetes.

Rehabilitation—A planned program in which disabled people progress toward, or maintain, the maximum degree of physical and psychological independence of which they are capable.

Reinforcement control—The identification and modification of the consequences of a target behavior. The goal is to increase a behavior's occurrence through positive reinforcement, which is the addition of something desired after the behavior, or by negative reinforcement, in which some aversive stimulus is removed following that behavior.

Relapse prevention—Relapse prevention helps to identify and deal successfully with high-risk situations by educating the client about the relapse process and using a variety of strategies to foster an effective coping response.

Relative humidity—A measure of the wetness of the air; the ratio of the amount of water vapor in the air to the maximum the air can hold at that temperature times 100%.

Relative leanness—The relative amount of body weight that is fat and nonfat. Also called body composition.

Relative weight—Reflection of the relationship of one's body weight to that recommended in height-weight tables. Calculated by dividing a person's body weight by the midpoint of the recommended weight range for a person that height.

Relax—To loosen or make less stiff or gain relief from work or tension.

Reliability—The degree to which the same test score will be achieved on separate administrations of a test.

Repetition maximum—The greatest number of muscle contractions before fatigue.

Repetitions—The number of muscle contractions executed during each set of exercises.

Repolarization—In the heart, the change from a working to a resting state. The T-wave on an ECG reflects the repolarization of the ventricle at the end of the systole and the beginning of the diastole.

Reproducibility—The degree to which a person is able to replicate performance exactly. For example, a reproducible work task is important in order to determine the progress a person makes as a result of a fitness program.

Rescue breathing—Artificial respiration; used to promote oxygenation of blood in an unconscious victim who is not breathing.

Residual volume—The volume of air remaining in the lungs at the end of maximal expiration.

Resistance—The amount of force applied opposite a movement.

Respiration—The act of breathing.

Respiratory exchange ratio—The ratio of the volume of carbon dioxide produced to the volume of oxygen utilized during a given period of time ($VCO_2 \cdot VO_2^{-1}$). Also called the "respiratory quotient (RQ)."

Respiratory shock—A condition in which the lungs are unable to supply enough oxygen to the circulating blood.

Resting metabolic rate—Number of calories needed to sustain the body in a normal, resting condition.

Reversibility—A corollary to the principle of overload; loss of a training effect with disuse.

Rheumatoid arthritis—Debilitating form of arthritis involving many joints.

Rhythm—In terms of the cardiac cycle, the sequence and regularity of events.

Risk factor—A characteristic, sign, symptom, or test score that is associated with increased probability of developing a health problem. For example, people with hypertension have an increased risk of developing CHD.

Role model—Someone who sets an example for similar people by behaving in accordance with the highest standards for a particular position.

Rotation—The movement of a bone around its longitudinal axis.

Rotational inertia—Reluctance to rotate; proportional to the mass and distribution of the mass around the axis.

Runner's high—A special emotional experience that transcends normal sensations; reported by some runners.

Running—Moving the whole body quickly by propelling the body off the ground during part of the movement.

Running shoes—Special athletic shoes offering good support and cushioning in the heel area to minimize trauma at impact.

S-wave—The first negative wave (after the R-wave) of the QRS complex in the ECG.

S–T segment—The part of the ECG between the end of the QRS complex and beginning of the T-wave. Depression below (or elevation above) the isoelectric line indicates ischemia.

S–T segment displacement—On an ECG, the depression or elevation of the portion of the ECG between the end of the QRS complex and the beginning of the T-wave; S–T segment displacement may indicate the development of myocardial ischemia.

Salt—A crystalline compound of sodium and chlorine, occurring as a mineral. High levels of salt intake have been associated with hypertension.

Sarcomeres—The basic units of muscle contraction; contain actin and myosin; tension is developed as the myosin cross bridges pull the actin toward the center of the sarcomere.

Sarcoplasmic reticulum—The network of membranes that surround the myofibril; stores calcium needed for muscle contraction.

Saturated fat—A fat that is not capable of absorbing any more hydrogen. These fats are solid at room temperature and are usually of animal origin, such as the fats in milk, butter, and meat.

Saturation pressure—Water vapor pressure that exists at a particular temperature when the air is saturated with water.

Scoliosis—An abnormal lateral curvature of the spine.

Screening—An examination used to select or reject. In fitness programs, potential participants are screened to determine whether they should be referred for medical attention prior to engaging in exercise.

Second wind—A phenomenon characterized by a sudden transition from a feeling of distress or fatigue during the early portion of a workout to a more comfortable, less stressful feeling later in the exercise.

Second-degree AV block—On an ECG, some but not all P-waves precede the QRS complex.

Secondary risk factor—A characteristic, sign, symptom, or test score that has a weak independent association with a health problem but increases the risk when other risk factors are present.

Sedentary—An inactive lifestyle, characterized by a lot of sitting.

Sequence of testing—The logical order in which tests are conducted.

Sets—The number of times the desired number of repetitions are performed in a strength training workout.

Shin splints—An inflammation of the musculotendinous unit of the anterior aspect of the lower leg caused by overexertion of muscles during weight-bearing activities.

Shock—A circulatory disturbance produced by severe injury or illness and largely caused by a reduction in blood volume, characterized by a fall in blood pressure, a rapid pulse, pallor, restlessness, thirst, and cold, clammy skin. A discrepancy exists between the circulating blood volume and the capacity of the vascular bed. The initial cause of shock is a reduction in the circulating blood volume; continuation is caused by vasoconstriction.

Simple fracture—Bone fracture without external exposure.

Sinus—On an ECG, refers to a regular sequence of electrical activity (i.e., SA node, atrium, AV node, ventricle).

Sinus arrhythmia—A normal variant with sinus rhythm in which the R-R interval varies by more than 10% per beat.

Sinus bradycardia—The normal rhythm (i.e., the sinus node is the pacemaker) and sequence, with slow heart rate (below 60 beats·min⁻¹ at rest). The occurrence of sinus bradycardia may indicate a high level of fitness or a mental problem, such as depression.

Sinus node—A mass of tissue in the right atrium of the heart, near the vena cava, that initiates the heartbeat.

Sinus rhythm—The normal timing and sequence of the cardiac events, with the sinus node as a pacemaker; resting rate is between 60 and 100 beats·min⁻¹.

Sinus tachycardia—The normal rhythm and sequence, with a fast heart rate (above 100 beats·min⁻¹ at rest). The occurrence of sinus tachycardia may indicate illness or stress.

Sit-and-reach test—A measure of hamstring muscle flexibility as one reaches forward in a seated position.

Sit-up—Not recommended. See curl-up.

Skinfold caliper—An instrument used to measure the thickness of folds of skin and fat that have been pinched away from the body.

Sliding filament theory—The theory that muscular tension is generated when the actin in the sarcomere slides over the myosin due to the action of the myosin cross bridges.

Slow twitch fiber—A muscle fiber characterized by its slow speed of contraction.

Smoking—Inhaling and puffing tobacco; a primary risk factor of CHD and lung cancer.

Social support—Verbal or tangible behavior of other people that prompts, reinforces, or supports a particular behavior.

Spasm—A sudden involuntary muscular contraction.

Special populations—People with physical or mental characteristics requiring special attention, often needing modified activities.

Specificity—Belonging to and characteristic of a particular thing. For example, skill is specific to a certain aspect of a sport.

Speed—Ability to move the whole body quickly.

Sphygmomanometer—A blood pressure measurement system composed of an inflatable rubber bladder, an instrument to indicate the applied pressure, an inflation bulb to create pressure, and an adjustable valve to deflate the system.

Spinal curves—Curves formed by the vertebrae of the spinal column: corvical, thoracic, lumbaar, sacral, and cocygeal.

Split routine—A mode of resistance training in which varying muscle groups are exercised on different days.

Spondylolisthesis—The vertebral body and transverse processes slip anteriorly (forward) on the vertebral body below; it is common for L4 to slip over L5.

Spot reduction—The myth that exercise emphasizing a particular body part will cause that area to lose fat quicker than the rest of the body.

Sprain—Stretching or tearing of ligamentous tissues surrounding a joint, resulting in discoloration, swelling, and pain.

Stability—The ease with which balance is maintained.

Stage—In exercise testing, a step in the levels of work going from light to hard.

Standard deviation—An indication of the variability of test scores based on the difference of each score from the group average.

State—A temporary condition. For example, a person's emotional state may change rapidly depending on the particular situation, as contrasted to a personality trait that is consistent and does not change quickly.

Static stretching—Flexing or extending a body part to the limit of its range of motion and holding it in that position.

Steady state—Unchanging, or changing very little. For example, during submaximal exercise, a person reaches a steady state (a leveling-off of VO_2, HR, and so on) after a few minutes.

Stethoscope—An instrument with ear pieces attached to a microphone used for listening to various body sounds, such as heart rate or the sound over the brachial artery while taking blood pressure.

Strain—The overstretching or tearing of a muscle or tendon.

Strength—The amount of force that can be exerted by a muscle group against a resistance.

Stress—A physiological or psychological response to a stressor beyond what is needed to accomplish a task.

Stress continuum—A characteristic extending along a continuous line from one extreme to another. Three continuums help describe stress, namely, functional response—severe stress; enjoyable—unpleasant; and results in development—deterioration.

Stress fracture—A defect in a bone that occurs because of an accelerated rate of remodeling to accommodate the stress of weight-bearing bones; results in a loss of continuity in the bone and periosteal irritation.

Stress management—The ability to cope with potential stressors so that there is a minimum stress response.

Stressor—Any stimulus or condition that causes physiological arousal beyond what is necessary to accomplish the activity.

Stretching—Extending the limbs through a full range of motion.

Stroke volume—The amount of blood pumped from the left ventricle each time the heart contracts.

Stroke—A vascular accident (embolism, hemorrhage, or thrombosis) in the brain, often resulting in sudden loss of body function. Also called "apoplexy."

Structural curves—Refers to the lack of ability to remove a spinal curve in normal movement due to chronically tight muscles; in this case, a functional curve becomes structural.

Submaximal—Less than maximal (e.g., an exercise that can be performed with less than maximal effort).

Substrate—A foodstuff used for energy metabolism.

Succinate dehydrogenase—A key enzyme involved in the generation of energy through the aerobic system.

Sulfur dioxide—A pollutant that can cause bronchoconstriction in asthmatics.

Summation—The additive effect of force generated during repetitive muscle contractions without complete muscle relaxation of the muscle between contractions.

Super set—The condition of exercising one muscle group to fatigue, then immediately exercising the opposing muscle group to fatigue. An example may consist of flexion and extension of the biceps and triceps muscles.

Superior vena cava—The upper main vein that discharges blood from the upper half of the body into the right atrium of the heart.

Supervised fitness program—A group of fitness activities conducted with instructor present.

Support—To uphold and aid. An important element in changing behavior or coping with stress is to have a group that provides encouragement. In an organization, the support-staff personnel provide needed technical and clerical assistance.

Sweat, perspiration—Moisture coming through the pores of the skin from the sweat glands, usually as a result of heat, exertion, or emotion.

Sympathetic nervous system—Part of the autonomic nervous system consisting of two groups of ganglia connected by nerve cords, one on either side of the spinal cord; it releases substances that cause a physiological arousal, such as increased heart rate and decreased activity of the digestive and reproductive organs; the opposite of the parasympathetic nervous system.

Symptom—A noticeable change in the normal working of the body that indicates or accompanies disease or sickness.

Synarthrodial joints—Immovable joints.

Syncope—Fainting.

Synovial membrane—The inner lining of the joint capsule.

Synovitis—Inflammation of the synovial membrane.

Systolic blood pressure (SBP)—The pressure exerted on the vessel walls during ventricular contraction, measured in millimeters of mercury by the sphygmomanometer.

T-wave—On an ECG, follows the QRS complex and represents ventricular repolarization.

Ta-wave—On an ECG, the result of atrial depolarization. The Ta-wave is not normally seen, because it occurs during ventricular depolarization and is hidden by the larger electrical forces generated by the ventricles (QRS).

Tachycardia—A heart rate greater than 100 beats·min^{-1} at rest. Tachycardia may be seen in deconditioned people or people who are apprehensive about a situation (e.g., an exercise test).

Tachypnea—Excessively rapid breathing which may be a sign of overexertion, shock, or hyperventilation.

Taper-down—Light activity after a workout, allowing a gradual return to normal, with leg muscles continuing to pump blood back to the heart, thus preventing pooling of blood in the lower extremities. Also called "cool-down."

Target heart rate (THR)—The heart rate zone recommended for fitness workouts.

Tendinitis—Inflammation of a tendon.

Tendon—A band of tough, inelastic, fibrous connective tissue that attaches muscle to bone.

Tennis elbow—Inflammation of the musculotendonous unit of the elbow extensors where they attach on the outer aspect of the elbow (lateral epicondylitis).

Tenosynovitis—Inflammation of a tendon sheath.

Testing protocol—A particular testing scheme, often the starting level, timing, and increments for each stage of an exercise tolerance test.

Testosterone—Primary male hormone responsible for skeletal muscle development.

Tetanus—Stimulation of skeletal muscle tension in response to very high stimulation frequencies.

Thermic effect of food—The energy needed to digest, absorb, transport, and store the food that is eaten.

Thermogram—Infrared measure of surface of body to locate "hot" spots associated with inflammation due to trauma.

Third-degree AV block—On an ECG, the QRS appears independently, P-R varies with no regular pattern, and heart rate less than 45 beats·min^{-1}.

Third-party payments—Reimbursement for services rendered by someone else. Third-party payments are usually some form of insurance payment.

Threshold—The minimum level needed for a desired effect. Often used to refer to the minimum level of exercise intensity needed to improve cardiorespiratory function.

Thrombosis—A blood clot in a blood vessel.

Tidal volume (TV)—The volume of air inspired or expired per breath.

Time to exhaustion—The time interval from the beginning of an exercise test until the participant is unable or unwilling to continue.

Timed vital capacity—The amount of the vital capacity that can be expelled in a certain time, usually 1 s.

Torque—The effect produced by a force causing rotation; the product of the force and length of force arm.

Total body water—Total amount of water in the body. This measure can be used to assess body composition.

Total cholesterol—This is the sum of all forms of cholesterol. Because LDL-C is the primary factor in the total amount, a high level of total cholesterol is also a risk factor for CHD.

Total cholesterol/HDL-C ratio—One of the best ways to determine risk of CHD in terms of cholesterol. High ratios of total cholesterol to HDL-C indicate a high risk of CHD.

Total fitness—Optimal quality of life, including social, mental, spiritual, and physical components. Also called wellness, or positive health.

Total lung capacity (TLC)—The sum of the vital capacity and the residual volume.

Total work—The amount of work accomplished during a workout.

Tourniquet—An apparatus used to control bleeding; placed above the site of bleeding.

Training—Physical conditioning through repeated bouts of exercise.

Training log—A daily record monitoring the training frequency, intensity, and sets performed.

Trait—A semipermanent characteristic that generally is true about a person and is resistant to change.

Tranquilizers—A class of medications that brings tranquillity by calming, soothing, quieting, or pacifying.

Transfer of angular momentum—Transfer of angular momentum from one body segment to another can be achieved by stabilizing the initial moving part at a joint.

Transtheoretical model—A general model of intentional behavior change in which behavior change is seen as a dynamic process that occurs through a series of interrelated stages. Basic concepts emphasize the individual's readiness to change, processes of change, self-efficacy, decisional balance (monitoring gains and losses from decisions), and the level of the problem.

Transverse tubule—Connects the sarcolemma (muscle membrane) to the sarcoplasmic reticulum; action potentials move down the transverse tubule to cause the sarcoplasmic reticulum to release calcium to initiate muscle contraction.

Treadmill—A machine with a moving belt that can be adjusted for speed and grade, allowing a person to walk or run in place. Treadmills are widely used for exercise-tolerance testing.

Tricuspid valve—A valve located between the right atrium and ventricle of the heart.

Trigeminy—In an ECG, every third beat is a premature ventricular contraction.

Triglycerides—The primary storage form of fats in the human body.

Tropomyosin—A protein in muscle that regulates muscle contraction; works with troponin.

Troponin—Binds calcium released from the sarcoplasmic reticulum and works with tropomyosin to allow the myosin cross bridge to interact with actin and initiate cross-bridge movement.

Twelve-lead ECG—A record of the electrical activity of the heart from different directions, with 6 limb leads and 6 chest leads.

Twelve-min run—A field test for cardiorespiratory endurance, scored by the distance run in 12 min.

Two-compartment model—Refers to body composition assessment models that divide the body in fat and fat-free component parts.

Two-mi run—A field test for cardiorespiratory endurance, scored by the time it takes to complete 2 mi.

Type A behavior—A label denoting a person who is hard-driving, time conscious, and impatient. Some evidence suggests that this type of behavior is a secondary risk factor of CHD. Type A is the opposite of Type B.

Type B behavior—Behavior that is relaxed, easy-going, or has no time urgency. The opposite of Type A behavior.

Type I (slow oxidative) fiber—A slow-contracting fiber generating a small amount of tension with most of the energy coming from aerobic processes; active in light to moderate activities; possesses great endurance.

Type I diabetes—Inability of tissues to use glucose because the pancreas no longer produces insulin (insulin-dependent diabetes).

Type II, non-insulin dependent diabetes—Occurs later in life than Type I diabetes and is linked to obesity. The Type II diabetic displays a resistance to insulin, which is usually available in adequate amounts.

Type IIa (fast oxidative, glycolytic) fiber—A fast-contracting muscle generating great tension that can produce energy aerobically as well as anaerobically; adds to Type I fiber's tension as exercise intensity increases.

Type IIb (fast glycolytic) fiber—A fast-contracting muscle generating great tension; produces energy by anaerobic metabolism; fatigues quickly.

U-wave—On an ECG, the wave occasionally seen after T-wave. The origin of the U-wave is unclear, and it is normally not a factor in interpreting the ECG for exercise prescription.

Universal precautions—Safety measures used to prevent occupational exposure to blood or other body fluids containing visible blood that may result in an infection.

Unsaturated fatty acids—The molecules of a fat that have one or more double bonds and are thus capable of absorbing more hydrogen. These fats are liquid at room temperature and usually are of vegetable origin.

Unsupervised program—A group of fitness activities conducted without qualified fitness personnel, for people with a low risk of health problems.

Validity—Evaluation of a test to determine if it measures what it is supposed to measure. Validity includes test consistency (reliability) and tester consistency (objectivity). Validity is determined by logic (content), comparison with a valid test (criterion), ability to accurately predict (predictive), and theoretical means (construct).

Valsalva maneuver—Increased pressure in the abdominal and thoracic cavities caused by breath holding and extreme effort.

Variable resistance—A condition in which the intensity of the load varies as the angle of the joint changes throughout the range of motion.

Vasoconstriction—The narrowing of a blood vessel.

Vasodilation—The opening or widening of a blood vessel.

Vein—A blood vessel that returns blood to the heart.

Ventilation—The process of oxygenating the blood through the lungs.

Ventilatory threshold—The intensity of work at which the rate of ventilation sharply increases.

Ventricle—The two (left and right) lower muscular chambers of the heart.

Ventricular arrhythmias—Irregular waveforms on the ECG caused by contractions originating in the ventricle rather than from the SA node.

Ventricular fibrillation—The heart contracts in an unorganized, quivering manner, with no discernible P or QRS complexes; requires immediate emergency attention.

Ventricular tachycardia—An extremely dangerous condition in which three or more consecutive premature ventricular contractions occur. Ventricular tachycardia may degenerate into ventricular fibrillation.

Vertigo—Dizziness.

Very low-density lipoproteins (VLDL)—Mainly triglycerides, a secondary risk factor for CHD.

Vigorous intensity—Greater than 6 METs.

Viscoelastic—The characteristic that allows a tissue to return to its original length following a quick stretch but to adapt when placed under prolonged slow stretch.

Vital capacity (VC)—The amount of air that can be expelled after a maximal inspiration.

Vital signs—The measurable essential bodily functions, such as pulse rate and temperature.

Vitamins—Organic substances essential to the normal functioning of the human body. They may be subdivided into fat-soluble and water-soluble categories.

VO_2max—The highest amount of oxygen that can be utilized by the body during hard work. (Also called "maximal oxygen uptake.")

Waist-to-hip ratio—Waist circumference divided by hip circumference. It is often used as an indicator of android-type obesity.

Walking—Moving the body in a set direction while maintaining foot contact with the ground or floor.

Warm-up—Physical activity of light to moderate intensity prior to a workout.

Water vapor pressure gradient—The difference between the water vapor pressure on the skin and the water vapor pressure in the air; the tendency for water to evaporate depends on this difference.

Water-soluble vitamins—Vitamins that are carried in water (B complex and C).

Wellness—Positive health that is more than simply being free from illness. See "total fitness."

Wenchebach AV block—See "Mobitz Type I AV block."

Wet-bulb temperature—Air temperature measured with a thermometer whose bulb is surrounded by a wick wetted with water; an indication of the ability to evaporate moisture from the skin.

Windchill—The coldness felt on exposed human flesh by a combination of temperature and wind velocity.

Work—The movement of a force through a distance; measured as foot-pound or kilogram-meter, as in the cycle ergometer.

Work rate—Power, or work done per unit of time (e.g., kilogram-meters per minute; watts).

Work-relief—The ratio of time spent in more- and less-intense exercise in an interval type of workout.

Workout—An exercise bout aimed at improving fitness or performance.

Wounds—Tearing, cutting, abrading, or penetration of skin.

Z line—The connective tissue of a sarcomere, the basic unit of muscle contraction.

Bibliography

Adrian, M.J., & Cooper, J.M. (1989). *Biomechanics of human movement*. Indianapolis: Benchmark Press.

Ainsworth, B.E., Haskell, W.L., Leon, A.S., Jacobs, D.S., Jr., Montoye, H.J., Sallis, J.F., & Paffenbarger, R.S., Jr. (1993). Compendium of physical activities: Classification by energy costs of human physical activities. *Medicine and Science in Sports and Exercise 25*, 71-80.

American Alliance for Health, Physical Education, Recreation and Dance. (1980). *Health-related physical fitness test manual*. Reston, VA: Author.

American Alliance for Health, Physical Education, Recreation and Dance. (1984). *Technical manual: Health-related physical fitness*. Reston, VA: Author.

American Association for Active Lifestyles. (1995). *Physical best and individuals with disabilities*. Reston, VA: AAHPERD.

American College of Obstetricians and Gynecologists. (1994). Exercise during pregnancy and the postpartum period. *American College of Obstetricians and Gynecologists Technical Bulletin #189*.

American College of Sports Medicine. (1975). Prevention of heat injuries during distance running. *Medicine and Science in Sport 7*, vii-viii.

American College of Sports Medicine. (1978). The recommended quality and quantity of exercise for developing and maintaining fitness in healthy adults. *Medicine and Science in Sports and Exercise 10*, vii-x.

American College of Sports Medicine. (1983). Proper and improper weight loss programs. *Medicine and Science in Sports and Exercise 15*, ix-xiii.

American College of Sports Medicine. (1985). The prevention of thermal injuries during distance running. *Medicine and Science in Sports and Exercise 19*, 529-533.

American College of Sports Medicine. (1990). The recommended quality and quantity of exercise for developing and maintaining fitness in healthy adults. *Medicine and Science in Sports and Exercise 22*, 265-274.

American College of Sports Medicine. (1993). Position stand: Physical activity, physical fitness, and hypertension. *Medicine and Science in Sports and Exercise 25*, i-x.

American College of Sports Medicine. (1994). *Exercise lite: A new recommendation for physical activity*. Indianapolis: Author.

American College of Sports Medicine. (1995). *Guidelines for exercise testing and prescription* (5th ed.). Philadelphia: Williams & Wilkins.

American Diabetes Association. (1990). Diabetes and exercise: Position statement. *Diabetes Care 13*, 804-805.

American Diabetes Association. (1994). Position statement: Nutritional recommendations and principles for people with diabetes mellitus. *Diabetes Care 17*, 519-522.

American Heart Association, National Cholesterol Education Program. (1988). *Physician's cholesterol education handbook*. Dallas: Author.

American Heart Association. (1989). *1989 heart facts*. Dallas: Author.

American Heart Association. (1992). Exercise standards: A statement for health care professionals from the American Heart Association. *Circulation 86*, 340-344.

American Red Cross. (1981). *Standard first aid and personal safety* (2nd ed.). New York: Doubleday.

Anderson, B. (1980). *Stretching*. Bolinas, CA: Shelter.

Åstrand, P.O., & Rodahl, K. (1970, 1977, 1986). *Textbook of work physiology* (1st, 2nd, and 3rd eds.). New York: McGraw-Hill.

Balke, B. (1963). A simple field test for assessment of physical fitness. *Civil Aeromedical Research Institute Report 63-66*. Oklahoma City: Civil Aeromedical Research Institute.

Balke, B. (1970). *Advanced exercise procedures for evaluation of the cardiovascular system.* [Monograph]. Milton, WI: Burdick.

Bassett, D.R., & Zweifler, A.J. (1990). Risk factors and risk factor management. In G.B. Zelenock, L.G. D'Alecy, J.C. Fantone, III, M. Shlafer, & J.C. Stanley (Eds.), *Clinical ischemic syndromes* (pp. 15-46). St. Louis: Mosby.

Berger, B.G. (1994). Coping with stress: The effectiveness of exercise and other techniques. *Quest 46*(1), 100-119.

Blair, S.N. (1995). Exercise prescription for health. *Quest 47*(3), 338-353.

Blair, S.N., Jacobs, D.R., & Powell, K.E. (1985). Relationships between exercise or physical activity and other health behaviors. *Public Health Reports 100*, 180-188.

Blair, S.N., Kohl, H.W., & Barlow, C.E. (1995). Changes in physical fitness and all-cause mortality: A prospective study of healthy and unhealthy men. *Journal of the American Medical Association 273*(14), 1093-1098.

Blair, S.N., Kohl, H.W., III, Paffenbarger, R.S., Jr., Clark, D.G., Cooper, K.H., & Gibbons, L.W. (1989). Physical fitness and all-cause mortality. *Journal of the American Medical Association 262*, 2395-2401.

Bond, V. (1997a). Endurance prescription for strength, endurance, and bone density. In E.T. Howley & B.D. Franks (Eds.), *Health fitness instructor's handbook* (3rd ed., pp. 291-313). Champaign, IL: Human Kinetics.

Bond, V. (1997b). Muscular strength and endurance. In E.T. Howley & B.D. Franks (Eds.), *Health fitness instructor's handbook* (3rd ed., pp. 229-246). Champaign, IL: Human Kinetics.

Borg, G.A.V. (1982). Psychological bases of physical exertion. *Medicine and Science in Sports and Exercise 14*(5), 377-381.

Bouchard, C., Shephard, R.J., & Stephens, T., (Eds.). (1994). *Physical activity, fitness, and health.* Champaign, IL: Human Kinetics.

Bouchard, C., Shephard, R.J., Stephens, T., Sutton, J.R., & McPherson, B.D., (Eds.). (1990). *Exercise, fitness, and health.* Champaign, IL: Human Kinetics.

Brownell, K.D. (1994). *The LEARN program for weight control.* Dallas: American Health.

Brownell, K.D., & Kramer, F.M. (1989). Behavioral management of obesity. *Medical Clinics of North America 73*, 185-201.

Brownell, K.D. (1988). Weight management and body composition. In S.N. Blair, P. Painter, R.R. Pate, L.K. Smith, & C.B. Taylor (Eds.), *Resource manual for guidelines for exercise testing and prescription* (pp.355-361). Philadelphia: Lea & Febiger.

Bruce, R.A. (1972). Multi-stage treadmill test of maximal and submaximal exercise. In American Heart Association (Ed.), *Exercise testing and training of apparently healthy individuals: A handbook for physicians* (pp. 32-34). New York: American Heart Association.

Buckworth, J. (1997). Behavior modification. In E.T. Howley and B.D. Franks (Eds.), *Health fitness instructor's handbook* (3rd ed., pp. 389-403). Champaign, IL: Human Kinetics

Canadian Association for Health, Physical Education, Recreation, and Dance. (1994). *The Canadian active living challenge.* Gloucester, Ontario: Author.

Carver, S. (1997). Injury prevention and treatment. In E.T. Howley and B.D. Franks (Eds.), *Health fitness instructor's handbook* (3rd ed., pp. 405-432). Champaign, IL: Human Kinetics

Caspersen, C.J., Powell, K.E., & Christenson, G.M. (1985). Physical activity, exercise, and physical fitness: Definitions and distinctions for health-related research. *Public Health Reports 100*, 126-131.

Center for Disease Control and Prevention. (1995). *Coordinated school health.* Atlanta: Author.

Center for Disease Control and Prevention. (1997a). *Guidelines for nutrition for adolescents.* Atlanta: Author.

Center for Disease Control and Prevention. (1997b). *Guidelines for physical activity for adolescents.* Atlanta: Author.

Chodzko-Zajko, W. (1996). Physical capabilities, psychological responses, and the aging process. *Quest 48*(3), 311-329

Cooper's Institute for Aerobics Research. (1992). *The Prudential FITNESSGRAM test administration manual.* Dallas: Author.

Cooper, K.H. (1977). *The aerobics way.* New York: Bantam.

Cureton, K.J., & Warren, G.L. (1990). Criterion-referenced standards for youth health-related fitness tests: A tutorial. *Research Quarterly for Exercise and Sports 61*, 7-19.

Cureton, T.K. (1965). *Physical fitness and dynamic health*. New York: Dial Press.

Deprés, J-P., Bouchard, C., & Malina, R.M. (1990). Physical activity and coronary heart disease risk factors during childhood and adolescence. *Exercise and Sports Sciences Reviews 18*, 243-261.

Drinkwater, B.L. (1994). Physical activity, fitness, and osteoporosis. In C. Bouchard, R.J. Shephard, & T. Stephens (Eds.), *Physical activity, fitness, and health* (pp. 724-736). Champaign, IL: Human Kinetics.

Duda, J. (1996). Goals: Process vs. outcome. *Quest 48*(3), 290-302.

Dunn, J. and Sherill, C. (1996). Movement and its implications for individuals with disabilities. *Quest 48*(3), 378-391.

Ekblom, B., Åstrand, P.O., Saltin, B., Stenberg, J., & Wallstrom, B. (1968). Effect of training on circulatory response to exercise. *Journal of Applied Physiology 24*, 518-528.

Ellestad, M. (1994). *Stress testing: Principles and practice*. Philadelphia: Davis.

Fagard, R.H., & Tipton, C.M. (1994). Physical activity, fitness, and hypertension. In C. Bouchard, R.J. Shephard, & T. Stephens (Eds.), *Physical activity, fitness, and health* (pp. 633-655). Champaign, IL: Human Kinetics.

Food and Nutrition Board. (1989). *Recommended dietary allowances*. Washington, DC: National Academy of Sciences, National Research Council.

Fox, E.L., Bowers, R.W., & Foss, M.L. (1993). *The physiological basis of physical education and athletics* (5th ed.). New York: Saunders College Publishing.

Franklin, B.A., Oldridge, N.B., Stoedefalke, K.G., & Loechel, W.E. (1990). *On the ball*. Carmel, IN: Benchmark Press.

Franks, B.D. (1979). Methodology of the exercise ECG test. In E.K. Chung (Ed.), *Exercise electrocardiography: Practical approach* (pp. 46-61). Baltimore: Williams & Wilkins.

Franks, B.D. (1989). *YMCA youth fitness test*. Champaign, IL: Human Kinetics.

Franks, B.D., & Gill, D.L., (Eds.). (1994). The Academy papers: Physical activity and stress. *Quest 46*(1), 1-148.

Franks, B.D., & Howley, E.T. (1989). *Fitness facts: The healthy living handbook*. Champaign, IL: Human Kinetics.

Garrick, J.G., & Requa, R.K. (1988). Aerobic dance—A review. *Sports Medicine 6*, 169-179.

Golding, L.A., Myers, C.R., & Sinning, W.E. (1989). *The Y's way to physical fitness*. Champaign, IL: Human Kinetics.

Gould, D. (1996). Personal motivation. *Quest 48*(3), 275-289.

Habgerg, J.M. (1990). Exercise, fitness, and hypertension. In C. Bouchard, R.J. Shephard, T. Stephens, J.R. Sutton, & B.D. McPherson (Eds.), *Exercise, fitness, and health* (pp. 455-466). Champaign, IL: Human Kinetics.

Hagberg, J.M. (1994). Physical activity, fitness, health, and aging. In C. Bouchard, R. J. Shephard, and T. Stephens (Eds.), *Physical activity, fitness, and health* (pp. 993-1005). Champaign, IL: Human Kinetics.

Haskell, W.L. (1994). Dose-response issues from a biological perspective. In C. Bouchard, R. J. Shephard, & T. Stephens (Eds.), *Physical activity, fitness, and health* (pp. 1030-1039). Champaign, IL: Human Kinetics.

Haskell, W.L. (1995). Physical activity in the prevention and management of coronary heart disease. *President's Council on Physical Fitness and Sports Physical Activity and Fitness Research Digest 2*(1).

Haskell, W.L. (1996). Background and definitions. In S. Blair (Ed.), *Surgeon General's report: Physical activity and health*. Washington, DC: U.S. Department of Health and Human Services.

Hill, J.O., Drougas, H.J., & Peters, J.C. (1994). Physical activity, fitness, and moderate obesity. In C. Bouchard, R.J. Shephard, & T. Stephens (Eds.), *Physical activity, fitness, and health* (pp. 684-695). Champaign, IL: Human Kinetics.

Holmer, I. (1980). Physiology of swimming man. *Exercise and Sport Sciences Reviews 7*, 87-123.

Howley, E.T. (1980). Effect of altitude on physical performance. In G.A. Stull & T.K. Cureton, Jr. (Eds.), *Encyclopedia of physical education, fitness, and sports: Vol. 2, Training, environment, nutrition, and fitness* (pp. 177-186). Salt Lake City: Brighton.

Howley, E.T. (1988). The exercise testing laboratory. In S.N. Blair, P. Painter, R.R. Pate, L.K. Smith, & C.B. Taylor (Eds.), *Resource manual for guidelines for exercise testing and prescription* (pp. 406-413). Philadelphia: Lea & Febiger.

Howley, E.T., & Franks, B.D. (1997). *Health fitness instructor's handbook* (3rd ed.). Champaign, IL: Human Kinetics.

Imrie, D., & Barbuto, L. (1988). The back-power program. In S.N. Blair, P. Painter, R.R. Pate, L.K. Smith, & C.B. Taylor (Eds.), *Resource manual for guidelines for exercise testing and prescription*. Philadelphia: Lea & Febiger.

Jackson, A.S., & Pollock, M.L. (1985). Practical assessment of body composition. *The Physician and Sportsmedicine 13*, 76-90.

Jacobsen, E. (1938). *Progressive relaxation*. Chicago: University of Chicago Press.

Jennings, G.L., Deakin, G., Korner, P., Meredith, I., Kingwell, B., and Nelson, L. (1991). What is the dose-response relationship between exercise training and blood pressure? *Annals of Medicine 23*, 313-18.

Johnson, C.C., & Slemenda, C. (1987). Osteoporosis: An overview. *The Physician and Sportsmedicine 15*(11), 65-68.

Kasch, F.W., Boyer, J.L., Van Camp, S.P., Verity, L.S., & Wallace, J.P. (1990). The effects of physical activity and inactivity on aerobic power in older men (a longitudinal study). *The Physician and Sportsmedicine 18*(4), 73-83.

Katch, F.I., & McArdle, W.D. (1977). *Nutrition, weight control, and exercise.* Boston: Houghton Mifflin.

Kline, G.M., Porcari, J.P., Hintermeister, R., Freedson, P.S., Ward, A., McCarron, R.F., Ross, J., & Rippe, J.M. (1987). Estimation of VO$_2$max from a one-mile track walk, gender, age, and body weight. *Medicine and Science in Sports and Exercise 19*, 253-259.

Kohl, H.W., & McKenzie, J.D. (1994). Physical activity, fitness, and stroke. In C. Bouchard, R.J. Shephard, & T. Stephens (Eds.), *Physical activity, fitness, and health* (pp. 609-621). Champaign, IL: Human Kinetics.

Kraus, H., & Raab, W. (1961). *Hypokinetic disease.* Springfield, IL: Charles C. Thomas.

Kreighbaum, E., & Barthels, K.M. (1990). *Biomechanics.* Minneapolis: Burgess.

Kriska, A.M., Blair, S.N., & Pereira, M.A. (1994). The potential role of physical activity in the prevention of non-insulin-dependent diabetes mellitus: The epidemiological evidence. In J.O. Holloszy (Ed.), *Exercise and sports sciences reviews, Vol. 22* (pp. 121-143). Baltimore: Williams & Wilkins.

Kuczmarski, R.J., Flegal, K.M., Campbell, S.M., & Johnson, C.L. (1994). Increasing prevalence of overweight among U.S. adults: The national health and nutrition examination surveys, 1960 to 1991. *Journal of the American Medical Association 272*, 205-211.

Lakka, T.A., Venalainen, J.M., Rauramaa, R., et al. (1994). Relation of leisure-time activity and cardiorespiratory fitness to the risk of acute myocardial infarction in men. *New England Journal of Medicine 330*, 1549-1554.

Landers, D.M., & Petruzzello, S.J. (1994). Physical activity, fitness, and anxiety. In C. Bouchard, R.J. Shephard, & T. Stephens (Eds.), *Physical activity, fitness, and health* (pp. 868-882). Champaign, IL: Human Kinetics.

Lee, I. (1995). Physical activity and cancer. *President's Council on Physical Fitness and Sports Physical Activity and Fitness Research Digest 2*(2).

Leon, A.S., & Norstrom, J. (1995). Evidence of the role of physical activity and cardiorespiratory fitness in the prevention of coronary heart disease. *Quest 47*(3), 320-337.

Lewis, J.L. (1997). Functional anatomy and biomechanics. In E.T. Howley & B.D. Franks, *Health fitness instructor's handbook* (3rd ed., pp. 79-110). Champaign, IL: Human Kinetics.

Liemohn, W.P. (1990). Exercise and the back. In T.C. Namey (Ed.), *Rheumatic disease clinics of North America: Vol. 16, Exercise and arthritis* (pp. 945-970). Philadelphia: Saunders.

Liemohn, W. (1997a). Flexibility and low-back function. In E.T. Howley & B.D. Franks, *Health fitness instructor's handbook* (3rd ed., pp. 247-262). Champaign, IL: Human Kinetics.

Liemohn, W. (1997b). Exercise prescription for flexibility and low-back function. In E.T. Howley and B.D. Franks, *Health fitness instructor's handbook* (3rd ed., pp. 315-329). Champaign, IL: Human Kinetics.

Lind, A.R., & McNicol, G.W. (1967). Muscular factors which determine the cardiovascular responses to sustained and rhythmic exercise. *Canadian Medical Association Journal 96*, 706-713.

Lohman, T.G. (1987). The use of skinfolds to estimate body fatness in children and youth. *Journal of Physical Education, Recreation and Dance 58*(9), 98-102.

Lohman, T.G. (1992). *Advances in body composition assessment.* Champaign, IL: Human Kinetics.

Londeree, B.R., & Moeschberger, M.L. (1982). Effect of age and other factors on maximal heart rate. *Research Quarterly for Exercise and Sport 53*, 297-304.

Mahler, D.A. (1993). Exercise-induced asthma. *Medicine and Science in Sports and Exercise 25*, 554-561.

Makker, H.K., & Holgate, S.T. (1994). Mechanisms of exercise-induced asthma. *European Journal of Clinical Investigation 24*, 571-585.

Martin, D., & Bassett, D.R., Jr. (1997). Exercise related to ECG and medications. In E.T. Howley and B.D. Franks (Eds.), *Health fitness instructor's handbook* (3rd ed., pp. 433-455). Champaign, IL: Human Kinetics

McArdle, W.D., Katch, F.I., & Katch, V.L. (1996). *Exercise physiology* (4th ed.). Baltimore: Williams & Wilkins.

McKenzie, D.C., McLuckie, M.L., & Stirling, D.R. (1994). The protective effects of continuous and interval exercise in athletes with exercise-induced asthma. *Medicine and Science in Sports and Exercise 26*, 951-956.

Metropolitan Life Insurance Company of New York. (1959). New weight standards for men and women. *Statistical Bulletin 40*, 1-4.

Montoye, H.J., Kemper, H.C.G., Saris, W.H.M., & Washburn, R.A. (1996). *Measuring physical activity and energy expenditure.* Champaign, IL: Human Kinetics.

Morgan, W.P. (1994). Physical activity, fitness, and depression. In C. Bouchard, R.J. Shephard, & T. Stephens (Eds.), *Physical activity, fitness, and health* (pp. 851-867). Champaign, IL: Human Kinetics.

Morrow, J.R., & Gill, D.L. (Eds.). (1995). The Academy papers: The role of physical activity in fitness and health. *Quest 47*(3), 1-140.

National Heart, Lung, and Blood Institute, & the Office of Medical Applications of Research, National Institutes of Health. (1996). *NIH consensus development conference on physical activity and cardiovascular health*. Washington, DC: Author.

National Institutes of Health. (1985). *Health implications of obesity: NIH consensus development conference statement*. Bethesda, MD: NIH.

National Institutes of Health. (1994a). *Bioelectrical impedance analysis in body composition measurement: NIH technology assessment conference statement*. Bethesda, MD: NIH.

National Institutes of Health. (1994b). *Optimal calcium intake: NIH consesus development conference statement*. Bethesda, MD: NIH.

National Research Council, Food and Nutrition Board. (1989). *Recommended dietary allowances* (10th ed.). Washington, DC: National Academy Press.

National Strength & Conditioning Association. (1995). Units of measurement and terminology. *Journal of Strength and Conditioning Research 9*(1).

Naughton, J.P., & Haider, R. (1973). Methods of exercise testing. In J.P. Naughton, H.R. Hellerstein, & L.C. Mohler (Eds.), *Exercise testing and exercise training in coronary heart disease* (pp. 79-91). New York: Academic Press.

New Games Foundation. (1976). *The new games book*. Garden City, NY: Dolphin.

Nieman, D.C. (1995). *Fitness and sports medicine: A health-related approach* (3rd ed.). Palo Alto, CA: Bull.

Norstrom, J. (1994). The activity pyramid. *Discover* (Summer), 3-4.

Park Nicollet Medical Foundation. (1995). *The activity pyramid*. Minneapolis: Author.

Park, R.S. (1989). *Measurement of physical fitness: An historical perspective*. Washington, DC: ODPHP National Health Information Center.

Pate, R.R., Pratt, M., Blair, S.N., Haskell, W.L., Marcera, C.A., and Bouchard, C. (1995). Physical activity and public health: A recommendation from the Centers for Disease Control and Prevention and the American College of Sports Medicine. *Journal of the American Medical Association 273*(5), 402-407.

Plowman, S.A. (1993). Physical fitness and healthy low back function. *President's Council on Physical Fitness and Sports Physical Activity and Fitness Research Digest 1*(3).

Plowman, S.A. (1994). Stress, hyperreactivity, and health. *Quest 46*(1), 78-99.

Pollock, M.L., Feigenbaum, M.S., & Brechue, W.F. (1995). Exercise prescription for physical fitness. *Quest 47*(3), 320-337.

Pollock, M.L., Schmidt, D.H., & Jackson, A.S. (1980). Measurement of cardio-respiratory fitness and body compositon in a clinical setting. *Comprehensive Therapy 6*, 12-27.

Pollock, M.L., & Wilmore, J.H. (1990). *Exercise in health and disease* (2nd ed.). Philadelphia: Saunders.

Powers, S.K., & Howley, E.T. (1997). *Exercise physiology* (3rd ed.). Dubuque, IA: Brown and Benchmark.

President's Council on Physical Fitness and Sports. (1995). *Presidential sports award*. Washington, DC: Author.

Rowland, T.W. (1990). *Exercise and children's health*. Champaign, IL: Human Kinetics.

Safrit, J. (1995). *Complete guide to youth fitness testing*. Champaign, IL: Human Kinetics.

Sallis, J.F., & Patrick, K. (1994). Physical activity guidelines for adolescents: Consensus statement. *Pediatric Exercise Science 6*(4), 302-314.

Seefeldt, V., & Vogel, P. (1986). *The value of physical activity*. Reston, VA: American Alliance for Health, Physical Education, Recreation and Dance.

Selye, H. (1956). *Stress of life*. New York: McGraw-Hill.

Selye, H. (1976). Stress and physical activity. *McGill Journal of Education 11*, 3-14.

Siri, W.E. (1956). Gross composition of the body. In J.H. Lawrence & C.A. Tobias (Eds.), *Advances in biological and medical physics, Vol. 4* (pp. 239-280). New York: Academic Press.

Sharkey, B.J. (1984, 1990). *Physiology of fitness* (2nd, 3rd eds.). Champaign, IL: Human Kinetics.

Shaw, J.M., & Snow-Harter, C. (1995). Osteoporosis and physical activity. *President's Council on Physical Fitness and Sports Physical Activity and Fitness Research Digest 2*(3).

Shephard, R.J. (1988). PAR-Q, Canadian home fitness test, and exercise screening alternatives. *Sports Medicine 5*, 185-195.

Shephard, R.J. (1996). Exercise, independence, and quality of life in the elderly. *Quest 48*(3), 354-365.

Sime, W.E., & McKinney, M.E. (1988). Stress management applications in the prevention and rehabilitation of coronary heart disease. In S.N. Blair, P. Painter, R.R. Pate, L.K. Smith, & C.B. Taylor (Eds.), *Resource manual for guidelines for exercise testing and prescription* (pp. 367-374). Philadelphia: Lea & Febiger.

Smith, E.L., & Gilligan, C. (1987). Effects of inactivity and exercise on bone. *The Physician and Sportsmedicine 15*(11), 91-102.

Smith, E.L., Smith, K.A., & Gilligan, C. (1990). Exercise, fitness, osteoarthritis, and osteoporosis. In C. Bouchard, R.J. Shephard, T. Stephens, J.R. Sutton, & B.D. McPherson (Eds.), *Exercise, fitness, and health* (pp. 517-528). Champaign, IL: Human Kinetics.

Soukup, J.T., & Kovaleski, J.E. (1993). A review of the effects of resistance training for individuals with diabetes mellitus. *Diabetes Education 19*, 307-312.

Tate, C.A., Hyek, M.F., & Taffet, G.E. (1994). Mechanism for the responses of cardiac muscle to physical activity in old age. *Medicine and Science in Sports and Exercise 26*, 561-567.

Thompson, D.L. (1997a). Body composition. In E.T. Howley and B.D. Franks (Eds.), *Health fitness instructor's handbook* (3rd ed., pp. 165-182). Champaign, IL: Human Kinetics.

Thompson, D.L. (1997b). Nutrition. In E.T. Howley and B.D. Franks (Eds.), *Health fitness instructor's handbook* (3rd ed., pp. 149-164). Champaign, IL: Human Kinetics.

Thompson, D.L. (1997c). Weight control. In E.T. Howley and B.D. Franks (Eds.), *Health fitness instructor's handbook* (3rd ed., pp. 183-198). Champaign, IL: Human Kinetics.

Thompson, P.D., & Fahrenbach, M.C. (1994). Risks of exercising: Cardiovascular including sudden cardiac death. In C. Bouchard, R.J. Shephard, & T. Stephens (Eds.), *Physical activity, fitness, and health* (pp. 1019-1028). Champaign, IL: Human Kinetics.

U.S. Department of Agriculture. (1992). *The Food Guide Pyramid.* Home and Garden Bulletin Number 252.

U.S. Department of Agriculture & U.S. Department of Health and Human Services. (1996). *Dietary guidelines for Americans* (4th ed.). Washington, DC: Authors.

U.S. Department of Health and Human Services. (1991). *Healthy people 2000: National health promotion and disease prevention objectives.* Washington, DC: DHHS publication PHS 91-50212.

U.S. Department of Health and Human Services. (1996). *Surgeon General's Report on Physical Activity and Health.*

U.S. Department of Health and Human Services, Public Health Service, Centers for Disease Control and Prevention, National Center for Chronic Disease Prevention and Health Promotion, Division of Chronic Disease Control and Community Intervention. (1996). *Promoting physical activity: A guide for community action.* Atlanta, GA: Center for Disease Control.

U.S. Public Health Service. (1985). Public health aspects of physical activity and exercise. *Public Health Reports 100*(2), 118-124.

U.S. Senate Select Committee on Nutrition and Human Needs. (1977). *Dietary goals for the U.S.* (2nd ed.). Washington, DC: U.S. Government Printing Office.

Vranic, M., & Wasserman, D. (1990). Exercise, fitness, and diabetes. In C. Bouchard, R.J. Shephard, T. Stephens, J.R. Sutton, & B.D. McPherson (Eds.), *Exercise, fitness, and health* (pp. 467-490). Champaign, IL: Human Kinetics.

Wadden, T.A., & Stunkard, A.J. (1993). Psychosocial consequences of obesity and dieting: Research and clinical findings. In A.J. Stunkard & T.A. Wadden. (Eds.), *Obesity: Theory and therapy* (2nd ed.). New York: Raven Press.

Wenger, N.K., & Hurst, J.W. (1984). Coronary bypass surgery as a rehabilitative procedure. In N.K. Wenger & H.K. Hellerstein (Eds.), *Rehabilitation of the coronary patient* (pp. 115-132). New York: Wiley.

Williams, M.H. (1988). *Nutrition for fitness and sport* (2nd ed.). Dubuque, IA: Brown.

Williams, P.C. (1974). *Low back and neck pain.* Springfield, IL: Charles C. Thomas.

Wilmore, J.H., & Costill, D.L. (1994). *Physiology of sport and exercise.* Champaign, IL: Human Kinetics.

Wolfe, L.A., Brenner, I.K.M., & Mottola, M.F. (1994). Maternal exercise, fetal well-being, and pregnancy outcome. In J.O. Holloszy (Ed.), *Exercise and Sport Sciences Reviews, Vol. 22* (pp. 145-194). Baltimore: Williams & Wilkins.

Wolfe, L.A., Hall, P., Webb, K.A., Goodman, L., Monga, M., & McGrath, M.J. (1989). Prescription of aerobic exercise during pregnancy. *Sports Medicine 8*, 273-301.

Young, J.C. (1995). Exercise prescription for individuals with metabolic disorders. *Sports Medicine 19*, 44-53.

Zwiren, L.D. (1993). Exercise prescription for children. In J.L. Durstine, A.C. King, P.L. Painter, J.L. Roitman, L.D. Zwiren, & W.L. Kenney (Eds.), *ACSM's resource manual for guidelines for exercise testing and prescription* (2nd ed., pp. 409-417). Indianapolis, IN: American College of Sports Medicine.

Credits

Figures

Figures 5.2, 5.3 Reprinted, by permission, from E.T. Howley and B.D. Franks, 1986, *Health fitness instructor's handbook* (Champaign, IL: Human Kinetics), 55.

Figure 6.1 Reprinted, by permission, from E.T. Howley and B.D. Franks, 1997, *Health fitness instructor's handbook,* 3rd ed. (Champaign, IL: Human Kinetics), 151.

Figure 7.4 Reprinted, by permission, from E.T. Howley and B.D. Franks, 1997, *Health fitness instructor's handbook,* 3rd ed. (Champaign, IL: Human Kinetics), 222.

Figure 8.8 Reprinted, by permission, from The President's Council on Physical Fitness, 1997, *1997-98 The president's challenge physical fitness program packet* (Washington D.C.: Author), **.

Figure 9.7 Reprinted, by permission, from E.T. Howley and B.D. Franks, 1997, *Health fitness instructor's handbook,* 3rd ed. (Champaign, IL: Human Kinetics), 327.

Figure 10.1 Adapted, by permission, from E.T. Howley and B.D. Franks, 1997, *Health fitness instructor's handbook,* 3rd ed. (Champaign, IL: Human Kinetics), 92.

Figures 10.3, 10.4 Reprinted, by permission, from E.T. Howley and B.D. Franks, 1997, *Health fitness instructor's handbook,* 3rd ed. (Champaign, IL: Human Kinetics), 329.

Figure 10.8 Reprinted, by permission, from E.T. Howley and B.D. Franks, 1997, *Health fitness instructor's handbook,* 3rd ed. (Champaign, IL: Human Kinetics), 245.

Figure 10.9 Reprinted, by permission, from E.T. Howley and B.D. Franks, 1997, *Health fitness instructor's handbook,* 3rd ed. (Champaign, IL: Human Kinetics), 262.

Figure 10.10 Reprinted, by permission, from the American Alliance for Health, Physical Education, Recreation and Dance, 1980, *Health related physical fitness test manual* (Reston, VA: Author), 70.

Figure 15.1 Reprinted, by permission, from E.T. Howley and B.D. Franks, 1997, *Health fitness instructor's handbook,* 3rd ed. (Champaign, IL: Human Kinetics), 392.

Figure 16.2 Reprinted, by permission, from E.T. Howley and B.D. Franks, 1997, *Health fitness instructor's handbook,* 3rd ed. (Champaign, IL: Human Kinetics), 61.

Figure 16.3 Reprinted, by permission, from E.T. Howley and B.D. Franks, 1997, *Health fitness instructor's handbook,* 3rd ed. (Champaign, IL: Human Kinetics), 62.

Figure 16.4 Reprinted, by permission, from E.T. Howley and B.D. Franks, 1997, *Health fitness instructor's handbook,* 3rd ed. (Champaign, IL: Human Kinetics), 63.

Figure 16.5 Reprinted, by permission, from E.T. Howley and B.D. Franks, 1997, *Health fitness instructor's handbook,* 3rd ed. (Champaign, IL: Human Kinetics), 65.

Figures 16.6-16.9 Reprinted, by permission, from B. Ekblom, P.O. Åstrand, B. Saltin, J. Stenberg, and B. Wallstrom, 1968, "Effect of training on circulatory response to exercise," *Journal of Applied Physiology* 24: 518-528.

Figures 16.10, 16.11 Reprinted, by permission, from E.T. Howley and B.D. Franks, 1997, *Health fitness instructor's handbook,* 3rd ed. (Champaign, IL: Human Kinetics), 65, 69.

Figure 16.12 "Muscular factors which determine the cardiovascular responses to sustained and rhythmic exercise"— Adapted from, by permission of the publisher, *CMAJ,* 1967; 96, pp. 706-713.

Figure 16.13 Adapted, by permission, from E.T. Howley and B.D. Franks, 1986, *Health fitness instructor's handbook* (Champaign, IL: Human Kinetics), 39.

Figure 16.14 Adapted, by permission, from E.T. Howley and B.D. Franks, 1997, *Health fitness instructor's handbook,* 3rd ed. (Champaign, IL: Human Kinetics), 92.

Figure 18.3 Reprinted, by permission, from E.T. Howley and B.D. Franks, 1997, *Health fitness instructor's handbook,* 3rd ed. (Champaign, IL: Human Kinetics), 410.

Tables

Table 2.1 Adapted, by permission, from E.T. Howley and B.D. Franks, 1997, *Health fitness instructor's handbook,* 3rd ed. (Champaign, IL: Human Kinetics), 277.

Table 3.1 Reprinted, by permission, from E.T. Howley and B.D. Franks, 1997, *Health fitness instructor's handbook,* 3rd ed. (Champaign, IL: Human Kinetics), 12.

Table 3.2 Reprinted, by permission, from E.T. Howley and B.D. Franks, 1997, *Health fitness instructor's handbook,* 3rd ed. (Champaign, IL: Human Kinetics), 34-36.

Table 4.1 Adapted, by permission, from E.T. Howley and B.D. Franks, 1997, *Health fitness instructor's handbook,* 3rd ed. (Champaign, IL: Human Kinetics), 33.

Table 4.2 Reprinted, by permission, from E.T. Howley and B.D. Franks, 1997, *Health fitness instructor's handbook,* 3rd ed. (Champaign, IL: Human Kinetics), 40-41.

Table 4.3 Reprinted, by permission, from E.T. Howley and B.D. Franks, 1997, *Health fitness instructor's handbook,* 3rd ed. (Champaign, IL: Human Kinetics), 44.

Tables 5.3, 5.4 Reprinted with permission. Pollack ML, Schmidt DH, Jackson AS. Measurement of cardiorespiratory fitness and body composition in the clinical setting. *Comp Ther.* 1980;6(9):12-27. ©American Society of Contemporary Medicine & Surgery. 4711 Golf Road, Suite 408, Skokie, IL 60076.

Tables 6.1, 6.2 Reprinted, by permission, from B.D. Franks and E.T. Howley, 1989, *Fitness facts: The healthy living handbook* (Champaign, IL: Human Kinetics), 39-40. © 1989 by B. Don Franks and Edward T. Howley.

Table 6.5 Adapted, by permission, from F.I. Katch and W.D. McArdle, 1977, *Nutrition, weight control, and exercise* (Baltimore: Lea & Febiger).

Table 7.1 Reprinted, by permission, from E.T. Howley and B.D. Franks, 1997, *Health fitness instructor's handbook,* 3rd ed. (Champaign, IL: Human Kinetics), 204.

Table 7.2 Reprinted, by permission, from American College of Sports Medicine, 1971, *Guidelines for exercise testing and prescription,* 4th ed. (Baltimore: Williams & Wilkins).

Table 7.3 Reprinted, by permission, from E.T. Howley and B.D. Franks, 1986, *Healt/fitness instructor's handbook* (Champaign, IL: Human Kinetics), 85.

Table 7.6 Reprinted, by permission, from American College of Sports Medicine, 1995, *Guidelines for exercise testing and prescription,* 4th ed. (Baltimore: Williams & Wilkins).

Table 7.7 Reprinted, by permission, from E.K. Chung, 1979, Methodology of the exercise ECG test. In *Exercise electrocardiography: Practical approach,* edited by E.K. Chung (Baltimore: Lea & Febiger), 46-61.

Table 7.8a Adapted, by permission, from J.P. Naughton and R. Haider, 1973, Methods of exercise testing. In *Exercise testing and exercise training in coronary heart disease,* edited by J.P. Naughton, H.R. Hellerstein, and L.C. Mohler (New York: Academic Press), 79-91.

Table 7.8c Adapted, by permission, from R.A. Bruce, 1972, Multi-stage treadmill test of maximal and submaximal exercise. In *Exercise testing and training of apparently healthy individuals: A handbook for physicians* (New York: American Heart Association), 32-34.

Table 7.12 Reprinted, by permission, from E.T. Howley and B.D. Franks, 1997, *Health fitness instructor's handbook,* 3rd ed. (Champaign, IL: Human Kinetics), 207.

Table 7.14 Reprinted, by permission, from E.T. Howley and B.D. Franks, 1997, *Health fitness instructor's handbook,* 3rd ed. (Champaign, IL: Human Kinetics), 213.

Table 11.1 Reprinted, by permission, from E.T. Howley and B.D. Franks, 1997, *Health fitness instructor's handbook,* 3rd ed. (Champaign, IL: Human Kinetics), 382.

Table 14.7 Adapted, from I. Holmer, 1979, "Physiology of swimming man," *Exercise and Sport Sciences Reviews* 7: 87-123.

Table 14.9 Adapted, by permission, from B.J. Sharkey, 1984, *Physiology of fitness* (Champaign, IL: Human Kinetics), **

Table 15.1 Adapted, by permission, from E.T. Howley and B.D. Franks, 1986, *Health/fitness instructor's handbook* (Champaign, IL: Human Kinetics), 200.

Table 16.1 Adapted, by permission, from W.D. McArdle, F.I. Katch, and V.L. Katch, 1986, *Exercise Physiology,* 2nd ed. (Baltimore: Williams & Wilkins), **

Table 16.2 Reprinted, by permission, from E.T. Howley and B.D. Franks, 1986, *Health/fitness instructor's handbook* (Champaign, IL: Human Kinetics), 43-45.

Table 18.1 Reprinted, by permission, from E.T. Howley and B.D. Franks, 1997, *Health fitness instructor's handbook,* 3rd ed. (Champaign, IL: Human Kinetics), 429.

Table 20.1 Reprinted, by permission, from C.B. Corbin and R. Lindsey, 1991, Concepts of physical fitness with laboratories, 7th ed. (Dubuque, IA: Wm. C. Brown), 41.

Table 20.2 Adapted, by permission, from B.J. Sharkey, 1984, *Physiology of fitness* (Champaign, IL: Human Kinetics), 191.

Table 21.4 Reprinted, by permission, from E.T. Howley and B.D. Franks, 1997, *Health fitness instructor's handbook,* 3rd ed. (Champaign, IL: Human Kinetics), 462.

Table 21.5 Reprinted, by permission, from E.T. Howley and B.D. Franks, 1997, *Health fitness instructor's handbook,* 3rd ed. (Champaign, IL: Human Kinetics), 472.

Tables A.1-A.3 Reprinted with permission from *Recommended dietary allowances,* 10th ed. © 1989 by the National Academy of Sciences. Courtesy of the National Academy Press, Washington, D.C.

Index

About the Authors

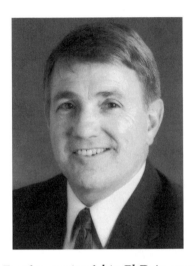

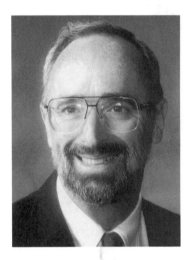

B. Don Franks received his PhD in exercise science from the University of Illinois at Urbana-Champaign (UIUC) in 1967, while working under fitness pioneer T.K. Cureton, Jr. He served on the UIUC faculty until 1970 and later taught at Temple University in Philadelphia and at the University of Tennessee in Knoxville. He was Senior Program Advisor for the President's Council on Physical Fitness and Sports in 1995. Currently he is a professor in and chair of the Department of Kinesiology at Louisiana State University.

Franks is a Fellow of the American College of Sports Medicine (ACSM), the American Academy of Kinesiology and Physical Education (AAKPE), and the Research Consortium of the American Alliance for Health, Physical Education, Recreation and Dance (AAHPERD). He is also a former president of AAKPE and the Research Consortium of AAHPERD, where he advocated a health-related approach to physical fitness and helped to develop the first health-related physical fitness test. Franks has received many honors, including the AAHPERD Physical Fitness Council Honor Award and the President's Council on Physical Fitness and Sports' Distinguished Service Award.

Edward T. Howley is a professor of exercise science at the University of Tennessee, where he frequently has been honored for his excellence in teaching. He received the university's College of Education John Tunstall Outstanding Professor Award in 1987 and 1995, the University of Tennessee Alumni Association Outstanding Teacher Award in 1987, and the George F. Brady Teaching Award in 1979 and 1986.

Howley holds a PhD in physical education from the University of Wisconsin at Madison and certification as a program director from ACSM. In addition, he has been active in ACSM as a Fellow, as president of the southeast chapter, as chair of the certification committee, as a faculty member in ACSM health fitness certification workshops, and as a member of the ACSM Preventive and Rehabilitative Committee, which developed the college's various certification programs.

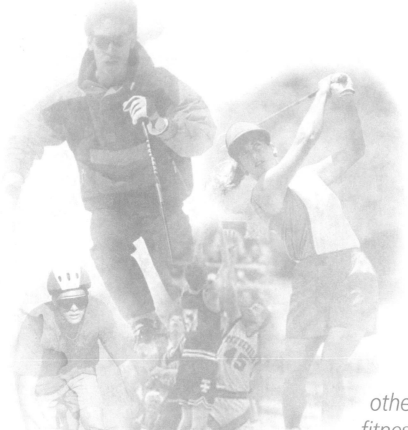